THIRD EDITION

Professionalization of Nursing

CURRENT ISSUES AND TRENDS

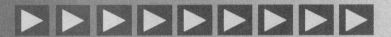

Patricia M. Schwirian, RN, PhD

Professor
College of Nursing
The Ohio State University
Columbus, Ohio

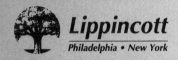

Lippincott

Philadelphia • New York

Acquisitions Editor: Lisa Marshall
Sponsoring Editor: Sandra Kasko
Project Editor: Sandra Cherrey Scheinin
Senior Production Manager: Helen Ewan
Production Coordinator: Michael Carcel
Design Coordinator: Nicholas Rook

Edition 3rd

9 8 7 6 5 4 3 2 1

Library of Congress Cataloging in Publications Data

Schwirian, Patricia M.
  Professionalization of nursing : current issues and trends.—3rd
ed. / Patricia M. Schwirian.
    p. cm.
  Rev. ed. of: Professionalization of nursing / Margaret M. Moloney.
2nd ed. c1992.
  Includes bibliographical references and index.
  ISBN 0–7817–1045–6 (alk. paper)
  1. Nursing—Practice. 2. Nursing—Study and teaching.
3. Professional practice. I. Moloney, Margaret M.
Professionalization of nursing. II. Title.
  [DNLM: 1. Education, Nursing—trends—United States. 2. Nursing—
trends—United States. 3. Professional Competence—nurses'
instruction. WY 16 S337p 1998]
RT86.7.M65 1998
610.73—dc21
DNLM/DLC
for Library of Congress   97–45687
                                                       CIP

Care has been taken to confirm the accuracy of the information presented and to describe generally accepted practices. However, the authors, editors, and publisher are not responsible for errors or omissions or for any consequences from application of the information in this book and make no warranty, express or implied, with respect to the contents of the publication.

The authors, editors, and publisher have exerted every effort to ensure that drug selection and dosage set forth in this text are in accordance with current recommendations and practice at the time of publication. However, in view of ongoing research, changes in government regulations, and the constant flow of information relating to drug therapy and drug reactions, the reader is urged to check the package insert for each drug for any change in indications and dosage and for added warnings and precautions. This is particularly important when the recommended agent is a new or infrequently employed drug.

Some drugs and medical devices presented in this publication have Food and Drug Administration (FDA) clearance for limited use in restricted research settings. It is the responsibility of the health care provider to ascertain the FDA status of each drug or device planned for use in their clinical practice.

♾ This Paper Meets the Requirements of ANSI/NISO Z39.48-1992 (Permanence of Paper).

This book is dedicated to my parents, Keith and Alice Millard, to The Schwirians (Kent, Julie, John, and Tom), and to students with whom I have had a continuing dialogue for 25 years regarding the nature and importance of nursing, professionalization, and their roles and responsibilities in making a contribution to the future of nursing and health care.

Preface

The third edition of *Professionalization of Nursing: Current Issues and Trends* is a complete revision of the first two editions of the book, which were authored by Margaret M. Maloney, PhD, RN, FAAN. My goals in writing the third edition have been to keep the strengths of the first two editions while adding fresh insights, cutting-edge information bearing on the continuing professionalization of nursing, and new features that enhance understanding and interest.

Professionalization of Nursing: Current Issues and Trends focuses on the link between the continuing professionalization process in nursing and the day-to-day problems faced in nursing in inpatient health care institutions, community health care delivery systems, and advanced practice settings.

Contents

PART I

This unit provides an overview of the professionalization process and how nursing is emerging to full professional status.

Chapter 1: Professions and the Professionalization of Nursing. Chapter 1 begins with a detailed discussion of four concepts: profession, professional, professionalism, and professionalization. It then turns to a discussion of nursing as a profession, including an assessment of where nursing stands on the occupation–profession continuum, as well as some of the needed transformations necessary for nursing to advance further professionalism in nursing. It concludes by focusing on some milestones in the professionalization of nursing.

PART II

This unit discusses nursing knowledge, nursing theory, and nursing research, as well as the current issues in the evolution of nursing knowledge and nursing science.

Chapter 2: Nursing Knowledge and Nursing Theory: Foundations of a Profession. The chapter begins with an overview of the nature of nursing knowledge. It contrasts the public's view of nursing knowledge with that of the discipline itself. Further, it evaluates the status of nursing as a scientific discipline. Next, the chapter deals with nursing theory. It assesses the role of imported theories, comprehensive deductive theories, and emerging practice-based nursing knowledge. The chapter concludes with nursing knowledge beyond empirics—that is, a discussion of ethics as knowledge, personal knowledge, and esthetic knowledge.

Chapter 3: Nursing Research: An Action Path to Professionalization. This chapter has two major foci. The first is an overview of the development and progress of the nursing research enterprise. It begins with the seminal work of Florence Nightingale and follows the development of nursing research into the 1990's and beyond. In doing so, it examines the changing foci of nursing research, the American Nurses Association's (ANA's) continuing support for nursing research, the university setting of nursing researchers, and the literature that supports nursing research. The second focus is on the relative contribution of quantitative and qualitative research methods and findings to the development of nursing knowledge and nursing science.

Chapter 4: Current Issues in the Evolution of the Knowledge Base for Nursing. The chapter begins with a discussion of the "trifurcation" among nursing theory, research, and practice, and how this slows the development of the nursing knowledge base. The discussion proceeds to a consideration of how gaps among these nursing activities can be overcome. Some possibilities include research utilization programs and the emergence of collaborative research projects. The chapter concludes with an in-depth examination of Nursing Information Classification Systems and emergent nursing taxonomies.

PART III

This unit focuses on nursing education and its central role in professionalization. It examines trends in basic nursing education and advanced education for nurses. It also deals with current issues and challenges facing nursing education today.

Chapter 5: Basic Nursing Education: An Evolving System. The chapter opens with a discussion of the role of Florence Nightingale in refocusing the direction of the preparation of nurses, and how that new focus became manifest in early nursing education in the United States. Next, the chapter compares and contrasts three nursing education programs: diploma schools, baccalaureate degree education, and associate degree preparation. The contribution of national nursing studies to nursing education is also considered. The chapter concludes with a discussion of new directions in nursing education, including critical thinking and nursing informatics utilization.

Chapter 6: Advanced Education for Nurses: A Hallmark of Professionalism. This chapter deals with both master's degree and doctoral degree preparation for nurses. Included are discussions of nurse practitioners, clinical nurse specialists, certified nurse midwives, and certified registered nurse anesthetists. Strategies that nurses should consider when preparing for master's and doctoral study are also considered. The chapter concludes with a look at postdoctoral education in nursing.

Chapter 7: Nursing Education: Issues and Challenges. The first topic addressed in this chapter is the "entry into practice" issue and its implications for preparing professional nurses. The second topic is the means whereby quality is assured in programs of nursing education. The central focus of this discussion is the role of accreditation. The chapter concludes with a discussion of diversity within and beyond nursing education. Topics include racial and ethnic minorities and the inclusion of men in nursing education and nursing practice.

PART IV

This unit deals with nursing practice itself and how it contributes to and reflects professionalization. It describes career opportunities for nurses as well as advanced nursing practice. Issues faced in nursing practice as our health care system changes also are examined.

Chapter 8: Nursing Career Opportunities. Nurses practice in several distinct settings. This chapter presents a detailed look at four of them: acute care hospitals, ambulatory care settings, the community, and long-term care facilities. The discussion of nursing in the community includes the broader base within which nurses work in the community including home health care, hospice care, school nursing, occupational health nursing, and parish nursing.

Chapter 9: Advanced Nursing Practice: Expanding Opportunities for Professionalization. The evolution of advanced nursing practice is described, including that of nurse anesthetists, nurse midwives, clinical nurse specialists, and nurse practitioners. Two models of advanced nursing practice are discussed: primary care and management of high-risk and vulnerable populations in the community. Role responsibilities of advanced practice nurses also are described.

Chapter 10: Issues in Nursing Practice: Changing Opportunities in a Changing Health Care Environment. The discussion in this chapter focuses on the managed care environment and what it means for nursing. Topics include what nurses are doing today in such diverse areas as home health care and perioperative nursing, as well as other areas of practice. The chapter also discusses what nurses should be doing in the managed health care environment to ensure patient safety and continued quality of nursing care. The chapter concludes with the argument that the changing American health care system offers changing opportunities for the growth of professional nursing practice.

PART V

This unit helps the student understand the various strategies necessary to enhance the process of professionalization in nursing. It deals with power, politics, and policy, as well as ethics and the law. The section concludes with a discussion of nursing in the future. In that discussion the link is shown between nursing and the broad forces of social change that are affecting all occupations and all people. As nursing continues to professionalize, it will be confronting the effects of these changes well into the 21st century.

Chapter 11: Power, Politics, and Policy: Advancing Nursing's Professionalization. The chapter begins with an in-depth consideration of the nature, sources, and use of power. It assesses the power of nursing in social, economic, and political matters as well as the strategies that nursing can use to further enhance its power and effectiveness. It describes the ANA's use of power in securing its agenda and concludes with advanced practice nursing as a critical area for political action.

Chapter 12: Nursing, Ethics, and the Law. Almost everything nurses do—both personally and professionally—involves ethical judgements. This chapter discusses the links between ethics and the law that nurses must consider. It distinguishes between everyday and technical ethics, and describes the fundamental values underlying codes of nursing ethics. These include justice, autonomy, fidelity, beneficence, veracity, and advocacy. The chapter also discusses how ethics can come into conflict as well as be a model for ethical decision-making. In addition, the chapter examines how advances in biotechnology have challenged nursing ethics, and how some of these challenges have been resolved. In addition, research ethics are examined, along with issues regarding patients as human subjects, and nurses' responsibilities to these patients. It concludes with a discussion of nursing and the law.

Chapter 13: Nursing for the Future: 2000 and Beyond. To understand where nursing is heading, one must understand both nursing's past, and the societal forces propelling the world, our country, and nursing into the future. The chapter describes how industrialization, bureaucratization, urbanization, globalization, and rationalization have created the social context in which nursing has evolved, developed, and continues to do so. Specific topics include: interactive care planning, nurse case manager roles, nursing management, information technology, and culturally competent care in nursing practice.

Features

A number of new features have been incorporated into this edition of *Professionalization of Nursing: Current Issues and Trends*. This was done in order to enhance students' level of interest and understanding of the nursing professionalization process and its centrality in practice, research, and education, and to assist instructors in providing focus for study and discussion.

Chapter Outlines at the beginning of each chapter allow the reader to quickly get a sense of the "whole" of the chapter and its content.

Key Terms are identified at the beginning of each chapter and are bolded the first time each one is defined in the text.

Learning Objectives appear at the beginning of each chapter to help students focus on what they should learn from reading the chapter.

Figures appear throughout the text and present visual interpretations of underlying processes, trends, and constructs.

Displays appear throughout the text and provide visual emphasis to important textual material.

Bulleted and Numbered Lists appear throughout the text and highlight important information.

Thinking Critically are special critical thinking in-text displays interspersed throughout all chapters. These special displays raise questions and challenges to engage the student in dialogue regarding content and ideas presented in each chapter.

Chapter Summaries provide the reader with a "wrap-up" of the overall goals embodied within the chapter content as it relates to the continuing professionalization of nursing and the challenges we confront.

Key Points appear at the end of every chapter and are organized and presented in such a way as to provide a brief "answer" to the learning objectives.

Recommended Readings appear at the end of every chapter, were identified and chosen in consultation with students, and are provided to encourage students to research the issues using current "readable" sources.

In sum, it is my hope that students who use this book will come to understand the proud heritage of nursing and realize that professionalization is an ongoing process, which is advanced by nurses' continually confronting and overcoming challenges. It also is important for students to understand that personal learning and advancement should never end if one is to be an effective nurse. In addition, it also is important that students recognize the necessity and value of supporting and affiliating with nursing organizations that promote the advancement of professionalism in nursing. Finally, it is my hope that students will learn to appreciate that further advancement of nursing as a profession is dependent on the willingness and commitment of every nurse to assume personal accountability and responsibility.

Patricia M. Schwirian, PhD, RN

Acknowledgments

While the author is ultimately responsible for a book's content and presentation, authors seldom work alone. There are many who contribute to the final version of any book. First and foremost, I would like to express my appreciation to Sarah Kyle, the editor with whom I worked most closely throughout the entire writing process. Sarah saw to it that every "i" was dotted, every "t" was crossed, and that every chapter attained its goals. Next, I would like to thank my two library research assistants, Terah Sproule and Adria Corbett, of The Ohio State University College of Nursing. They efficiently combed the university libraries in search of readings of particular value to students.

Special thanks go to my daughter, Julia Schwirian George, for her remarkable ability to troubleshoot computer problems and decode Windows 95 for me. Last, but not least, I would like to thank my husband, Kent Schwirian, for his editorial assistance with the whole project and for his contributions to the material dealing with social change and nursing.

Contents

▶ PART I
Introduction to Professionalization and Nursing

CHAPTER 1

Professions and the Professionalization of Nursing • • • • • • • • • • • • • • • 3

Profession • 4
Professional • 7
Professionalism • • • • • • • • • • • • • • • • • • • 8
Professionalization • • • • • • • • • • • • • • • 8
Nursing as a Profession • • • • • • • • • • • 11
Milestones in the Professionalization
of Nursing • • • • • • • • • • • • • • • • • • • 17

Barriers to the Emergence of Full
Professional Status • • • • • • • • • • • • • 24
Chapter Summary • • • • • • • • • • • • • • • • 25
Key Points • 26
References • 27
Classic References • • • • • • • • • • • • • • • • 28
Recommended Readings • • • • • • • • • • • 29

▶ PART II
A Knowledge Base for Nursing: A Work in Progress

CHAPTER 2

Nursing Knowledge and Nursing Theory:
Foundations of a Profession • 33

Nursing Knowledge • • • • • • • • • • • • • 34
Theory for Nursing
Knowledge • • • • • • • • • • • • • • • • • • • 39
Knowledge for Nursing: Beyond
Empirics • 48

Chapter Summary • • • • • • • • • • • • • • • • 52
Key Points • 52
References • 53
Classic References • • • • • • • • • • • • • • • • 54
Recommended Readings • • • • • • • • • • • 56

CHAPTER 3

Nursing Research: An Action Path to Professionalization • • • • • • • • 58

Development and Progress of Nursing
Research • 59
Types of Research Contributing
to Nursing Science • • • • • • • • • • • • • 69
Chapter Summary • • • • • • • • • • • • • • • • 81

Key Points • 81
References • 82
Classic References • • • • • • • • • • • • • • • • 83
Recommended Readings • • • • • • • • • • • 84

CHAPTER 4

Current Issues in the Evolution of the Knowledge Base for Nursing • 85

Development and Use of Nursing
Knowledge • • • • • • • • • • • • • • • • • • • 86
Fostering the Development of Nursing
Knowledge: Nursing Information
Classification Systems • • • • • • • • • • 100

Chapter Summary • • • • • • • • • • • • • • 109
Key Points • 109
References • 109
Classic References • • • • • • • • • • • • • • 111
Recommended Readings • • • • • • • • • 112

▶ PART III
Nursing Education: At the Heart of Professionalization

CHAPTER 5

Basic Nursing Education: An Evolving System • • • • • • • • • • • • • • • • • 115

Development of Nursing
Education • • • • • • • • • • • • • • • • • • • 116
Types of Basic Nursing Education
Programs • 119
National Nursing Studies: Impact
on Nursing Education • • • • • • • • • • 128
New Directions in Nursing Education:
Enhancing Skills for Professional
Nursing • 131

Chapter Summary • • • • • • • • • • • • • • 135
Key Points • 135
References • 136
Classic References • • • • • • • • • • • • • • 138
Recommended Readings • • • • • • • • • 138

CHAPTER 6

Advanced Education for Nurses:
A Hallmark of Professionalism • 140

The Need for Advanced
Education • • • • • • • • • • • • • • • • • • • 141
Master's Degree Preparation
for Nurses • • • • • • • • • • • • • • • • • • • 142
Doctoral Degree Preparation
for Nurses • • • • • • • • • • • • • • • • • • • 151

Chapter Summary • • • • • • • • • • • • • • 155
Key Points • 156
References • 157
Classic References • • • • • • • • • • • • • • 158
Recommended Readings • • • • • • • • • 158

CHAPTER 7

Nursing Education: Issues and Challenges • 160

Entry Into Practice • • • • • • • • • • • • • 161
Accreditation • • • • • • • • • • • • • • • • • 166
Diversity • 170
Other Issues • • • • • • • • • • • • • • • • • • 180
Chapter Summary • • • • • • • • • • • • • • 180

Key Points • 181
References • 183
Classic Reference • • • • • • • • • • • • • • 184
Recommended Readings • • • • • • • • • 184

▶ **PART IV**
Nursing Practice and Professionalization

CHAPTER 8
Nursing Career Opportunities • **189**

Nursing in Acute
Care Hospitals • • • • • • • • • • • • • • • 191
Nursing in Ambulatory
Care Settings • • • • • • • • • • • • • • • • 196
Nursing in the Community • • • • • • • 199
Nursing in Long-Term
Care Facilities • • • • • • • • • • • • • • • • 208

Chapter Summary • • • • • • • • • • • • • • 210
Key Points • 211
References • 212
Recommended Readings • • • • • • • • • • 213

CHAPTER 9
Advanced Nursing Practice: Expanding Opportunities
for Professionalization • **215**

Evolution of Advanced Nursing
Practice • 218
Models of Advanced
Nursing Practice • • • • • • • • • • • • • • 226
Role Responsibilities
of APNs • 231

Chapter Summary • • • • • • • • • • • • • • 234
Key Points • 234
References • 236
Classic References • • • • • • • • • • • • • • 237
Recommended Readings • • • • • • • • • 237

CHAPTER 10
Issues in Nursing Practice: Changing Opportunities in a Changing
Health Care Environment • **239**

The Managed Care
Environment • • • • • • • • • • • • • • • • • 241
The Managed Care Environment
and Nursing • • • • • • • • • • • • • • • • • • 245
Thriving in the Managed Care
Environment • • • • • • • • • • • • • • • • • 254

Chapter Summary • • • • • • • • • • • • • • 259
Key Points • 260
References • 262
Recommended Readings • • • • • • • • • 264

▶ **PART V**
Strategies to Enhance Professionalization in Nursing

CHAPTER 11
Power, Politics, and Policy:
Advancing Nursing's Professionalization • **267**

Power: The Concept • • • • • • • • • • • • • 269
Nursing and Politics • • • • • • • • • • • • • 275

Policy to Further
Professionalization • • • • • • • • • • • • 283

Chapter Summary · · · · · · · · · · · · · · · · 285
Key Points · 286

References · 288
Recommended Readings · · · · · · · · · · 289

CHAPTER 12
Nursing, Ethics, and the Law · 290

Ethics and Codes of Ethics · · · · · · · · 291
Biotechnology and Nursing
   Ethics · 296
Research Ethics and Human
   Subjects · 301
The Law and Nursing
   Professionalization · · · · · · · · · · · · 306

Chapter Summary · · · · · · · · · · · · · · · · 309
Key Points · 309
References · 311
Recommended Readings · · · · · · · · · · 311

CHAPTER 13
Nursing for the Future: 2000 and Beyond · 313

The Great Social
   Transformation · · · · · · · · · · · · · · · 314
Nursing and the Great Social
   Transformation · · · · · · · · · · · · · · · 320

Chapter Summary · · · · · · · · · · · · · · · · 340
Key Points · 340
References · 342
Recommended Readings · · · · · · · · · · 343

Index · 344

PART I

Introduction to Professionalization and Nursing

1

Professions and the Professionalization of Nursing

CHAPTER OUTLINE

Profession
Professional
Professionalism
Professionalization
Nursing as a Profession
Milestones in the
   Professionalization of Nursing

Barriers to the Emergence of Full
   Professional Status
Chapter Summary
Key Points
References
Classic References
Recommended Readings

LEARNING OBJECTIVES

▶ **1** Discuss the characteristics that differentiate professions from occupations.

▶ **2** Understand the process of professionalization.

▶ **3** Recognize how nursing has progressed toward full professional status.

▶ **4** Examine the challenges nursing must meet to achieve professionalization.

▶ **5** Examine the role of the American Nurses Association, other professional organizations, and research studies in terms of their contribution to the professionalization process.

▶ **6** Discuss the barriers that slow the professional development of nursing.

KEY TERMS

autonomy   profession   professionalizers
Flexner report   professional   traditionalizers
Goldmark report   professionalism   utilizers
occupation   professionalization

Isabel Hampton Robb, one of the great nursing leaders of the early 1900s, observed that "medicine has taken the decision out of our hands, and has made trained nursing a profession, but how soon we shall attain to the full professional level depends upon ourselves entirely" (Robb, 1975, p. 326). It seems ironic, but if Robb were to evaluate the nursing scene today—almost a century later—she might conclude that her observation is as pertinent today as it was in 1900.

There is much debate among nurses as to whether full professional status has been achieved in nursing. Many nurses enjoy being called professionals. However, many nurses question whether full professional status has been achieved. Much of the confusion among nurses as to nursing's professional status is due in large measure to inadequate definitions of profession. More than 30 years ago, Martha Rogers, an esteemed nurse leader and educator, pointed out that "a philosophy of nursing as a learned profession demands a major reorientation for the bulk of nurses [and] . . . loose usage of the prestigious word 'professional' must give way to more precise definition."(Rogers, 1964, p. 10).

Therefore, to determine whether nursing has reached full professional status, we must first define "profession," "professional," "professionalism," and "professionalization" and then determine how these concepts apply to nursing.

Profession

It is important to make the distinction between profession and occupation. An **occupation** is a job or a career. All professions are occupations, but not all occupations are professions. For example, a person who has the occupation of physician is a member of the medical profession; on the other hand, a person whose occupation is construction worker does not belong to the construction profession. Perhaps there are no more than 30 or 40 professions altogether (Wilensky, 1962). The characteristics that differentiate profession from occupation are examined in detail below and are followed by a definition of profession.

Characteristics of a Profession

What characteristics do professions have in common that differentiates them from other occupations? One of the earliest and most important discussions of the characteristics of a profession was presented by Abraham Flexner, a noted educator of the early 20th century. In 1915, he argued that the characteristics of a profession were:

- ▶ Basically intellectual, carrying with it high responsibility
- ▶ Learned in nature, because it is based on a body of knowledge
- ▶ Practical rather than theoretical

- ▶ Technique can be taught through educational discipline
- ▶ Well organized internally
- ▶ Motivated by altruism. (Flexner, 1915)

Flexner listed intellectual endeavor as the first criterion, viewing it as the *core* of professions. He clearly reasserted the importance of learning 15 years later in the following statement:

> How are we to distinguish professions that belong to universities from vocations that do not belong to them? The criteria are not difficult to discern. Professions are, as a matter of history—and very rightly—"learned professions"; there are no unlearned professions; unlearned professions—a contradiction in terms—would be vocations, callings, or occupations. (Flexner, 1930)

More recently, sociologists have added the notions of self-regulation, self-control, and self-identification to the definition of a profession (Etzioni, 1969; Goode, 1960; Greenwood, 1962; Parsons, 1954). According to them, a profession is characterized by the following:

1. *A lengthy, rigorous education is required preparation.* Often the requirements include graduate school, internships, residencies, and postdoctoral training. Typically, an examination admits one to full membership in the profession and the privilege to practice that profession independently.
2. *The educational component is firmly grounded in theory.* Education to profession is not simply technical in nature.
3. *Professions are self-regulating.* The members themselves claim the exclusive knowledge to set professional standards and certify those who are qualified to enter the profession (and those whose actions should prompt decertification). As sociologist Ernest Greenwood put it, "Anyone can call himself a carpenter, locksmith, or metal-plater if he feels so qualified. But a person who assumes the title of physician or attorney without having earned it conventionally becomes an impostor" (Greenwood, 1962, p. 211).
4. *Professionals have authority over clients.* They claim this on the basis of their specialized education and theoretical understanding. It is the client's obligation to follow the professional's instructions (Henslin, 1995, p. 396).
5. *Altruism is a driving motivation.* Members of a profession hold as their highest calling service to people, not self-interest.
6. *There is strong identification with peers in the profession.* This extent of identification may surpass even the extent to which they identify with their employers.

Occupational Prestige
In addition to the six characteristics that distinguish a profession from an occupation, there is the matter of social prestige. Society holds professional people in esteem because of the importance of their knowledge to the smooth functioning of society and the well-being of people, the difficulty of acquiring the knowledge, and the ability of the profession itself to control access to the profession. Society's esteem for a profession is seen in our widespread desire to be professionals, the extent to which we are pleased to find relatives and friends entering professions, the respect we accord members of the professions, and the fact that members of most professions make more money than the rest of the population (Curry, Jiobu, & Schwirian, 1997). The 10 most prestigious occupations, all of which are considered professions, are listed in Box 1-1.

BOX 1-1

Most Prestigious Occupations

- ► Supreme Court Justice (lawyers by training)
- ► Physician
- ► Lawyer
- ► College professor
- ► Physicist
- ► Computer scientist
- ► Architect
- ► Chemist
- ► Biologist

(Adapted from Curry T, Jiobu R, Schwirian K [1996]. *Sociology for the 21st Century.* Upper Saddle River, NJ: Prentice-Hall.)

 CRITICALLY THINKING ABOUT . . .

When you think of the term "profession," what characteristics—in addition to those discussed in the text—come to mind?

Definition of Profession

Based on the characteristics that differentiate profession from occupation, **profession** can be defined as a prestigious occupation with a high degree of identification among the members that requires a lengthy and rigorous education in an intellectually demanding and theoretically based course of study; that engages in rigorous self-regulation and control; that holds authority over clients; and that puts service to society above simple self-interest.

Occupation–Profession Continuum

Although professions can be differentiated from occupations, it is important to understand that there actually is a continuum, a continuous dimension, on which all occupations may be placed. This continuum is anchored at one end by "occupation" and at the other by "profession." To be at the full profession end, an occupation must manifest all the characteristics of a profession. If some of the characteristics are absent, then the occupation is considered a semiprofession. It may well be in a transitional status from occupation to profession, or society may have locked it into a permanent semiprofessional status by denying it such things as legal control over the practice of its members. If few or none of the characteristics of a profession are present, the occupation is at the occupation end. Medicine, law, the ministry, and university teaching have claimed professional status for centuries. By the 19th century, architecture, dentistry, and some branches of engineering were professionalized. More recently, several scientific and engineering fields, along with certified public accountants, have come to be recognized as professions (Goode, 1969). Some occupations are still in progress toward full professional status; these include social work,

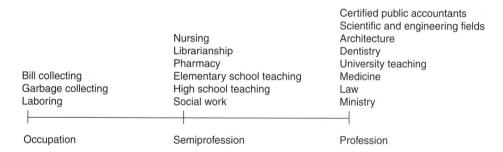

Figure 1-1. The occupation–profession continuum.

elementary and secondary school teaching, librarianship, pharmacy, and (perhaps) nursing. Other occupations, such as laborers, bill collectors, and garbage collectors are at the occupation end of the continuum (Fig. 1-1). **Professionalization**, the process by which professions move up the occupation–profession continuum, is discussed later in the chapter.

Impact of Bureaucracies on Professions

Among the major changes in the last century has been the rise of the large-scale bureaucracy as the form of organization in which society conducts its business in all institutional arenas. Bureaucracies are characterized by a complex division of labor; a hierarchy of authority, with few people at the top and many at the bottom; explicit rules that govern all aspects of the organization down to the smallest detail; a system of rewards based on performance; and an extensive system of written rules and records (Curry, Jiobu, & Schwirian, 1997). In health care, it is the hospital, the health maintenance organization, and the clinic.

Bureaucracies exert pressures that undermine the independent status of professions and semiprofessions. In a bureaucratic system, professionals and semiprofessionals are converted to employees, as a result losing a large part of their professional autonomy and control. For example, nurses are usually employees of hospitals and in many instances have felt the need to organize for collective bargaining—an activity not normally expected of members of a profession. Thus, the net effect of this organizational shift toward bureaucratization is to move many professions toward the occupation end of the occupation–profession continuum.

Professional

The term **professional**, whether used as a noun or as an adjective, refers to the degree to which the characteristics of a profession are present (Hughes, 1965). As a noun, a professional is someone who is a member of an established learned profession. For example, a physician is considered a professional because his or her line of work (medicine) is considered a profession. As an adjective, professional is used to describe a person or activity that characterizes or conforms to the technical and ethical standards of a profession. For example, a physician who treats patients in a way consistent with the expectations for physicians would be considered professional.

However, if a physician gives a premature or false diagnosis, is haphazard in prescribing treatment or evaluating its effect, or is uncaring to patients, he or she would be considered unprofessional.

To be considered truly professional, a person's behavior must be professional within the profession and outside of the profession within the larger community. For example, if a physician is a respected member of the local school board, it serves to reinforce his or her professional status in the eyes of community members. On the other hand, if a physician cheats on his or her spouse, neglects the children, publicly gambles, or drinks to excess, his or her status as a professional is diminished in the eyes of the public.

As stated earlier, professions are self-regulating. Therefore, breaches of the profession's behavioral norms by its members—whether they occur within the practice of the profession or outside in the larger community—are usually treated with severe negative sanctions leveled by an investigative board. If the violations are judged to be extreme, the violator may be expelled from the profession and prohibited from further practice.

Professionalism

Professionalism refers to the conduct, goals, or qualities that characterize or mark a profession or a professional person. A significant portion of one's educational preparation for entry into a profession is the development of qualities, behaviors, and even appearances that embody professionalism. Professions usually develop codes of ethics that describe expected behaviors that reflect professionalism among its members.

Professionalism is often seen in the extent to which professionals develop a sense of calling to the profession (Olesen & Whittaker, 1968). Some identify with the profession to such a degree that they experience a "role/self merger." *Role* refers to the behaviors associated with a position (eg, doctor, nurse, or teacher) within society. *Self-concept* is the set of labels (eg, son, wife, female, male) people use to identify themselves. A role/self merger has taken place if a fundamental part of a person's self-concept is the professional role that he or she fulfills. For example, if a person cannot think of himself or herself without identifying as a nurse or physician, a role/self merger has occurred. Professionals who have experienced this merger have a very difficult time leaving the profession for another, retiring from the profession, or becoming disinterested in professional matters.

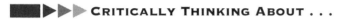 **CRITICALLY THINKING ABOUT . . .**

What types of behaviors reflect professionalism among nurses?

Professionalization

Professionalization is the process occupations go through as they move to the profession end of the occupation–profession continuum. Aaronson described it as a "dynamic process, whereby many occupations can be observed to change certain crucial characteristics in the direction of profession—an exchange process between society and an occupational group striving for professional status" (Aaronson, 1989, p. 274). In the exchange between society and the occupational group, society recognizes the professional status of the occupation and the profession performs the important tasks for society for which it was recognized. For example, medicine is recognized by society as a profession; therefore, medicine takes on itself, among other things, the massive burden of diagnosing and treating physical illness, training prospective members of the profession, conducting basic research into cures for disease, and regulating the professional behavior of its members.

Process of Professionalization

The process of professionalization is generally described as a series of stages characterized by specific events or changes in the structure of the occupation as it strives to achieve professional status (Wilensky, 1962). In studying established professions and occupations in the process of professionalization, Wilensky observed that a series of events occur as occupations move toward professionalism:

- ▶ People begin doing the work full-time and stake out a jurisdiction.
- ▶ Early masters of the technique or adherents of the movement become concerned about standards of training and practice and set up a training school, which, if not lodged in universities at the start, makes academic connections within two or three decades.
- ▶ Teachers and activists achieve success in promoting more effective organization—first local and then national.
- ▶ Legal protection appears.
- ▶ A formal code of ethics is adopted. (Wilensky, 1964, pp. 143–144)

The "natural history" of professionalization refers to the chronologic occurrence of these events throughout the stages of professionalization. Table 1-1 presents a comparison of the natural history of professionalization of selected professions and occupations in the process of becoming professionalized. It reveals the sequence of events that has characterized the development of professions in this country.

In examining Table 1-1, it is clear that there are differences among medicine, nursing, librarianship, law, school teaching, and social work in regard to the dates in which the first training and university schools were established and when the first national professional associations were organized. National professional associations were established before university schools in social work, school teaching, nursing, and librarianship; university schools were established before national professional associations in medicine and law.

Wilensky (1994) explains the significance of these differences in the natural history of professionalization by stating that "a clue to the obstacles to any marked growth of professionalism is in the difference between the process by which the established professions have achieved their position and the process pursued by occupations aspiring to professional status." He adds, "in the recent history of professionalism, the organization push comes before a solid technical and institutional base is formed; the professional association, for instance, typically precedes university-based training schools, and the whole effort seems more an opportunistic struggle for the rewards of monopoly than a natural history of professionalism."

TABLE 1-1   THE PROCESS OF PROFESSIONALIZATION

Profession	Became Full-Time Occupation	First Training School	First University School	First National Professional Association	First State License Law	Formal Code of Ethics
Law	17th century	1784	1817	1878	1732	1908
Medicine	1700	1765	1779	1847	Before 1780	1912
School teaching	17th century	1823	1879	1857	1781	1929
Librarianship	1732	1887	1897	1876	Before 1919	1938
Nursing	17th century	1861	1909	1897	1903	1950
Social work	1898	1898	1904	1874	1940	1948

(Modified from Wilensky HL [1964]. The Professionalization of Everyone? *Am J Sociology* 70:2 [September]: 143. Reprinted by permission of the University of Chicago Press. Copyright © 1964, University of Chicago Press.)

▶▶▶ **CRITICALLY THINKING ABOUT . . .**

How does the importance of nursing to society contribute to its professionalization?

Nursing as a Profession

Now that the concepts of profession, professional, professionalism, and professionalization have been defined and discussed, it is possible to examine how these concepts apply to nursing and to determine whether nursing has reached full professional status. In doing so, nursing's position on the occupation–profession continuum will be determined, the progress nursing has made over the years in relation to professionalization will be discussed, and challenges that still face the professionalization of nursing will be examined.

Nursing's Position on the Occupation–Profession Continuum

Earlier in this chapter, the concept of a continuum extending from occupation to profession on which any occupation could be evaluated was presented. Ronald Pavalko (1971) constructed one such continuum consisting of eight characteristics or dimensions that differentiate occupations from true professions. By inserting a column for nursing, the extent to which nursing has advanced toward the professional end of the continuum in terms of each of Pavalko's eight dimensions can be determined (Table 1-2). Although this table was created in 1971, nursing's position on the occupation–profession continuum has not changed significantly overall. However, as discussed below, much progress has been made.

TABLE 1-2	**POSITION OF NURSING ON THE OCCUPATION– PROFESSION MODEL**		
Dimension	**Occupation**	**Nursing**	**Profession**
1. Theory	Absent	Present (limited)	Present
2. Relevance to social values	Not relevant	Relevant	Relevant
3. Training period	Short, not specialized	Varied in length; some specialization	Long and specialized
4. Motivation	Self-interest	Service	Service
5. Autonomy	Absent	Incomplete	Complete
6. Commitment	Short-term	Varies; relatively short	Long-term
7. Sense of community	Low	Minimal	High
8. Code of ethics	Undeveloped	Highly developed	Highly developed

(Adapted from Pavalko RM [1971]. *Sociology of Occupations and Professions.* Itasca, IL: FE Peacock, p. 26. Reprinted by permission of the publisher.)

The data in Table 1-2 show that when nursing is compared with professions in general, it scores very well in relevance to social values, service motivation, and a code of ethics. However, nursing theory is still in the process of being developed and refined; its education is still not standardized with university preparation as a minimum requirement; control over its practice is limited; many of its members are not wholly committed to their work; and a sense of community and cohesion has yet to be fully realized. Because some of nursing's professional characteristics are not as highly developed as those of the established professions, it continues to rank just slightly above the midpoint on the Pavalko continuum—thus, it is classified as a semiprofession.

Nursing's Progress Toward Professionalism

Although nursing has not yet been recognized as a full profession, it has made remarkable progress over the years, especially within the past 20 years. Most nurses would agree that the occupation of nursing continues to improve its position on the occupation–profession continuum. This is evidenced by certain observable changes in the characteristics required of professions—upgraded educational requirements, advances in research, successful efforts in legislation, and improved distribution of manpower. In addition, tremendous improvements have been made in schools of nursing, in scholarly research productivity, in state nursing boards, and in the educational preparation of nursing service administrators.

Because of vigorous collective bargaining activities, the American Nurses Association (ANA) has obtained significantly improved salaries and improved working conditions for its members. However, not everyone would agree that following a union model is the "professional" thing to do. Moreover, some nurses feel that state nurses associations have been burdened with the task of collective bargaining under the new federation model of the ANA. They believe that other programs (eg, staff support for panels, councils, and commissions) have suffered because of funds being used for collective bargaining. However, many other nurses are very much in favor of supporting the state nursing association's collective bargaining program.

Another area of considerable progress that most would agree is consistent with increased professionalism is significant (and often hard-won) changes in nurse practice acts all over the country. These nurse practice acts provide legal sanction and greater flexibility and autonomy for nurses in assuming expanded roles. This movement will be discussed more fully in Chapter 10. In addition, the current attempt of the American Association of Colleges of Nursing to become the accrediting body for baccalaureate and higher degree programs is a significant step toward self-governance and self-management in nursing education (American Association of Colleges of Nursing, 1996).

Another way that nursing is evolving toward full professional status is through development of nursing leaders. The lack of qualified leaders in nursing was cited as a barrier to progress in the professionalization of nursing in an earlier edition of this book (Moloney, 1992). For the most part, this barrier has been overcome, largely because of the development of strong doctoral programs in nursing at major universities across the country. Graduates of these programs are strongly committed to their careers, are highly educated, are firmly grounded in the sciences, and have been educated in highly professionalized environments. They have had role models and mentors who are true professionals. Thus, the cadre of qualified, dedicated leaders is growing dramatically. These well-prepared nurses are regularly assuming leadership in nursing organizations at local, state, and national levels in accord with the professional role expectations of the institutions of higher education where they go on to contribute to nursing as teachers, researchers, and administrators.

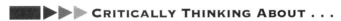 **CRITICALLY THINKING ABOUT . . .**

Does it matter to you whether nursing is considered a profession or a semiprofession? Why or why not?

Challenges to the Professionalization of Nursing

The progress toward full professionalization of nursing is hampered by several significant factors. The first three are extremely important and interrelated characteristics of a true profession—a unique, theoretically sound knowledge base; autonomy over education and practice; and a monopoly over services. Of these, the primary characteristic is the knowledge base; the other two characteristics can emerge from the knowledge base. Without a knowledge base, little progress in either autonomy or monopoly of services is likely. However, the knowledge base must not only exist, but it also must be recognized, validated, and valued by nurses, other health professionals, health administrators, and the general public.

Two other challenges to be met to achieve full professionalization of nursing are increasing the level of commitment to nursing and limiting the number of professionals.

Specialized Knowledge Base

Because professional knowledge is held by only a few, it is distinguished from more common knowledge. The new professional is given access to confidential information or information of an intimate nature particular to the profession. The three most firmly established professions—medicine, law, and the ministry—have a strong claim to such knowledge. Thus, clients observe in the tasks performed by professionals an air of mystery the ordinary man or woman does not possess (Wilensky, 1964).

An occupation aspiring to full professionalism must be be able to control a substantial body of unique knowledge that is not controlled by other occupations (Goode, 1969), but having such a unique body of knowledge is not enough. For occupations to justify their claim to autonomy, this knowledge base must be recognized by other professionals and the general public (Goode, 1966).

A body of knowledge unique to nursing is still developing (see Chaps. 2 and 3). However, most nurses would agree that society does not yet understand the significance of this developing body of knowledge or the unique contributions to health care provided by the body of knowledge. Unfortunately, nursing knowledge is primarily viewed as ancillary to medicine—in other words, that it is medical knowledge in a lesser amount than that possessed by physicians (Hughes, 1980).

One may think that nursing alone should be the judge of the validity of its own knowledge base. However, the professionalization process is greatly influenced by whether or not society accepts nursing's claim of special knowledge and expertise in health care and whether or not society supports and values the services provided by nurses. Therefore, nursing is striving diligently to alter the public's outdated view of nursing knowledge. The issues concerning nursing knowledge and theory are discussed in great detail in Chapter 2.

Increasing nursing's knowledge base implies an increase in the number of people performing specialized intellectual work as compared with those doing manual labor or unspecialized routine activities. As nursing's body of knowledge advances, an increase in the number of professional nurses having baccalaureate, master's, and doctoral degrees in nursing should occur, giving nursing the intellectual leadership and professional knowledge required for professional practice.

Autonomy in Nursing

Autonomy means independence. Some characteristics of autonomy among professions are control of practice, control of entry into the profession, and determination of the qualifications needed by those seeking entry and the organization of their training, thus deciding who will be one's colleagues (Gross, 1962). In addition, autonomy allows a profession to control its services by control of competition and influence on state and federal lawmakers. This is done through professional associations and other pressure groups and by controlling the behavior of the members of the profession. Thus, the profession can enforce standards and maintain whatever values it thinks are desirable (Gross, 1962).

Many registered nurses are convinced that they have professional autonomy because they possess a license to practice. However, licensure is simply a mandate related to the government's responsibility to protect its citizens from harm. Licensure has little relation to what is required of professionals. In fact, effective professional autonomy is granted only when society is convinced that the group has a unique and valuable knowledge base and thus can exert self-control over its own education and practice (Goode, 1960).

Autonomy or independence in nursing refers to "freedom to make decisions and clinical judgements within their (nurses') scope of practice" (Oermann, 1997). Because it is not a full profession, nursing does not yet have true autonomy. Even if nursing were to have a specialized knowledge base recognized by society, there are two major threats to the development of true autonomy.

The first threat centers on the issue of the difference in occupational prestige between physicians and semiprofessionals (including nurses). In 1964, Wilensky described hospitals as a working environment where members of semiprofessions were inevitably placed in the "stultifying shadow of medicine" (Wilensky, 1964, p. 156). Moreover, as Katz pointed out, medicine, by legal and informal means, offers resistance to anyone encroaching on its authority—in other words, "the caste-like system" places a wall that is impossible to scale between the physician and semiprofessionals in the hospital (Katz, 1969, p. 69). This issue is very important to understanding nurses' autonomy and is relevant to the concept of occupational prestige discussed earlier. Those with high prestige enjoy a great deal of autonomy; those of lesser prestige have their autonomy constrained. Semiprofessions enjoy less freedom from being supervised than do the more prestigious professions (Simpson & Simpson, 1969). Semiprofessionals are frequently told exactly what to do and how it is to be done.

Although the general nature of the relation between persons of greater and lesser occupational prestige remains very much the same as in the 1960s when these observations were made, many changes have occurred in both the health care system and in society in general that alter the autonomy factors for nurses. First, with the advent of large-scale cost-saving measures in hospitals of all kinds, the all-powerful role that physicians once routinely enjoyed has been diminished in the name of controlling expenses considered unnecessarily burdensome by hospital administrators. In effect, the occupational prestige of many physicians in hospital settings has decreased, so the discrepancy between the status of physicians and nurses is not so great. Another factor affecting autonomy is the increasing numbers of nurses who are obtaining educational preparation in graduate programs of study, increasing both their level of function and their status as both clinicians and scientists. This is leading to increased opportunities for nurse–physician collaboration and in turn to mutual respect for abilities and the idea of division of labor between colleagues rather than the direct supervision of a nurse by a physician-ordered task.

A third important factor is the movement of many care functions from inpatient hospital settings to the community. Nurses began their history of direct care in this country by providing independent nursing care to persons and families in their own homes and community centers. This pattern is reemerging, and the autonomy of nurses in their practice is bound to benefit.

The second significant threat to the development of autonomy of nurses who practice in hospitals comes simply from being an employee of a firmly entrenched bureaucracy. As pointed out earlier, bureaucracies provide a direct challenge to professionalism—including autonomy and colleague authority (Monnig, 1978). Interestingly, as health maintenance organizations and managed care environments have established more and more power in the health care industry, even established professionals are beginning to experience unprecedented bureaucratic threats to their heretofore unchallenged autonomy.

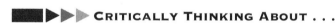 CRITICALLY THINKING ABOUT . . .

Will nursing ever attain professional autonomy as long as nurses work for health care bureaucracies? Why or why not?

Monopoly Over Services

Monopoly over services is achieved when social and economic rewards are given to a profession in exchange for the profession's specialized knowledge base. Professions further acquire a monopoly over services by keeping their essential services in scant supply. Occupations desiring to use professional authority to gain a monopoly over services must locate a technical basis for it, state their exclusive jurisdiction, connect skill and jurisdiction to standards of training, and persuade the public of its uniquely trustworthy services.

Nursing is in the process of redefining its function to claim a monopoly over its services. To date, nursing has not succeeded in establishing a special knowledge base acquired through an intellectually rigorous, intense period of training. Additionally, nursing lacks the power to control the supply of nurses. However, establishing a specialized body of knowledge and controlling the supply of nurses alone will not enable nursing to claim a monopoly over services. It is only by controlling its unique services, which society wants and deems necessary, that nursing can acquire a monopoly.

Level of Commitment

Another challenge in the professionalization of nursing is the lack of lifetime commitment of many nurses to their work. Many nurses view nursing as a temporary job rather than as a full-time career. When compared with members of established professions—lawyers, engineers, university professors—nurses tend to leave their occupation at a much higher rate. The fact that a lifetime commitment is stronger in established professions is due in part to the higher rewards, the ideology of the profession, the longer period of professional socialization, and strong colleague orientations. These factors make members less likely to leave their professions.

Furthermore, semiprofessionals usually obtain rewards from their position in the organization, not from performance of work. In addition, semiprofessionals frequently require more supervision and encouragement than professionals. As a result, they tend to be less resistant to bureaucratic control, more accepting of orders from administrators or supervisors, and less inclined to seek autonomy in their work situation.

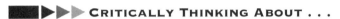 CRITICALLY THINKING ABOUT . . .

What are things a nurse should do to demonstrate a commitment to nursing?

Limiting the Number of Professionals

Almost a half-century ago, economist Eli Ginzberg offered suggestions to nurses concerned about the professional status of their occupation. He suggested that nursing should begin to develop a fixed group of graduates from good college and university programs who could properly be called professionals (Horgan, 1960, p. 50). To ensure that nurses would understand his meaning of a professional, he defined professionals as a group that:

1. Possesses extensive training
2. Provides "intellectual leadership" recognized in its field
3. Conducts research of worth
4. Has independence in defining its specific area of worth.

Ginzberg stated that nursing should recruit and educate only the number of professional nurses that nursing believes are needed. He was convinced that there were too many registered nurses (RNs) for the economy to support at the salary level of a professional. By limiting the group to a maximum of 70,000, the occupation could hope to receive professional pay. According to Ginzberg, nursing could concentrate on developing a group of professional nurses and still encourage licensed practical nurses, associate degree nurses, and diploma graduates to move upward if they so desired.

Despite the fact that numerous nursing groups have suggested similar ideas, the concept of developing an "elite corps" of professional nurses has not been well received and has not been implemented in any way. In fact, it is impossible to raise the knowledge and skill level required for professional nursing unless an economic status that will attract highly qualified people can be achieved. In addition, to restrict the labor supply of professional nurses, the occupation of nursing needs power. Nursing's power base continues to stay at a very low level due in part to the disunity that exists over professional preparation of its practitioners. Therefore, nursing cannot control the number of admissions to all types of nursing programs.

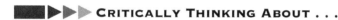 CRITICALLY THINKING ABOUT . . .

> Do you think that enrollments in schools and colleges of nursing should be limited as a means of promoting professionalization? Why or why not?

Needed Transformations

To meet the challenges described above and accomplish the professionalization of nursing, nurses must undergo transformation within their nursing role. They must go beyond seeking socioeconomic advantages to assume greater responsibility in the professional role. Nurses have started, and must continue, to realize that they must act as professionals, attend professional meetings, assist in policy formulation, and take responsibility for their professional lives. The important question is whether or not most nurses are willing to pay the cost of such a transformation. They will have to decide how much of themselves and their time, energy, and resources they will be willing to invest to achieve full professionalism. If nurses decline to act, the goal of full professional status for nursing will be delayed.

Milestones in the Professionalization of Nursing

The existence of professional organizations and the development of research studies within nursing are two important factors that have helped to advance nursing as a profession. In fact, each has brought about important milestones throughout the years. However, neither factor has been able to advance nursing to the full level of profession. The strengths and weaknesses of professional organizations and research studies are discussed below.

Professional Organizations

There are rare humans, such as Florence Nightingale, who—through farsighted vision, personal commitment and determination, favorable social position and connections, and charismatic personality—can have a major impact on the professionalization of an occupation. However, most persons on their own can do little to influence the course of a profession's development. It is through the collective actions of many members' individual efforts that much can be attained. The force of collective action may be limited by only the number of persons working together. Collective action is reflected in the establishment and development of professional organizations within nursing.

American Nurses Association

The Nurses Associated Alumnae of the United States and Canada was established in 1896, and by 1911 it came to be known as the American Nurses Association (ANA). The purpose of the organization was to provide a professional home for nurses working for professionalization (Ellis & Hartley, 1995; Kelly & Joel, 1996). The activities of the ANA have included:

- ◘ Development of uniform and improved nursing standards in practice and nursing education
- ◘ Registration and licensure of all nurses in accordance with nursing standards
- ◘ Welfare of nurses in working conditions and economic matters
- ◘ Collective bargaining.

Despite all its activities, the ANA has yet to reach its full potential as nursing's flagship organization. Low membership is the main reason: only 10% to 15% of all RNs are ANA members. A major factor in low ANA membership is cost. ANA membership fees exceed $200, and many nurses feel that the ANA does not return an amount of service equal to that fee to individual members. The exception, of course, is nurses for whom the ANA is the collective bargaining organization with their hospital employers. To many nurses, specialty nursing groups (eg, American Association of Critical Care Nurses, American Association of Nurse Anesthetists, and Association of Operating Room Nurses) seem closer to their daily practice activities than does the ANA, and limited personal budgets make many nurses choose membership in their practice speciality group over membership in the ANA. However, far too many nurses do not belong to any professional organizations, and this limits the impact organizations have on the professionalization of nursing.

IMPORTANT ANA INITIATIVES

In an effort to provide a means of reaching agreement and promoting action on issues of common concern to the nursing profession, the ANA sponsored the first meeting of the Nursing Organization Liaison Forum (ANA, 1984). This forum was held to provide an arena for the development of consensus on the following issues:

- ◘ Federal funding for nursing education and research
- ◘ Access to quality health care services, including nursing services
- ◘ Role of the government in meeting basic human needs and protecting the environment and public health. (ANA, 1985)

In December 1987, in an effort to strengthen itself, the ANA Board of Directors established a 23-member Commission on Organizational Assessment (COAR) to conduct a national study of its professional association. The commission sent out a survey to state nurse associations and other nursing groups that addressed issues and interrelated problems confronting the association. In June 1989, the ANA House of Delegates implemented the COAR recommendations and adopted a new set of by-laws that would restructure the professional association (Selby, 1989, p. 1).

At the ANA House of Delegates meeting in June 1990, a Congress of Nursing Practice and a Congress on Nursing Economics were formed. The focus of each congress was on long-range policy development, standard setting, program development, and evaluation in their area of expertise (Selby, 1989, p. 16). Another notable change in the bylaws suggested ways to involve specialty organizations in the ANA House of Delegates and the Congress of Nursing Practice. In addition to these efforts to strengthen the organization—and thus the voice of nursing—the ANA has issued a broad range of important position statements since 1994 (Box 1-2). These

---

Box 1-2

ANA Position Statements

- ▶ Assisted suicide
- ▶ Active euthanasia
- ▶ Lead poisoning and screening
- ▶ Childhood immunization
- ▶ Informal caregiving
- ▶ Long-term care
- ▶ Cessation of tobacco
- ▶ Health promotion and disease prevention
- ▶ Drug testing for health care workers
- ▶ National nursing database to support clinical nursing practice
- ▶ Polygraph testing of health care workers
- ▶ Restructuring
- ▶ Work redesign
- ▶ Job and career security of registered nurses

(Kelly, LY, Joel LA [1996]. *The Nursing Experience: Trends, Challenges, and Transitions,* 3d ed. New York: McGraw-Hill.)

---

position statements have made important contributions to the national debate on the future of health care and, in doing so, have contributed to the professional stature of nursing.

 CRITICALLY THINKING ABOUT . . .

Imagine that the ANA had never been established. Would nursing be where it is today? Explain.

Other Organizations

In addition to the ANA, other organizations have contributed to the professionalization of nursing. The *National League for Nursing*, established in 1893, has played an important leadership role in improving and standardizing nursing education (see Chap. 5). The *American Academy of Nursing* was established in 1973 to recognize excellence in professional achievement in nursing. Nurses selected for their contributions to the profession by the Academy are designated as Fellows and are entitled to use the initials FAAN (Fellow of the American Academy of Nursing) as part of their professional title. The *American Nurses Foundation* was established in 1955 as a nonprofit organization to support nursing research. It solicits, receives, and administers grants for a wide variety of projects covering almost all areas of nursing scholarship. An organization specifically for nursing students is the *National Student Nurses Association*. Established in 1953, it serves as the voice of nursing students in matters of nursing education, nursing practice, and health care reform.

To advance the political agenda of the ANA, a political action committee was established in 1974. Known as the *American Nurses Association Political Action Committee*, the organization aims to improve American health care through both educational activities and support of political candidates who work or will work to help attain its agenda.

As noted earlier, there are many organizations that focus on specific practice areas (eg, American Association of Critical Care Nursing). In addition, as nursing has developed and moved toward professional status, organizations for specific nurse populations have been formed to meet the needs of that population. For example, the *National Association of Colored Graduate Nurses* existed from 1924 through 1951 to support African-American nurses as they encountered racial barriers to education and employment and discrimination in practice. The *Men Nurses Section* of the ANA was formed in 1941 to support male nurses and address sexual prejudice, discrimination, and other problems that men face in employment in nursing (Kalisch & Kalisch, 1995).

 CRITICALLY THINKING ABOUT . . .

What can the National Student Nurses' Association do to promote progress toward true professionalization in nursing?

Important Research Studies

Research studies serve as important milestones in the professionalization of nursing because they critically examine the strengths and weaknesses within nursing. Typically, these studies have been conducted by high-profile, knowledgeable professionals with the support and resources of professional organizations, private foundations, or agencies who identified the need for information in a significant area. Consequently, such studies usually have far-reaching impacts on the profession.

The Flexner Report: Medicine's Impetus to Professionalism

The **Flexner report**, although directed at medical education, served as the template for nursing studies. Abraham Flexner discovered a deplorable lack of standards and facilities in medical education in the United States. Lack of standards was particularly noticeable in relation to admission and curriculum requirements. As a result of the Flexner report, published in 1910 by the Carnegie Foundation for the Advancement of Teaching, 65 medical schools were closed by 1915 (Flexner, 1910; Brubacher & Rudy, 1958). Consequently, the number of graduating physicians declined markedly. Through the combined efforts of the American Medical Association and the American Public Health Association, a veritable revolution in medical education took place. Within only 10 years, most of the reforms outlined in the report, including educational requirements and licensure of physicians, were completed due to the strong leadership of the medical association and the cooperation of medical educators and practitioners, who welcomed the need for change.

Flexner's reforms for the medical profession reflected his philosophy of the importance of university-based education for medical practitioners. By raising the standards of medical schools as well as limiting their numbers and thereby reducing the number of graduating physicians, it was possible to obtain a monopoly over medical services. Physicians would always be in demand and thus could charge higher fees for their services. As a result of these reforms, the prestige, status, income, and power of the medical profession were enhanced far beyond what the reformers had ever anticipated. Between 1910 and 1920, power and money were required to raise educational standards in medicine, but such an investment increased the physician's prestige, the profession's power in legislation, and the average doctor's income (Goode, 1969).

Flexner's report, which produced epochal changes in medical education, was the first instance of a survey of higher education that was national in scope. Although it had no direct bearing on nursing at the time, it continues to challenge nursing, demonstrates the impact of strong leadership, and illustrates how acceptance of its recommendations quickly standardized university preparation as the educational requirement for medical practitioners.

The Goldmark Report

Shortly after Flexner's work, efforts to upgrade nursing education were initiated by the Rockefeller Foundation. In 1919, the Foundation organized the Committee for the Study of Nursing Education to conduct a comprehensive study of nursing, similar to what Flexner did in medicine. This committee identified the inadequacies of nursing schools, most of which were controlled and financed by hospitals, and published the **Goldmark report** in 1923. The report recommended that all nursing schools should be supported independently of hospitals and that more schools of nursing offering 5-year programs should be established as independent units in universities (Goldmark, 1923). In addition, it listed standards of university education with strong recommendations for the inclusion of the fundamental sciences and liberal arts, as well as professional training. The committee was convinced that the system of nursing education would have to be drastically altered if nursing practice were to be improved.

Unfortunately, the Goldmark report, unlike the Flexner report in medicine, was largely ignored and provided little impetus for needed change. The vast majority of nurses continued to be educated in hospital-based programs. In fact, enrollment in hospital-based programs showed no significant decline until the 1950s, with the introduction of 2-year associate degree programs—a direction that was actually contrary to the Goldmark recommendations.

Although the Goldmark report was issued more than 70 years ago, its main recommendation for sound educational policy and standardization of nursing education has still not been heeded. Flexner's report changed the face of medicine in the United States and worldwide, but Goldmark's report had virtually no impact on the direction of nursing. The 1,760 hospital schools of nursing in existence were either unable or unwilling to take specific action on these recommendations, thus preventing nursing from acquiring full professional status at that period and for many years to come. One reason nursing schools may have been unable to change is because at the time of the Goldmark report, nurses and nursing were dominated by hospital administrators and physicians. Nursing units were staffed primarily by student nurses, and the expectation that hospital-based diploma programs must continue was high: it simply was part of the economics of health care.

Studies and Reports of the 1920s, 1930s, and 1940s

The Goldmark report, however, stimulated other nursing studies. The Committee on the Grading of Nursing Schools, directed by May Ayres Burgess, published several significant reports between 1927 and 1934 on the status of nursing schools and nursing service. One report focused on the economics of hospital-based nursing schools, the supply and demand for graduate nurses, working conditions, salaries, and the geographic distribution of nurses throughout the country (Burgess, 1928).

In 1934, the same committee published the results of a study by Blanche Pfefferkorn and Ethel Johns entitled *An Activity Analysis of Nursing*. This study described the activities engaged in by nurses in various health care institutions (Johns & Pfefferkorn, 1934) and helped nurse educators correlate theory and practice in a more realistic manner. However, theory, at that time, was concerned only with disease, pathology, and illness care. Nursing theory as it is currently known was not developed until the 1960s.

The Committee on the Grading of Nursing Schools recognized the increasing responsibilities that were required of nursing and the lack of a collegiate level of education in the hospital-based nursing schools. Therefore, in its final report, *Nursing Schools: Today and Tomorrow,* the committee recommended that nursing education be placed on a true professional level (Committee on the Grading of Nursing Schools, 1934). Despite this report, still no changes were made.

With the growing concern over the poor quality of nursing education programs, another study was conducted shortly after World War II. The Russell Sage Foundation supported a study by social anthropologist Esther Lucille Brown entitled *Nursing for the Future* (Brown, 1948). Brown focused on nursing service and nursing education, and, like so many before her, stressed the importance of collegiate preparation for nursing:

> Almost without a dissenting voice, those who are conversant with the trend of professional education in the United States agree that preparation of the professional nurse belongs squarely within the institution of higher learning. . . . [W]ithin a democratic society there is no person, group of persons, or organized voluntary body that has power to order sudden and drastic change. Such changes as are effected will result from long and careful planning at the conference table of national, state, and local nursing associations and other bodies. (Brown, 1948, p. 138, 140)

Mid-Century Calls for Improvements in Nursing Education

Around the middle of the century, several other nursing reports were published:

1. A 1948 report by the Committee on the Function of Nursing, chaired by Eli Ginzberg, entitled *A Program for the Nursing Profession* (Committee on the Function of Nursing, 1948)
2. A 1951 study by Mildred Montag describing an educational program to prepare nursing technicians (Montag, 1951)
3. Margaret Bridgeman's critique of collegiate education for nurses in 1953 (Bridgeman, 1953).

Each of these studies echoed similar calls for drastic changes in the prevailing system of nursing education.

In 1958, Hughes and colleagues published *Twenty Thousand Nurses Tell Their Story,* in which they confirmed the existence of considerable discontent among the nation's nurses (Hughes, Hughes, & Deutscher, 1958). Five years later, the Surgeon General's Consultant Group on Nursing published a report emphasizing the need for a national study of nursing that would focus on the profession's needs and resources. It recommended upgrading the nursing profession by increasing the number of schools of nursing in universities and colleges, by emphasizing research, and by increasing enrollment for minority students, males, and older adults (Surgeon General's Consultant Group on Nursing, 1963).

A landmark for nursing was reached in 1965 when the ANA Committee on Education issued its first position paper on educational preparation for professional nursing and for those assisting them. This paper recommended that education for nursing take place in institutions of higher learning within the general system of education rather than in hospitals. They further recommended that a baccalaureate degree in nursing should be considered minimum preparation for beginning professional nursing practice and an associate degree in nursing should be the minimum preparation for beginning technical practice (ANA, 1965).

The Lysaught Reports
In 1970, a committee appointed by the Secretary of Health, Education, and Welfare to study extended roles for nurses determined that many nurses lacked the educational preparation for such roles (U.S. Department of Health, Education, and Welfare, 1971). This report had a considerable impact on nursing education and nursing practice. The earlier Surgeon General's Consultant Group (1963) had recommended a national study of nursing. Accordingly, funds were obtained from the Avalon and W.K. Kellogg Foundations in 1966 for a 3-year investigation. A final report of the National Commission for the Study of Nursing and Nursing Education (NCSNNE) entitled *An Abstract for Action* was the product (Lysaught, 1970). The Lysaught group concluded that the delivery of health care would be improved by analyzing and improving nursing, and they too emphasized redirecting nursing education into the mainstream of general education. A follow-up study by the NCSNNE from 1970 to 1973 resulted in a full report in 1973, *From Abstract into Action,* detailing the outcome of activities carried out to strengthen the recommendations of the 1970 report (Lysaught, 1973).

From 1977 to 1979, Lysaught pursued yet another longitudinal study with funds from the W.K. Kellogg Foundation to determine what progress had been made on some of the NCSNNE's 1970 recommendations to improve nursing. Findings and conclusions from this study appeared in *Action in Affirmation: Toward an Unambiguous Profession of Nursing* (Lysaught, 1981). The report indicated that considerable progress had been achieved by nursing in most of the recommendations for nursing roles and nursing education: of the 21 specific proposals, some were fully achieved, some progress had been made on most, and little or no progress was made on only a few.

ANA Studies: Entry Into Practice and Credentialing
In 1978 (following the directives of the recommendations issued 13 years earlier), the ANA House of Delegates passed resolutions on entry into practice. They supported two levels of nursing practice by 1985—the professional nurse, requiring a baccalaureate education, and an unnamed category, requiring associate degree education. Additional resolutions emphasized that competencies for both levels were to be developed by 1980 and opportunities for career mobility to facilitate movement from the unnamed level to the professional level were to be increased (ANA, 1978). Competencies for both levels have been identified and reviewed by nurse educators and practitioners since 1980. However, the entry into practice resolutions have gone

largely ignored. Graduates of all three basic nursing programs—associate degree, diploma, and baccalaureate degree—still qualify to take examinations and be licensed as RNs. For many, the entry into practice debate is a professionalization problem that simply will not go away; others, however, consider it a dead issue.

The Study of Credentialing in Nursing: A New Approach, published in 1979 and sponsored by the ANA, included a history of the credentialing movement, an account of the adequacy of credentialing mechanisms in nursing for accreditation, certification, and licensure, and the need for a national credentialing center. The Committee for the Study of Credentialing in Nursing, composed of 10 nurses and 5 other persons and chaired by Margretta Styles, former Dean of the School of Nursing at the University of California, San Francisco, made several recommendations, which were forwarded to the national nursing organizations for their review and approval. However, there was no consensus among these various organizations; thus, no further action on the committee's recommendations was taken (Committee for the Study of Credentialing in Nursing, 1979).

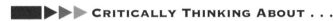 CRITICALLY THINKING ABOUT . . .

How has the Goldmark report made a difference in the way students are educated to practice nursing?

Barriers to the Emergence of Full Professional Status

It is clear from the previous section that many well-intentioned persons and groups have been concerned for years about enhancing the professional status of nursing. The vast majority of these people and committees have focused on the element of educational preparation for practice, and their recommendations have much in common. If there has been so much agreement among studies and reports such as these, one can only surmise that powerful barriers to change have been (and still are) in existence within nursing.

Disunity and Divisiveness

A major barrier—some would say the most serious—to nursing's drive toward professionalism is that of persisting disunity and divisiveness within nursing (Bowman & Culpepper, 1974). Nursing continues to experience dissension within its own ranks, which has compromised its distinction as a profession. There can be no professional nursing identity without consensus about nursing's competencies and purpose (Mundinger, 1980). Examples of disunity within nursing include:

- ▣ Conflicting positions regarding basic education and licensing issues
- ▣ Competition over accreditation rights
- ▣ Division and resultant flattening of the power base under the guise of decentralization
- ▣ Controversies over collective bargaining as a means of self-determination and access to economic rewards

▶ Dimensions and standards of practice
▶ Artificial bifurcation of nursing service and nursing education. (Styles, 1976)

Although these examples of divisiveness within nursing were expressed more than 20 years ago, most of them are still accurate today.

Alternative Understandings and Motivations

Another major barrier is the work orientation of many nurses. Habenstein and Christ (1955) formulated three descriptors to illustrate differences in motivation among nurses carrying out their nursing responsibilities: traditionalizers, utilizers, and professionalizers.

Traditionalizers see nursing as low-status, self-sacrificing, personal service of clients based on past generations of experience, rather than on complex knowledge and skills. Traditionalizers consider expediting physicians' orders to be a primary responsibility and the significant reason for their positions.

Utilizers lack motivation in their work and are uninvolved in activities to improve nursing's status. They view nursing solely as a job and often use their nursing position to further their own personal gains. These nurses expect to be evaluated on their work by the limits of individual tasks or procedures and not on how their performance affects the larger scene.

Professionalizers are concerned with achieving occupational advancement. They advance their own professional status—and that of nursing—by means of the political process. Professionalizers are dedicated to inquiry and scholarship; to designing and offering new approaches to preparing nurse practitioners, administrators, educators, and investigators; and to planning and evaluating innovative means for delivering high-quality nursing care (Schlotfeldt, 1982, p. 1).

Many share the opinion that nursing has too many traditionalizers and utilizers and not nearly enough professionalizers. Nursing must endeavor to increase the number of its professionalizers to ensure that the goal of professionalism will be achieved. Although this is a challenge to nursing and to nurses as a whole, it is of particular importance to nursing educators, who have the primary responsibility for professional socialization of future generations of nurses. This issue will be addressed in Chapters 5 and 7.

 CRITICALLY THINKING ABOUT . . .

What do you think about the claim that nurses are their own worst enemies when it comes to professionalization?

▶ CHAPTER SUMMARY

Although full professionalization of nursing has not yet been reached, nursing has made tremendous progress toward achieving full professional status. Before the turn of the next century, the predominant accrediting body for baccalaureate and higher degree programs will be the American Association of Colleges of Nursing, a body committed to high standards of excellence and rigor in educational preparation of nurses. The phenomenal growth in Ph.D. programs in nursing has fostered the development of nurse scholars prepared to teach new generations with content and methods on the cutting edge of nursing education and to generate the new knowledge required to develop a satisfactory knowledge base for an established, recognized nursing science. In addition, the dramatic changes in the American health care system provide both significant challenges to nursing and tremendous opportunities to nurses who are adequately prepared and visionary enough to meet the challenges and seize the opportunities to better themselves and nursing.

It is important for nurses to build on these achievements and also transform themselves. Commitment to professional behaviors and courses of action is essential. Nurses must join their professional and community organizations in support of nursing and health, and they must seek leadership in those organizations. Nurses must commit themselves to a program of lifelong learning that will benefit themselves, their patients, their peers, and their profession. If nurses accept those responsibilities, which are indeed the responsibilities of professionals, the time when nursing is accorded full professional status is not far in the future.

KEY POINTS

▶ 1 Professional occupations have distinct characteristics that differentiate them from nonprofessional occupations: a lengthy, rigorous educational requirement; a unique knowledge base with strong theoretical foundations; self-regulation of preparation, entry, and practice; a monopoly over practice; authority over clients; altruism as the driving motivation; and strong identification with professional peers.

▶ 2 Occupations can be placed on an occupation–profession continuum depending on the extent to which they have achieved the characteristics of a profession. Progression from occupation status to profession status occurs over time through the process known as professionalization.

▶ 3 Nursing is above the midpoint and closer to the profession end on the occupation–profession continuum. Nursing has made considerable progress over the years. Examples include upgraded educational requirements, advances in research, successful efforts in legislation, and improved distribution of manpower. In addition, nursing has achieved improvements in salaries and working conditions through collective bargaining. Significant changes in nurse practice acts have been achieved. Steps toward self-governance and self-management in education have been made. The number of qualified, dedicated nursing leaders has grown dramatically.

▶ 4 Nursing has not yet fully achieved certain characteristics of a true profession. Several challenges that nursing must meet include development of a unique, theoretically based knowledge base; autonomy over practice and educational preparation; a monopoly over practice; mechanisms for restricting the number and types of practicing nurses; personal commitment to nursing as a lifelong career; and strong identification with nursing peers.

▶ 5 The American Nurses Association has worked for the betterment of nurses and nursing for almost a century and has played a major role in the continuing professionalization of nursing. Many other organizations have contributed to professionalization as well. Since the Goldmark report of 1923, committees, reports, and organizations have repeatedly called for the improvement and professionalization of nursing by improving the rigor of nursing education and placing it in the university environment, thereby incorporating the humanities, the arts, and the sciences as well as education for nursing practice.

▶ 6 Some of the barriers to achieving full professionalization exist within nursing itself. These barriers are disunity and diversity among nurses and the lack of understanding or motivation of nurses to be professionalizers.

REFERENCES

Aaronson L (1989). A challenge for nursing: Re-reviewing a historic competition. *Nursing Outlook 37,* 274–279.

American Association of Colleges of Nursing (1996). Unpublished press release, Nov. 5, 1996.

American Nurses Association (1978). Resolutions. *American Nurse 10*(9), 9–10.

American Nurses Association (1984). Forty-nine groups attend nursing organization liaison forum. *American Nurse 16,* 5.

American Nurses Association (1985). *Facts About Nursing 1984–85.* Kansas City: American Nurses Association.

Bowman R, Culpepper R (1974). Power: Rx for change. *AJN 74,* 1054–1056.

Committee for the Study of Credentialing in Nursing (1979). *The Study of Credentialing in Nursing: A New Approach.* Kansas City: American Nurses Association.

Curry T, Jiobu R, Schwirian K (1997). *Sociology for the 21st Century.* Upper Saddle River, NJ: Prentice-Hall.

Ellis JR, Hartley CL (1995). *Nursing in Today's World* (5th ed.). Philadelphia: JB Lippincott.

Henslin JM (1995). *Sociology: A Down-to-Earth Approach* (2nd ed.). Boston: Allyn and Bacon.

Kalisch PA, Kalisch BJ (1995). *The Advance of American Nursing,* (3rd ed.). Philadelphia: JB Lippincott.

Kelly LY, Joel LA (1996). *The Nursing Experience: Trends Challenges and Transitions* (3rd ed.). New York: McGraw-Hill.

Lysaught J (1981). *Action in Affirmation: Toward an Unambiguous Profession of Nursing.* New York: McGraw-Hill.

Moloney MM (1992). *Professionalization of Nursing: Current Issues and Trends* (2nd ed.). Philadelphia: JB Lippincott.

Monnig G (1978). Professionalism of nurses and physicians. In Chaska N (Ed.), *The Nursing Profession: Views Through the Mist.* New York: McGraw-Hill.

Mundinger M (1980). *Autonomy in Nursing.* Germantown, MD: Aspen Systems Corp.

Oermann MH (1997). *Professional Nursing Practice.* Stamford, CT: Appleton-Lange.

Popenoe D (1993). *Sociology* (9th ed.). Englewood Cliffs, NJ: Prentice-Hall.

Schlotfeldt R (1982). *A Brave New Nursing World.* Washington DC: American Association of Colleges of Nursing.

Segal E (1985, June 15). Is nursing a profession? *Nursing '85, 6,* 40–43.

Selby T (1989). House adopts new structure for ANA. *American Nurse 21*(7), 1–20.

Starr P (1982). *The Social Transformation of American Medicine.* New York: Basic Books.

Styles M (1976). *Declaring our future.* Paper presented at the Indiana League for Nursing annual meeting, Indianapolis, IN, October 9, 1976.

Classic References

American Nurses Association (1965). *A Position Paper: Educational Preparation for Nurse Practitioners and Assistants to Nurses.* Kansas City: American Nurses Association.

Bridgeman M (1953). *Collegiate Education for Nursing.* New York: Russell Sage Foundation.

Brown E (1948). *Nursing for the Future.* New York: Russell Sage Foundation.

Brubacher J, Rudy W (1958). *Higher Education in Transition.* New York: Harper & Row.

Burgess M (1928). *Nurses, Patients and Pocketbooks: A Report of a Study on the Economics of Nursing.* New York: The Commonwealth Fund.

Carr-Saunders A, Wilson P (1933). *The Professions.* Oxford: Clarendon Press.

Cogan M (1953). Toward a definition of profession. *Harvard Educational Review* 23.

Committee on the Function of Nursing (1948). *A Program for the Nursing Profession.* New York: MacMillan.

Committee on the Grading of Nursing Schools (1934). *Nursing Schools: Today and Tomorrow.* New York: National League of Nursing Education.

Dibble V (1962). Occupations and ideologies. *Am J Sociology 61,* 229–241.

Etzioni AE (Ed.) (1969). *The Semi-Professions and Their Organization: Teachers, Nurses, Social Workers.* New York: The Free Press.

Flexner A (1910). *Medical Education in the United States and Canada.* Carnegie Foundation for the Advancement of Teaching Bulletin No. 4. Boston: Merrymount Press.

Flexner A (1915). Is social work a profession? In *Proceedings of the National Conference of Charities and Corrections.* Chicago: Hildermann, pp. 578–581.

Flexner A (1930). *Universities: American, English, German.* New York: Oxford University Press.

Goldmark J (1923). *Nursing and Nursing Education in the United States.* New York: Macmillan.

Goode W (1960). Encroachment, charlatanism and the emerging profession: Psychology, sociology and medicine. *Am Sociological Rev 25,* 902–913.

Goode W (1966). Librarianship. In Vollmer HJ, Mills DL (Eds.) *Professionalization.* Englewood Cliffs, NJ: Prentice-Hall.

Goode W (1969). The theoretical limits of professionalization. In Etzioni AE (Ed.), *The Semi-Professions and Their Organizations: Teachers, Nurses, Social Workers.* New York: The Free Press.

Greenwood E (1957). Attributes of a profession. *Social Work 2,* 44–55.

Greenwood E (1962). Attributes of a profession. In Nosow S, Form WH (Eds.) *Man, Work and Society.* New York: Basic Books, pp. 206–218.

Gross E (1962). When occupations meet: Professions in trouble. *Hospital Administration 7,* 40–59.

Habenstein K (1963). Critiques of profession as a sociological category. *Sociological Quarterly 4,* 291–300.

Habenstein R, Christ E (1955). *Professionalizer, Traditionalizer and Utilizer.* Columbia: University of Missouri.

Horgan PD (1960). Is nursing really a profession? *RN 23,* 48–51.

Hornsby JA, Schmidt RE (1914). *The Modern Hospital: Its Inspiration, Its Architecture, Its Equipment, Its Operation.* Philadelphia: WB Saunders.

Hughes E (1965). Professions in K. Lynn and the editors of Daedalus, *The professions in America.* Boston: Houghton Mifflin.

Hughes E, Hughes H, Deutscher D (1958). *Twenty Thousand Nurses Tell Their Story.* Philadelphia: JB Lippincott.

Johns E, Pfefferkorn B (1934). *An Activity Analysis of Nursing: A Report of the Second Study Sponsored by the Committee on the Grading of Nursing Schools.* New York: National League of Nursing Education.

Katz F (1969). Nurses. In Etzioni AE (Ed.), *The Semi-Professions and Their Organization: Teachers, Nurses, Social Workers.* New York: The Free Press.

Kast F, Rosenzweig J (1970). *Organization and Management.* New York: McGraw-Hill.

Lysaught J (1970). *An Abstract for Action.* New York: McGraw-Hill.

Lysaught J (1973). *Abstract into Action.* New York: McGraw-Hill.

Montag M (1951). *The Education of Nursing Technicians.* New York: GP Putnam's Sons.

Nightingale F (1860). *Notes on Nursing: What It Is and What It Is Not.* New York: Appleton.

Olesen V, Whittaker E (1968). *The Silent Dialogue.* San Francisco: Jossey-Bass.

Parsons T (1954). The professions and social structure. In Parsons T (Ed.), *Essays in Sociological Theory,* rev. ed. New York: The Free Press.

Pavalko R (1971). *Sociology of Occupations and Professions.* Itasca, IL: FE Peacock.

Robb I (1975). A general review of nursing forces. In Flanagan L (Ed.), *One Strong Voice: The Story of the American Nurses Association.* Kansas City: American Nurses Association.

Rogers M (1964). *Reveille in Nursing.* Philadelphia: FA Davis.

Simpson R, Simpson I (1969). Women and bureaucracy in the semi-professions. In Etzioni AE (Ed.), *The Semi-Professions and Their Organization: Teacher, Nurses, Social Workers.* New York: The Free Press.

Surgeon General's Consultant Group on Nursing (1963). *Toward Quality in Nursing: Needs and Goals.* U.S. Department of Health, Education and Welfare (Pub. No. 992). Washington DC: DHEW.

U.S. Department of Health Education and Welfare (1971). *Extending the Scope of Nursing Practice.* Washington DC: U.S. Government Printing Office.

Vollmer H, Mills D (1966). *Professionalization.* Englewood Cliffs, NJ: Prentice-Hall.

Wilensky H (1962). The dynamics of professionalization: The case of hospital administration. *Hospital Administration 7,* 6–24.

Wilensky H (1964). The professionalization of everyone? *Am J Sociology 70,* 137–187.

RECOMMENDED READINGS

Allen CE (1991). Holistic concepts and the professionalization of public health nursing. *Public Health Nursing 8*(2), 74–80.

Bullough B (1995). Professionalization of nurse practitioners. *Ann Rev Nursing Res,* pp. 239–265.

Carter H (1994). Confronting patriarchal attitudes in the fight for professional recognition. *J Adv Nursing 19,* 367–372.

Esterhuizen P (1996). Is the professional code still the cornerstone of clinical nursing practice? *J Adv Nursing 23,* 25–31.

Forsyth S (1995). Historical continuities and constraints in the professionalization of nursing. *Nursing Inquiry 2,* 164–171.

Harris BL (1990). Becoming deprofessionalized: One aspect of the staff nurse's perspective on computer-mediated nursing care plans. *Adv Nursing Sci 13,* 63–74.

Hart E (1996). Action research as a professionalizing strategy: Issues and dilemmas. *J Adv Nursing 23,* 454–461.

Lawler TG, Rose MA (1987). Professionalization: A comparison among generic baccalaureate and RN/BSN nurses. *Nurse Educator 12*(3), 19–22.

Mosley MOP (1996). A new beginning: The story of the national association of colored graduate nurses 1908–1951. *Journal of National Black Nurses Association 8*(1), 20–32.

Parkin PAC (1995). Nursing the future: A re-examination of the professionalization thesis in light of some recent developments. *J Adv Nursing 21,* 561–567.

vanMaanen HMT (1990). Nursing in transition: An analysis of the state of the art in relation to the conditions of practice and society's expectations. *J Adv Nursing 15,* 914–924.

PART II

A Knowledge Base
for Nursing:
A Work in Progress

CHAPTER

2

Nursing Knowledge and Nursing Theory: Foundations of a Profession

CHAPTER OUTLINE

Nursing Knowledge
Theory for Nursing Knowledge
Knowledge for Nursing: Beyond
    Empirics
Chapter Summary

Key Points
References
Classic References
Recommended Readings

LEARNING OBJECTIVES

▶ **1** Explain how the definitions and parameters of nursing knowledge have evolved over time.

▶ **2** Discuss the idea of nursing as a science.

▶ **3** Examine how society views nursing knowledge.

▶ **4** Compare and contrast imported theory, deductive theory, and inductive theory as they relate to nursing knowledge.

▶ **5** Discuss ethics, personal knowing, and esthetics and their contribution to nursing knowledge.

KEY TERMS

adaptation theory	developmental theory	ethics
advocacy	empirics	general systems theory
centering	engaging	imported theory
clarifying	envisioning	inductive theory
deductive theory	esthetics	intuiting
		nursing

(continued)

KEY TERMS (CONTINUED)

nursing knowledge	opening	role theory
Nursing's Social Policy Statement	personal knowing	valuing
	realizing	

Most scholars agree that a unique body of knowledge is one of the indispensable characteristics of a profession. If professional health practitioners are to be able to control the tasks they must perform and be consistent in predicting the outcomes of their actions, they must have at their disposal a well-defined body of knowledge that will enable them to comprehend the bases and consequences of their actions. Indeed, the very autonomy of a profession rests most firmly on the uniqueness, recognition, and recognized validity of its knowledge. Unique knowledge is the foundation for attaining the respect, recognition, and power accorded a fully developed profession.

Most of nursing knowledge development has been in the realm of empirical knowledge—knowledge that is observed and experienced; concrete knowledge that can be tested and proven. The development of empirical knowledge is vital to the full professionalization of nursing because it is knowledge that can be recognized by society and other professional groups. A theoretical foundation for empirical nursing knowledge is also essential to the professionalization of nursing because it explains, supports, and helps to develop the scientific body of nursing knowledge. The holistic discipline of nursing does not have one theoretical foundation; instead, imported theory, deductive theory, and inductive theory all help to support the discipline.

In addition to empirical knowledge, three other types of knowledge lend valuable information to nursing—ethics, personal knowing, and esthetics. These types of knowledge are not based on observation and physical experience; rather, they are based on moral principles, perception of self and the external world, and the vision of possibilities.

All types of knowledge are important to the development of a complete nursing knowledge base; one is not more important than the others. In fact, all four types of knowledge are often used simultaneously in daily nursing practice. Therefore, it is important to acquire an accurate and thorough understanding of the different types of nursing knowledge.

Nursing Knowledge

In the previous chapter, the need for a scientific body of knowledge was emphasized as a means to acquire autonomy and provide direction for nursing practice. Many argue that the development of nursing knowledge has been an extremely slow process. **Nursing knowledge** was originally limited to specific nursing tasks and procedures. It changed gradually to have a strong illness and disease orientation because most nurses were educated in hospital-based schools of nursing. In the mid-1970s, Dorothy E. Johnson expressed the opinion that "nursing stands today as a field of practice without a scientific heritage—an occupation created by society long ago to offer a distinctive service, but one still ill-defined in practical terms, a profession without the theoretical base it seems to require" (Johnson, 1974, p. 373).

Things have changed a great deal since Johnson's pronouncement. Nursing knowledge is centered more and more on health, health promotion, and wellness. The number of nurse scholars who are contributing significantly to the advancement of nursing knowledge is steadily increasing, as is the quality of their work. Accelerated growth in both knowledge and theory development by nurse scholars and in the use of this systematic knowledge by clinicians in nursing practice has occurred throughout the 1990s. This progress must continue if nursing is to professionalize further.

To gain insight into the realm of nursing knowledge, it is a good idea to understand the definition and nature of nursing, the current status of nursing as a scientific discipline, and society's view of nursing knowledge.

Definition and Nature of Nursing

From Nightingale's time until today, nurses have worked to provide a definition of nursing that would clarify its position in the health care system. Broad definitions are the most general and certainly capture the range of both nursing goals and activities, and thereby they have the greatest appeal for nurses. But such definitions might be the hardest for the public to understand because broad definitions might muddle the distinction between nursing and medicine in the public's mind. Narrow definitions might be easier for the public to grasp, but they tend to oversimplify the range of goals and activities nurses pursue. Whichever definition of nursing is used—broad or narrow—the definition must convey the idea that nursing is based on specialized, systematized, and scientifically sound knowledge unique to nursing. If the professionalization of nursing is to be advanced, the public and the other health care professions must come to see nursing knowledge for what it is: the unique and cumulative body of knowledge on which nursing is based.

The practice of nursing exists within a societal context, and societies change over time. The definition of **nursing** has also changed throughout history, but two elements are always inherent: a set of actions that are considered "nursing" and a statement of goals to be achieved. Also implicit in most definitions is the idea that the nurse's actions are carried out in the context of nurse–client interaction. Table 2-1 provides a historical perspective on the definition of nursing.

The most recent efforts to define nursing occurred in 1992 when the American Nurses Association Congress of Nursing Practice appointed a second task force, led by Linda Cronenwett, to continue the work of clarifying the nature and focus of nursing. The task force produced a document called ***Nursing's Social Policy Statement*** (ANA, 1995). In addition to the following definition of nursing, this statement defines the social context of nursing, identifies underlying values and assumptions, and delineates the knowledge base for nursing practice. It also addresses the scope of practice for basic nursing and advanced nursing and the regulation of nursing practice. Rather than providing a single, succinct definition of nursing like the definition presented in the 1980 statement (ANA, 1980), this document characterized the features that are part of definitions of nursing in general. "Since 1980, nursing philosophy and practice have been influenced by a greater elaboration of the science of caring and its integration with the traditional knowledge base for diagnosis and treatment of human response to health and illness" (ANA, 1995, p. 6). The authors go on to identify the four essential features of definitions of contemporary nursing practice:

TABLE 2-1	DEFINITION OF NURSING—AN HISTORICAL PERSPECTIVE

Year	Nurse Theorist	Definition
1859	Florence Nightingale	"A service to humankind aimed at alleviating pain and suffering." The nursing action she called for to put the patient in the best condition for nature to act on him or her was the provision of the proper environment, including light, fresh air, cleanliness, warmth, and good nutrition.
1952	Hildegard Peplau	"Nursing is a therapeutic interpersonal process involving two people [nurse and client] who share a common goal."
1966	Virginia Henderson	"The unique function of the nurse is to assist the individual, sick or well, in the performance of those activities contributing to health or its recovery (or to peaceful death) that he would perform unaided if he had the necessary strength, will, or knowledge, and to do this in such a way as to help him gain independence as rapidly as possible."
1972	Martha Rogers	"Nursing is concerned with people, all people— well and sick, rich and poor, young and old, wherever they may be, at work and at play."
1973	Abdellah, Beland, Martin, & Matheney	"Nursing is a service to individuals that helps them cope with their health needs—whether they are well or ill."
1980	ANA Congress for Nursing Practice; chairperson: Norma Lang	Nursing defined in *Nursing: A Social Policy Statement*. **Nursing:** The diagnosis and treatment of human responses to actual or potential health problems **Phenomena of concern:** The phenomena of concern to nurses are human responses to actual or potential health problems. Any observable manifestation, need, condition, concern, event, dilemma, difficulty, occurrence, or fact that can be described or scientifically explained and is within the target area of nursing practice is of interest to nurses.

1. Attention to the full range of human experiences and responses to health and illness without restriction to a problem-focused orientation
2. Integration of objective data with knowledge gained from an understanding of the patient's or group's subjective experience
3. Application of scientific knowledge to the processes of diagnosis and treatment
4. Provision of a caring relationship that facilitates health and healing. (ANA, p. 6)

▶▶▶ CRITICALLY THINKING ABOUT . . .

If you were to write your own definition of nursing, what would it be?

Status of Nursing as a Scientific Discipline

Science is defined as a body of knowledge consisting of interrelated concepts and conceptual schemes. It is obtained by observation and experimentation and the formulation and testing of hypotheses. In regard to nursing, it has also been defined as "the process and the result of ordering and patterning the events and phenomena of concern to nursing" (Jacobs & Huether, 1978, p. 66). Commitment to science is essential if nursing is to be recognized as a full profession and to contribute accountably to society's needs. Johnson declared that a profession cannot exist for any length of time without clearly stating its theoretical base for practice so that its knowledge can be communicated, tested, and expanded (Johnson, 1959, p. 291).

The history of nursing science in recent decades has undergone several shifts of emphasis. Early theorists explored the interpersonal relationships between patient and nurse. More recently, theorists have emphasized the definition and nature of nursing practice and the movement of patients from illness to health. At present, health is considered to be a dynamic process, moving back and forth over a person's lifetime. The need to refine factors observed in the relation between the patient and the environment is a vital one (Newman, 1983).

Nursing is rapidly becoming a scientific discipline because nurse theorists and researchers are using scientific methods to explain, predict, and apply new knowledge in the practice of professional nursing. However, many nurses still do not understand or appreciate the value of theory for practice and why nursing should be diligently pursuing its development to advance professionalism. In addition, there is a major tension between nursing as science and nursing as practice. Nursing practice is still identified as procedure- and task-oriented, with routines determined by policies, directives, and physicians' orders rather than by actions based on the findings of nursing research.

Despite this tension, nursing will be greatly influenced in its progress toward professionalism over the next decade by the continuing work of nurse theorists and researchers, who are accepting the challenge of developing nursing as a scientific discipline. These scholars recognize the importance of developing the theoretical and scientific base for nursing to facilitate the emergence and recognition of nursing as a true profession. "[T]he emergence of nursing science as an independent professional discipline valued by society parallels the professional and social demands to assume full responsibility for nursing decisions, actions, and resulting consequences" (Bilitski, 1981).

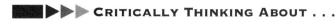 CRITICALLY THINKING ABOUT . . .

Does the tension between nursing as science and nursing as practice negatively or positively affect the professionalization of nursing? Why?

Society's View of Nursing Knowledge

Despite the developments in nursing knowledge and use of this knowledge, society does not recognize the unique contributions of nursing knowledge to health care. In fact, society often is not even aware of the existence of nursing knowledge. Society's image of nurses and their knowledge is an obstacle to achieving full professional status because, as stated in Chapter 1, the knowledge base itself is important to profes-sionalization and full professional status will not be reached without the recognition of the unique knowledge base by society.

More than 20 years ago, Beletz (1974) commented that society's perception of the nurse was in sex-linked, task-oriented terms: a female who performs unpleasant technical jobs and functions as an assistant to the physician. Unfortunately, in many instances this is still the general perception. Nursing care is frequently conceived of in terms of task performance and not as using independent thought or decision-making skills to fulfill its responsibilities.

In addition, the public's appreciation for the field of medicine is far greater than for that of nursing. Both medicine and nursing require a great deal of knowledge and skill on the part of practitioners. However, the privileges and rewards expected by physicians and afforded them by society clearly are superior to those generally ex-pected by nurses and accorded by those they serve. The work of Campbell-Heider, Hart, and Bergren (1994) has demonstrated that the differences have persisted; nurses are seen as nice and caring but not particularly well educated. Until the public recognizes the value of nursing services to the extent that it recognizes the value of physician services, the image of nursing will not change substantially. If the public lacks understanding of the contributions nurses make to health care or the benefits received from nursing care, it will not grant nursing full professional status. There-fore, the public needs to be made aware of these contributions and to be more ac-cepting of nursing as an important health discipline.

Media portrayal of contemporary views about women and women's professions influences this limited, negative, and subservient image of nursing. Indeed, even in "our own" literature, the nursing image often is subverted. Aber and Hawkins (1992) studied how nurses were portrayed in advertisements in medical and nursing journals. All too often those portrayals were stereotypical and demeaning—depen-dent, passive minor figures on the health care scene. As nurses assume more respon-sibility for patient care and health promotion, they are becoming dissatisfied with society's image because it does not incorporate the realities of modern nursing, in-cluding the expanded role of nursing and the independence that is beginning to characterize the profession.

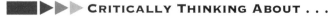 CRITICALLY THINKING ABOUT . . .

What do nurses do or know that is different from physicians?

Changing Society's View of Nursing Knowledge

Is society's image of the nurse doomed to be static? Can nursing effect changes to alter such stereotypes? Perhaps if the public understood the meaning of nurses' profession-alism, some significant changes in their views about nursing might occur. Nurses must make their vital contributions to health care known to enhance the public's awareness and demand for nursing services. Programs to educate consumers about nursing and the real value of its services are increasing. The writings of Philip and Beatrice Kalisch (1980, 1981, 1982, 1986) have made a significant contribution to awakening nurses and the public about nursing's poor public image and the need to improve it.

However, to project a more acceptable professional image to the public, a simple publicity campaign will not be enough. Images are usually a byproduct of the deeper social reality of the occupation; therefore, significant changes must occur within nursing itself. Nurses must first identify a distinct body of knowledge that would justify nursing's claim to full professional status; this would enhance the public's image of nursing. As stated in Chapter 1, part of being accorded true professional status is that the public must agree to that status. Therefore, it is important to develop a knowledge base that is not only scientifically sound but is also recognized and understood by the public as being unique and valuable (Goode, 1961).

Theory for Nursing Knowledge

Theory often is referred to as an explanation or description of a body of specific knowledge. Scientific disciplines are characterized by their theoretical foundations. Past efforts in nursing theory development have resulted in controversy over whether nursing science is basic or applied, unique or borrowed from other disciplines. Nursing is a holistic discipline and therefore requires a theoretical foundation that is broad, eclectic, and uniquely articulated. The history of any science and its theoretical foundations is a developmental process, usually irregular in its progress and characterized by considerable scholarly controversy all along the way. The development of theory and science for nursing is no exception. A base or theoretical foundation for nursing knowledge has always been in existence but has evolved over time.

For the theoretical foundation to contribute to the professionalization of nursing, it must be understood and valued by nurses themselves, their nonnursing colleagues, and society in general. This presents a tremendous challenge with which nursing scholars have struggled mightily since the 1950s. Indeed, to date, there is no single answer or perspective regarding what constitutes nursing's theoretical foundation. Instead, it is generally accepted that many theories are essential to the full development of the body of scientific knowledge for nursing. Three general categories of theory are essential to the support of the discipline:

1. Imported theories
2. Deductive theories (comprehensive)
3. Inductive theories (practice-based or grounded).

The deductive theories and their derivation have received the most attention and have been deemed the most important in the last half of the 20th century. However, the other two categories still persist as an integral part of nursing education and nursing practice, and they are undeniably important. Indeed, it is likely that inductive theory, which is developed *from* practice, will emerge as an increasingly important aspect of nursing knowledge in the 21st century. This will continue to strengthen nursing's knowledge base and contribute substantially to its uniqueness and subsequent recognition, thus moving nursing further toward full professional status.

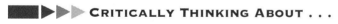 CRITICALLY THINKING ABOUT . . .

Can you identify things you have learned in your nursing study that come from the three categories of nursing knowledge theory?

Imported Theories for Nursing

Emphasis on integrating concepts from the biologic and behavioral sciences began in the 1950s, and nursing is greatly indebted to several of these **imported theories**. In fact, much of nursing knowledge and practice is built on principles of these theories, adapted to nursing. Some of these theories include biologic science theory, general systems theory, role theory, adaptation theory, and developmental theory.

Biologic Science Theory

Theories from the firmly established biologic sciences, such as biology, physiology, and pathophysiology, have been useful to nursing for many years. These theories are considered foundational information at all levels of nursing education and provide the rationale for a host of nursing interventions. In physiology, for example, nurses learn about the processes and "loops" that occur in all living systems, both simple and complex. Physiologic theory also explains the complexity and amazing interdependence of human body systems and the importance of control systems in maintaining healthy functioning. Theory and knowledge from the sciences must be a part of the scientific practice of nursing; therefore, they are appropriately part of the scientific theory for nursing (Guyton & Hall, 1996; West, 1990; Vander, Sherman, & Luciano, 1994).

General Systems Theory

General systems theory (or simply systems theory), imported from the realm of social and behavioral sciences, makes a significant contribution to the development of a scientific knowledge base for nurses. It is similar to the physiologic theory because of the emphasis on system interdependency. However, this theory extends far beyond the limits of the body into environmental and interpersonal interaction, group function, organization, and society (up to and including national and supranational systems) (Miller, 1978).

Systems theory is not entirely outside the realm of nursing. The process and terminology of systems theory underlie many nursing models, and elements of it appear in many nursing textbooks and the professional nursing literature (Catalano, 1996).

The basic concept of a system is a set of objects with relations between the objects and between their attributes (Hall & Fagen, 1968). Systems may be open or closed—that is, they may or may not exchange matter, energy, or information with the environment. However, there is some doubt that a totally closed system could exist: "It is difficult to imagine a system that is totally impervious to its environment" (Tappen, 1995, p. 5). Systems are hierarchical in nature—in other words, there are multiple levels of systems within systems. The smaller systems within systems are subsystems, and the larger system surrounding the target system is the suprasystem (Lazlo, 1972) (Fig. 2-1).

Open systems function and interact with their environment in a manner shown in Figure 2-2. Input (in the form of matter, energy, or information) is obtained from the environment. The system processes that act on and use that input are referred to as throughput. The product returned to the environment is output. This output serves to change the environment, which via the feedback loop provides a new kind of input to the system. Thus, the functioning of open living systems is cyclical: it is in constant exchange with its constantly changing environment.

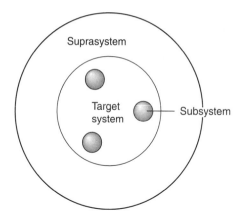

Figure 2-1. Hierarchical nature of systems.

Role Theory

Role theory is another imported theory useful to nursing. An understanding of the nature, components, and processes inherent to role theory helps nurses in clarifying and enacting their own professional roles appropriately and effectively. Much of the frustration of being members of a semiprofession striving for full professional status and recognition has its roots in the different statuses accorded to nursing and medicine and how that status difference plays out in role enactment. Understanding role theory also helps nurses in enhancing their therapeutic effectiveness in nurse–client interactions.

The origins of role theory date back to the work of "pre-role" psychologists and social philosophers but took form in the 1930s and 1940s in the work of social theorist George Herbert Mead (1934), anthropologist Ralph Linton (1936), and psychiatrist Jacob Moreno (1945). Mead developed one of the most influential theories about socialization. He believed that social, not biologic, forces are the primary source of human behavior. He conceptualized the self as the capacity of mind and organism to be an object to itself. Mead also argued that the self develops through social process when persons learn to evaluate themselves as social objects. Thus, the absence of social interaction precludes the development of the self.

Linton linked the ideas of role and status. A role is the behavior of someone with a given status, and status is a socially defined position in a group or society—a collec-

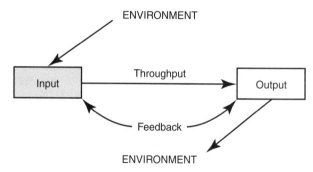

Figure 2-2. Function of open systems.

tion of rights and duties. According to Linton, one *occupies* a status, but *plays* a role; moreover, there are no roles without statuses or statuses without roles. Moreno added an element of control to the process of learning to enact one's role properly. As a psychiatrist, his goal was to alter maladaptive enactment of roles using psychodrama and sociodrama. He believed that learning occurs through experiencing and observing interactions with others in a controlled group context.

Nurses learn from role theory that all of us—ourselves, our colleagues, and our patients—play multiple roles; this is part of the complexity of everyone's daily life. Nurses also profit from understanding that if the different roles we play are incompatible, we can experience role conflict, producing competing demands on our time, energy, resources, and loyalties.

Adaptation and Developmental Theories

Nurses also learn about and routinely use other imported theories in a comprehensive practice. **Adaptation theory** is the dynamic adjustment of living matter to other living things and to environmental conditions. Adaptation for humans involves interaction and response and occurs on three levels: inner self, social, and physical. Adaptation theories for stress and coping are frequently used in nursing (Holmes & Rahe, 1967; Antonovsky, 1979; Selye, 1976).

Effective nursing practice also incorporates an understanding of developmental theories. Beginning in the early 20th century, researchers developed classic **developmental theories** to explain human behavior and development responses that occur at various ages throughout life. Examples of developmental theories imported into nursing include psychoanalytic theory (Freud, 1938), psychosocial theory (Erikson, 1950), cognitive development theory (Piaget, 1926, 1969), moral development theory (Kohlberg, 1981, 1984), and theory of human needs (Maslow, 1954).

 CRITICALLY THINKING ABOUT . . .

Does it make a difference where you learn about the theories that have been imported into nursing—in a nursing course or in the specific discipline? Why?

Deductive Nursing Theories

The imported theories discussed above substantially advanced the scientific knowledge for nursing practice. However, they failed to provide answers to the questions and challenges regarding the uniqueness of nursing science and its knowledge base. In short, nurses were still basing their practice on someone else's science. By the middle of the 20th century, many nursing scholars were expressing the belief that nursing knowledge and practice should not be developed simply by applying basic principles from other disciplines. Rather, they urged the nursing community to develop its own knowledge base and theory for nursing practice—**deductive theory** (Wald & Leonard, 1964).

Dorothy Johnson's work provided something of a transition from strictly borrowed theory to exclusively nursing theory. Johnson viewed nursing science as an applied science in which findings from several fields are synthesized and provide a perspective for nursing. She defined nursing science as "a synthesis, reorganization, or extension of concepts drawn from the basic or other applied sciences which in their reformulation tend to become 'new' concepts" (Johnson, 1959, p. 292).

Johnson provided an interesting perspective on the nature of the knowledge required for nursing practice. In her view, nursing theory should address knowledge of order, knowledge of disorder, and knowledge of control. Knowledge of order refers to order in nature and describes the normal state and natural schema of things. Knowledge of disorder provides understanding of undesirable events that could threaten the well-being of persons or society. Finally, knowledge of control allows the prescribing of a course of action, which, if and when performed, could change the sequence of events in a desired way toward specific outcomes. In her opinion, this third type of knowledge represents what others have described as "prescriptive" theory. Johnson also believed that nurse theorists would have to develop their own theory and ask questions about events and phenomena in the universe that are of specific concern to nursing, and she stressed the need for knowledge to go beyond simple description and even prediction to that of prescription if it were to be of use in guiding nursing practice. Moreover, Johnson stressed the fact that the phenomena of interest to nursing differ from those of the basic sciences; thus, a knowledge base unique to nursing would develop (Johnson, 1968).

In their response to a proposal for nursing practice theory, Dickoff and James produced a four-level model of theory in a practice discipline:

1. Factor-isolating theory: involves naming and classifying phenomena of interest
2. Factor-relating theory: examines relations among phenomena
3. Situation-relating theory: allows one to predict outcomes when phenomena are treated or manipulated
4. Situation-producing theory: theory that will lead to producing a desired change in a nursing client or a nursing situation. (Dickoff & James, 1968)

The main difference between situation-relating theory and situation-producing (or prescriptive) theory is in commitment to a goal (Meleis, 1985, p. 98). Situation-producing theory is considered by Dickoff and James to be the highest level of theory for a practice discipline; they maintain that because nursing is a practice discipline, then it needs prescriptive theory to determine the goals to be achieved and the activities needed to meet these goals.

More recent writers such as Diers (1983), Fawcett (1983), and Beckstrand (1978) have taken a different position from that of Dickoff and James. Essentially, they hold the opinion that descriptive, explanatory, and predictive theories—along with ethical knowledge—are adequate for practice. Therefore, prescriptive theory is generally unnecessary for practicing nurses. (As noted earlier, the developmental history of a science always includes scholarly debate, and this is one of those debates in the development of nursing science.)

In the meantime, nursing theorists toiled diligently to explicate the fundamental concepts, constructs, and processes that characterize the appropriate theoretical foundations for nursing practice. These theories usually address and define four fundamental concepts (person, environment, health, and nursing) and delineate the functional interrelations between and among them. Various theories developed from 1952 to 1980 are presented in Table 2-2.

Among the more recent in this series of theory development is the work of Rosemarie Rizzo Parse (1981). Parse developed a philosophical model focusing on the inseparable concepts of man, living, and health as the concern of nursing. Using an existential approach, she derived three principles that center on the idea of man, living, and health always moving toward greater diversity and "becoming." Parse's principles are:

TABLE 2-2	NURSING THEORISTS AND THEORIES

Theorist	Year	Theory
Hildegard Peplau	1952	Nursing is an interpersonal process focusing on patients with felt needs.
Ida Jean Orlando	1961	Emphasized the nurse–patient relationship using a "deliberative" nursing approach, which focused on "care for the needs of the patients who are distressed, with consideration for perception, thought, and feeling through deliberate action" (Meleis, 1985, p. 175).
Virginia Henderson	1966, 1971	Conceptualized nursing as assisting patients with 14 essential functions toward independence, including "breathe normally," "eat and drink adequately," "eliminate body wastes," and "sleep and rest."
Myra Extrin Levine	1967, 1973	Defined four conservation principles of nursing: conservation of energy and conservation of structural, personal, and social integrity.
Martha Rogers	1970, 1980	Developed the science of unitary man, incorporating the concepts of energy fields, openness, pattern, and organization.
Imogene King	1971, 1975, 1981	Proposed theory of goal attainment through nurse–client interactions.
Sister Callista Roy	1970, 1976, 1980, 1984	Proposed the adaptation model, in which the nurse's role is to adjust the patient's stimuli (focal, contextual, or residual).
Betty Neuman	1980	Proposed her health care systems model, which she conceptualized as a total person approach.
Madeleine Leininger	1978, 1984, 1991	Introduced the notion of transcultural nursing and caring nursing.
Jean Watson	1979, 1985	Discussed the philosophy and science of caring and humanistic nursing.
Dorothy Johnson	1980	Presented a complete behavioral system theory model for nursing. "Clients behave in an integrated, systematic, patterned, ordered and predictable way, and that behavior is goal-oriented. Moreover, behavior is the sum total of biological, social, cultural, and psychological behaviors." To Johnson, nursing's specific contribution to patient welfare is through identification of a behavioral subsystem or subsystems that are threatened or could potentially be threatened by illness or hospitalization (Meleis, 1985, p. 198).

▶ *Meaning*: Arises from any interrelation with the world; refers to happenings to which we attach varying degrees of significance

▶ *Rhythmicity*: Movement of humans and the environment toward greater diversity

▶ *Co-transcendence*: Process of moving toward future possibilities. (Creasia & Parker, 1996, p. 162)

Considerably less esoteric is the work of Nola Pender (1982, 1987, 1992), whose development of a health promotion model has prompted a vigorous line of solid nursing research efforts. Afaf Meleis, herself a respected scholar in nursing theory, presented an excellent and thorough discussion of the history of this progression of theory (Meleis, 1985).

From reviewing the literature on nursing theory development, it is apparent that nursing should continue to define its focus and unique perspective if theories for practice are to be generated. Using these theories, specific research questions pertaining to observed phenomena should be addressed to develop nursing's knowledge base. Developing key questions about phenomena of interest to nursing provides directions for research activities and ultimately aids in research development and the development of a unique, generally respected knowledge base for nursing science.

Nursing has developed a powerful and fruitful body of nursing theory that has proved very useful in the further development of nursing as a science. Theory of this type is a work in progress, as are the other forms of nursing knowledge. The early decades of the 21st century should prove to be an explosive period in the development of ever more comprehensive theories. The prospects are very good that development of theory of this type will increasingly be informed by advances in practice-based knowledge as clinicians, theorists, and researchers coordinate their efforts—a mark of a true profession.

Problems with Deductive Nursing Theories

Many see the theories discussed above as too remote for application in "the real world" (Fawcett, 1995; Fitzpatrick & Whall, 1989; King, 1994; Koziol-McLain & Maeve, 1993, Maeve, 1994). This perceived remoteness is reflected in the change of terminology by some writers and researchers—a change from the use of the term "theories" of nursing to the term "models" or "theoretical models" of nursing.

Often "theory" and "model" are used interchangeably, but there is a distinction between the two. Theories have a common structure; they are composed of component concepts that must be logically related to each other by a series of theoretical statements or propositions. Theories may be broad or limited. Most importantly, theories can be tested and can be linked to the real world (Ellis, 1982). In contrast, conceptual models are broader and more abstract than theories. The statements of relations among and between concepts often are not clearly stated and may even be missing. Such models can be considered pretheoretical and have not yet made links to the real world (Oermann, 1997). Thus, many writers now refer to "nursing models" rather than "nursing theories" because they do not perceive the models as being connected to or part of the real world of nursing.

 CRITICALLY THINKING ABOUT . . .

Many nurses fail to see any connection between general nursing theories and day-to-day nursing practice. What should be done and by whom to overcome this gap?

Inductive Nursing Theories

Although much attention has been paid to nursing theories such as those discussed in the previous section, not all nurses value them as the best answer to the need for a respected nursing knowledge base. This is in large part due to their perceived remoteness. In the four decades during which the theories discussed in the earlier section were being developed, promulgated, refined, and researched, another category of theory was being strengthened by nursing scholars and researchers—**inductive theory**. This theory is composed of a knowledge base inductively derived from practice; nursing practice informs nursing theory, rather than the other way around. Inductive theories differ from deductive theories, which are intended as theory to inform nursing practice. These positions are not necessarily antithetical, but rather their recognition and creative articulation contribute to the uniqueness and viability of the total knowledge base of the discipline of nursing.

Practice-based nursing knowledge is inextricably bound to the care nurses deliver every day. It is generated by practitioners and nursing scholars in the many diverse settings in which nurses deliver care. Practice-based nursing knowledge is not removed from the realities of patient–nurse interaction; rather, it is derived with the participation of the many diverse clients nurses serve. Finally, practice-based nursing knowledge may be derived using both traditional quantitative research methods and qualitative methods as well. Hildegard Peplau, almost 40 years after she first presented her considerations of interpersonal relationships in nursing, noted that although nursing practice is not widely considered a research endeavor, it is in part a scientific and scholarly endeavor (Peplau, 1988).

Pamela Reed has conducted a revisionist analysis of Peplau's early work from a postmodernist perspective:

> A closer look at Peplau's theory demonstrates an approach to knowledge development through the scholarship of practice; nursing knowledge is developed *in* practice as well as *for* practice. . . In this postmodern era, knowledge development is no longer only a concern of theoretical nursing; it is a concern in practice. Knowledge development increasingly is recognized not merely as a product to apply in practice, but as an activity in the everyday life of the practicing nurse. (Reed, 1996, pp. 29–30)

Reed describes a three-step strategy for linking knowledge development and practice:

1. Knowledge development begins with observations made in the context of practice.
2. Theoretical explanations of those observations are "peeled out"—that is, concepts are abstracted from one's clinical knowledge and from existing scientific theories, whatever those theories may need to be. These concepts then represent the phenomena observed in practice.
3. Through the application of one's esthetic perspective, intellectual competencies, and clinical judgment, the nurse transforms practice knowledge into nursing knowledge. (Peplau, 1988, p. 13)

"Nursing knowledge is developed in the context of practice through synthesis of existing scientific theories, clinical observation, and judgement of nurses, and knowledge and active participation of the patients" (Reed, 1996, p. 31).

Abundant literature attests to the existence, viability, and importance of nursing knowledge emerging from practice. One example of nursing knowledge emerging from the practice setting through quantitative research methods is given in the following example. Nurses in the neonatal special care unit of a community hospital observed that the tiny infants in their care came to the unit with round little heads. However, by the time the infants were ready to be discharged, those who had long stays on the unit showed distortion of their original head shape—a flattening on both sides of the head and a narrowing and apparent elongation of the face. The experienced nurses realized that parents of premature infants are at high risk for bonding problems with their babies and were concerned with maintaining a normal head appearance of these babies to promote bonding between infant and parents. The nurses tried various techniques for relieving the pressure on the babies' heads that was producing the distortion. Eventually they hit on one that they believed was effective—the use of a water pillow made from a common, inexpensive plastic cervical ice collar. However, they had no systematic means of testing its effectiveness. Accordingly, they sought help from the hospital's clinical nursing research consultant. The clinical research team designed and conducted an empirical, quasiexperimental study. The results of the study demonstrated that infants placed on water pillows showed less head shape distortion that those cared for in the customary manner (Schwirian, Eesley, & Cuellar, 1986).

Nurse researchers using qualitative methods in practice environments also are making significant contributions to nursing's knowledge base. For example, Morse and Doberneck (1995) used interviews with hospitalized patients to delineate the concept of hope. They interviewed heart transplant patients (before the procedure), patients with spinal cord injury, breast cancer survivors, and breast-feeding mothers intending to continue nursing while employed. Nurses know that patients' general attitudes and beliefs contribute substantially to their recovery; thus, an understanding of hope is an important part of nursing's knowledge base.

Jenny and Logan (1996) used inductive theory to examine the meaning of metaphors used by hospitalized critical care patients about the ventilator weaning experience. In explaining the clinical implications of their findings, they noted:

> Examining patients' metaphors is a valuable approach to understanding the experiential world of patients in critical care so that nursing actions can be directed toward personal needs that may not be expressed openly. Providing interventions aimed at these personal needs will help patients find suitable levels of physical and emotional comfort. (p. 349)

A high degree of excitement comes with the discovery of nursing-based knowledge. It is rewarding to see interventions designed by nurses bring improvement for patients. The professional challenge when such an advance takes place is to pass it along systematically to other nurses in practice so that it may find a place in treatment and care protocols. Professional meetings and publications are available for such reports, and nurses in practice must keep abreast of the knowledge available in such outlets.

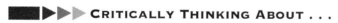 **CRITICALLY THINKING ABOUT . . .**

What have you observed in a practice setting that you think merits research that can contribute to nursing's knowledge base?

Knowledge for Nursing: Beyond Empirics

To this point, much of the nursing knowledge we have studied is what has been called **empirics** (Chinn & Kramer, 1995)—that is, knowledge that draws on observation and experience. This knowledge is then incorporated into systematic descriptions and theories relevant to nursing. Indeed, formal knowledge has been considered foundational to nursing practice ever since Nightingale first established formal education as a requirement for nurses. However, scientifically derived knowledge is not the only knowledge essential to nursing. There are three additional types of knowledge that, along with empirics, constitute the whole of nursing knowledge:

▶ Ethical knowledge or ethics
▶ Personal knowing
▶ Esthetic knowing.

Figure 2-3 shows a model of the whole of knowing that incorporates the four patterns. The four patterns are not totally separate and distinct from each other. In some areas of the model the patterns are separate from the others, and in others they overlap; often all four types overlap simultaneously. This way of viewing nursing knowledge helps us perceive the complexity and uniqueness of the knowledge that supports our discipline.

Ethics

Ethics is the moral knowledge within nursing. Over the course of a day, nurses ask many questions, including:

▶ "Is this action right?"
▶ "For whom is this right and for whom is this wrong?"
▶ "What should I do in this situation to be doing the right thing?"
▶ "Who is responsible here? Are we responsible?"

To lead a moral life, we must determine how to apply values, norms, and moral codes to a specific situation. This is often difficult because norms, values, and principles frequently conflict with each other.

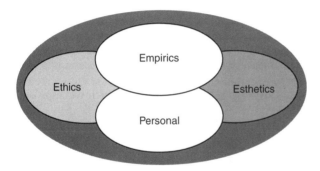

Figure 2-3. The whole of knowing. (Chinn PL, Kramer MK [1995]. *Theory and Nursing: A Systematic Approach* (4th ed.) St. Louis: Mosby.)

Consider the nurse on the cancer unit caring for a patient who is in terrible pain. The attending physician's orders prohibit further medication for at least 2 more hours. The physician is unavailable and has not left orders covering this situation. The resident who is covering has not yet responded to the nurse's page of 30 minutes ago. Should the nurse adhere to the usual hospital norms of the situation of doing nothing until the physician responds? Or should he or she undertake humane actions to relieve the patient's pain, even though they could result in a severe reprimand or even the loss of the nurse's job? Many nurses have faced this situation, and through the years a general norm for this situation has developed that calls for restraint of independent action by the nurse until the physician acts. The resolution of this dilemma—acting to relieve pain versus adhering to the role definitions of nurse and physician in the hospital bureaucracy—reflects Chinn and Kramer's observation that "ethical knowing nursing requires both an implicit knowledge on which difficult on-the-spot decisions are based and knowledge of the formal principles and ethical theories of the discipline and society" (Chinn & Kramer, 1995, p. 8).

There are three creative processes of ethical knowing in nursing: clarifying, valuing, and advocating. **Clarifying** is the process by which unclear or conflicting values and norms are made explicit and sharpened. **Valuing** helps us see the different moral weights attached to alternative values and norms. Together, clarifying and valuing help form an ethical foundation that directs **advocacy** by nurses for themselves or others. Advocacy entails valuing an individual's self-determination and assuring an individual's independence and right to decision making to the greatest extent possible. Chinn and Kramer (1995) argue that these three creative processes assist in developing ethical principles, guidelines, and theory that provide insight into the relative ethics of possible courses of action.

 CRITICALLY THINKING ABOUT . . .

What would nursing's code of ethics say about physician-assisted suicide?

Personal Knowing

As humans develop, we encounter experiences and significant persons, some major and some minor. These encounters contribute to our development of self-concept, our view of others (specific and general), our perception of the world in which we operate, and our concept of the worlds in which others operate. This knowledge is accumulated over the course of a lifetime; in effect, a person is the ultimate work in progress. So although there is in a sense a continuity to the core self, there is an ongoing reconfiguration of orientation to self and to the external world as our knowledge base expands, corrects past observations, and is resorted and reinterpreted.

Personal knowing is not limited to simple perceived facts but may also include spiritual and metaphysical forms of knowing. Indeed, each human is a complex system of mind, body, and spirit. Personal knowledge is accumulated about each realm.

Personal knowing is of critical importance: it is the basis on which we approach each other, relate to others, and interpret others' response to us. The accumulation of personal knowing keeps us balanced throughout life. This is true in life in general, and it is certainly true as nurses relate to clients. As nurses progress through their careers, they acquire an enormous amount of experientially based knowledge. As a result, they begin to change as persons and as valued colleagues. The experienced nurse's view of the world in general, of nursing, and of appropriate relations with clients, physicians, and other health care professionals is often very different from that of the new nurse graduate. Many of the differences reflect the differences in personal knowing between the two.

Chinn and Kramer (1995) argue that there are three creative processes in personal knowing: opening, centering, and realizing.

Opening refers to taking in the fullness of experiences with a conscious awareness. If humans are not open to experiences, they cannot enhance their personal knowing. At one time or another, most people pass through life's experiences in a closed fashion, thereby losing the opportunity to enhance their personal knowing. The person who remains open grows as a person, as a friend, and as a valued colleague. One of the things that happens in stressful nursing situations is that to cope with the stress and perhaps avoid burnout, nurses close themselves to the ongoing experiences around them. Remaining closed to the world potentially stunts personal growth and limits personal knowing.

Centering consists of the processes in which people seriously contemplate their experiences. In centering, people ask such basic questions of themselves as, "What do I really know?" or "Do I know what it is that I actually do?" The process of centering leads to the development of a personal meaning for the experiences we accumulate. The hectic nature of industrial society provides limited opportunity for centering; a person must carve out a time and select a place where such undisturbed introspection can take place. Without centering, our experiences may remain unclear, disconnected, and unexamined, thereby contributing little to personal knowing.

 CRITICALLY THINKING ABOUT . . .

How important is centering for nursing students when they are working and learning in clinical settings?

Realizing is the third creative process of personal knowing. **Realizing** is the process by which people express their whole self, consistent with the experienced inner life that results from opening and centering. By expressing the self, people come to know their genuine self to an even greater extent, and as people come to know themselves, they are better able to have authentic, positive, and productive relationships with others.

Personal knowing typically has not been recognized or explored as a legitimate or formal source of new knowledge in the same way that empirics and ethics have. However, personal knowing has long been recognized as an important component of nursing practice because it allows nurses to develop interpersonal relationships that are genuinely therapeutic—that is, the therapeutic use of self.

Esthetics

Each form of knowing has its own defining question (Table 2-3), and for esthetics the question is, "What does this mean?" According to Chinn and Kramer (1995), "**Esthetic** knowing in nursing is the comprehension of meaning in a singular, particular, subjective expression . . . (that) makes it possible to move beyond the limits and

TABLE 2-3	DEFINING QUESTIONS: WAYS OF KNOWING
Type of Knowing	**Defining Question**
Empirics	"What is this and how does it work?"
Ethics	"Is this right?"
Personal knowing	"Do I know what I do and do I do what I know?"
Esthetics	"What does this mean?"

circumstances of a particular moment, to sense the meaning of the moment, and to envision what is possible but not yet real" (p. 10). In interaction with others—patients, physicians, patient family members, and others on the health care team—the nurse makes esthetic knowing visible through his or her actions, physical bearing, attitudes, and verbal and nonverbal communication. Esthetic knowing permits us to act at once, without protracted deliberation; it permits us to see what is most important in a given situation; it allows us to understand the gravity of a situation and therefore what requires immediate attention and direct action. Without this type of knowing, a nurse would not be able to respond rapidly to the demands of diagnosis and treatment in a health care setting.

There are three creative processes in esthetic knowing: engaging, intuiting, and envisioning. **Engaging** is the total involvement of the self in the situation. By doing this, the meaning of the situation becomes defined on the basis of past subjective experiences. In effect, we intuitively understand the nature of the situation and what action is required. **Intuiting** is the process that allows us to see the unique nature of the situation. The third process, **envisioning**, allows us to think of or dream up new and creative responses to the situation. Esthetic knowing is the art of nursing in which the nurse creates unique and meaningful solutions to difficult problems.

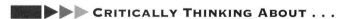 CRITICALLY THINKING ABOUT . . .

How would you describe the art of nursing?

These three ways of nonempirical knowing contribute to the understanding that nurses develop about their practice. With understanding, the nurse comprehends the practice experience as a whole, sees the interconnection between the nurse's responsibilities and actions and the responsibilities and actions of others on the health care team, and comes to see the patient in a holistic manner—that is, as a fellow human embedded in a network of social and family relations that can have either positive or negative effects on the patient's progress toward wellness. In these ways, personal knowledge increases the nurse's professionalism and contributes to the further professionalization of the field.

Clearly ethics, personal knowing, and esthetics are important forms of nursing knowledge. However, things work best in the development of nursing when the three are wed to the empiric form of knowledge. All are necessary, and in their unique combination they give nursing a distinct knowledge domain, a domain that permits nursing to stand independently of all other fields of professional knowledge.

▶ CHAPTER SUMMARY

In the past 100 years, nursing has come a long way in terms of systematically developing and defining a unique, scientifically sound body of knowledge and theoretical foundation to establish nursing as a fully acknowledged profession. Nursing knowledge has emerged from being physician-directed and task-oriented to focus on the maintenance and wellness of clients, a perspective and body of knowledge unique to nursing. In addition, a theoretical foundation for nursing knowledge is still developing. Nursing theory consists of a synthesis of knowledge from three primary sources: theory borrowed from other sciences and disciplines, deductively derived theory specific to nursing science, and inductively derived theory specific to nursing science. Also important to the complete body of nursing knowledge is knowledge that goes beyond empirics: ethical, personal, and esthetic knowledge.

When woven together, these knowledge sources become a rich tapestry that serves as a fitting background to the practice of a discipline that is at the same time holistic and diverse. Nursing scholars, researchers, and clinicians have all contributed to the weaving of that tapestry. As more nurses develop their scholarship and enhance the quality of their practice, new insights and understandings will be engendered to add to the richness and uniqueness of the intellectual foundation of our discipline.

KEY POINTS

▶ 1 There are many definitions of nursing, but most include two elements: a set of actions that are considered nursing and a set of goals for those nursing actions to achieve.

▶ 2 Nursing is moving rapidly into becoming a scientific discipline because nurse theorists and researchers are using scientific methods to explain, predict, and apply new knowledge in the practice of professional nursing.

▶ 3 Although developments in nursing knowledge have occurred, society does not yet truly recognize the unique contributions of nursing knowledge to health care. This is due to dated perceptions of the nurse and nursing knowledge as accessory to medical knowledge, and media reinforcement of this perception. To change this image, nurses must promote their existing knowledge and services as unique. However, most importantly, they must fully develop a unique, sound body of nursing knowledge.

▶ 4 Three categories of theoretical foundations support the body of scientific nursing knowledge: imported theories, deductively derived theories, and knowledge inductively derived from nursing practice. Imported theories, such as biologic, general systems, role, adaptive, and developmental, are borrowed from other disciplines and adapted as an integral aspect of nursing. Nurses themselves have developed numerous deductive theories of nursing, the common elements of which are person, environment, health, and nursing, and the nature of the interrelations among these elements. Nurses have also developed inductive theories grounded in the situations and environments in which they practice.

▶ **5** Beyond empirics (the science of nursing), nurses have three important ways of knowing: ethical knowing, personal knowing, and esthetic knowing. Ethical knowing is the moral knowledge of nursing and addresses the question, "What should I do in this situation to be doing the right thing?" Personal knowing is the knowledge of themselves that nurses develop over time and serves as the basis on which they can relate therapeutically to others. Esthetic knowing is the art of nursing from which nurses create unique and meaningful solutions to difficult problems.

REFERENCES

Aber CS, Hawkins JW (1992). Portrayal of nurses in advertisements in medical and nursing journals. *Image: Journal of Nursing Scholarship 24,* 289–293.

American Nurses Association (1980). *Nursing: A Social Policy Statement.* Kansas City, MO: Author.

American Nurses Association (1995). *Nursing's Social Policy Statement.* Washington DC: Author.

Bilitski J (1981). Nursing science and the laws of health: The test of substance as a step in the process of theory development. *Advances in Nursing Science 4*(1), 15–29.

Campbell-Heider N, Hart CA, Bergren MD (1994). Conveying professionalism: Working against the old stereotypes. In Bullough B, Bullough V (Eds.) *Nursing Issues for the Nineties and Beyond.* New York: Springer.

Catalano JT (1996). *Contemporary Professional Nursing.* Philadelphia: FA Davis.

Chinn PL, Kramer MK (1995). *Theory and Nursing: A Systematic Approach* (4th ed.). St. Louis: Mosby.

Creasia JL, Parker B (1996). *Conceptual Foundations of Professional Nursing Practice* (2nd ed.). St. Louis: Mosby.

Diers D (1983). *Research in Nursing Practice.* Philadelphia: JB Lippincott.

Ellis R (1982). Conceptual issues in nursing. *Nursing Outlook 30,* 406–420.

Fawcett J (1983). Contemporary nursing research: Its relevance to nursing practice. In Chaska N (Ed.), *The Nursing Profession: A Time to Speak.* New York: McGraw-Hill.

Fawcett J (1995). *Analysis and Evaluation of Nursing Theories.* Philadelphia: FA Davis.

Fitzpatrick JJ, Whall AL (1989). *Conceptual Models of Nursing: Analysis and Evaluation.* Norwalk, CT: Appleton-Lange.

Freud S (1938). *The basic writings of Sigmund Freud* (A.A. Brill, Trans.). New York: Modern Library.

Guyton A, Hall J (1996). *Textbook of Medical Physiology* (6th ed.). Philadelphia: WB Saunders.

Jenny J, Logan J (1996). Caring and comfort metaphors used by patients in critical care. *Image: Journal of Nursing Scholarship 28,* 349–352.

Kalisch PA, Kalisch BJ (1980). Perspectives on improving nursing's public image. *Nursing and Health Care 1,* 138–164.

Kalisch PA, Kalisch BJ (1982a). The image of the nurse in motion pictures. *AJN 82,* 605–611.

Kalisch PA, Kalisch BJ (1982b). Nurses on prime time television. *AJN 82,* 264–270.

Kalisch PA, Kalisch BJ (1982c). The image of the nurse in novels. *AJN 82,* 1220–1224.

Kalisch PA, Kalisch BJ (1986). A comparative analysis of nurse and physician characters in the entertainment media. *J Adv Nursing 11,* 179–195.

Kalisch BJ, Kalisch PA, Scobey M (1981). Reflections on a television image: The nurses 1962–1965. *Nursing and Health Care 2,* 248–255.

King M (1994). Nursing theories outdated [letter to the editor]. *J Psychosocial Nursing 32,* 6.

Kohlberg L (1981). *The Philosophy of Moral Development: Moral Stages and the Idea of Justice*, Vol. 1. San Francisco: Harper & Row.

Kohlberg L (1984). *The Psychology of Moral Development: Moral Stages and the Life Cycle*, Vol. 2. San Francisco: Harper & Row.

Koziol-McLain J, Maeve MK (1993). Nursing theory in perspective. *Nursing Outlook 41*, 9–82.

Leininger M (1991). *Culture Care Diversity and Universality: A Theory of Nursing* (NLN Publication No. 15-2402). New York: National League for Nursing.

Maeve MK (1994). The carrier bag theory of nursing practice. *Adv Nursing Science 16*(4), 9–22.

Meleis AI (1985). *Theoretical Nursing: Development, Progress*. Philadelphia: JB Lippincott.

Morse JM, Doberneck B (1995). Delineating the concept of hope. *Image: Journal of Nursing Scholarship 27*, 277–285.

Newman M (1983). The continuing revolution: A history of nursing science. In Chaska N (Ed.), *The Nursing Profession: A Time to Speak*. New York: McGraw-Hill.

Oermann MH (1997). *Professional Nursing Practice*. Stamford, CT: Appleton-Lange.

Parse R (1981). *Man–Living–Health: A Theory of Nursing*. New York: John Wiley & Sons.

Pender NJ (1982). *Health Promotion in Nursing Practice*. Norwalk, CT: Appleton-Century-Crofts.

Pender NJ (1987). *Health Promotion in Nursing Practice* (2nd ed.). Norwalk, CT: Appleton-Century-Crofts.

Pender NJ, Barkauskas VH, Hayman L, Rice VH, Anderson ET (1992). Health promotion and disease prevention: Towards excellence in nursing practice and education. *Nursing Outlook 40*, 106–112.

Reed PG (1996). Transforming practice knowledge into nursing knowledge: A revisionist analysis of Peplau. *Image: Journal of Nursing Scholarship 28*, 29–33.

Schwirian PM, Eesley T, Cuellar L (1986). Use of water pillows in reducing head shape distortion in preterm infants. *Research in Nursing and Health 9*, 203–207.

Tappen R (1995). *Nursing Leadership and Management: Concepts and Practice* (3rd ed.). Philadelphia: FA Davis.

Vander AJ, Sherman JH, Luciano DS (1994). *Human Physiology: The Mechanisms of Body Function* (6th ed.). New York: McGraw-Hill.

Watson J (1985). *Nursing: Human Science and Health Care*. Norwalk, CT: Appleton-Century-Crofts.

West J (1990). *Best and Taylor's Physiological Basis of Medical Practice* (12th ed.). Baltimore: Williams & Wilkins.

Classic References

Abdellah FG, Beland IL, Martin A, Matheney RV (1973). *New Directions in Patient-Centered Nursing: Guidelines for Systems of Service Education and Research*. New York: Macmillan.

Antonovsky A (1979). *Health, Stress and Coping*. San Francisco: Jossey-Bass.

Beckstrand J (1978). The notion of a practice theory and the relationship of scientific and ethical knowledge to practice. *Research in Nursing and Health 1*, 131–136.

Beletz E (1974). Is nursing's public image up-to-date? *Nursing Outlook 22*, 432–435.

Dickoff J, James P (1968). Theory in a practice discipline, Part I. *Nursing Res 17*, 415–435.

Erikson EH (1950). *Childhood and Society*. New York: Norton.

Goode W (1961). The librarian: From occupation to profession? *Library Quarterly 3*(4), 306–320.

Greene J (1979). Science, nursing and nursing science: A conceptual analysis. *Adv Nursing Science 2*(1), 57–64.

Hall AD, Fagen RE (1968). Definition of system. In Buckley W (Ed.), *Modern Systems Research for the Behavioral Scientist*, pp. 81–92. Chicago: Aldine Publishing.

Henderson V (1966). *The Nature of Nursing: A Definition and Its Implications for Practice Research and Education*. New York: Macmillan.

Henderson V (1971). Health is everybody's business. *Canadian Nurse 67*, 31–34.

Holmes T, Rahe R (1967). The social adjustment rating scale. *J Psychosomatic Research 11*, 213–218.

Jacobs M, Huether S (1978). Nursing science: The theory–practice linkage. *Adv Nursing Science 1*(1), 63–74.

Johnson DE (1959). The nature of a science of nursing. *Nursing Outlook 7*, 291.

Johnson DE (1968). Theory in nursing: Borrowed and unique. *Nursing Research 17*, 206–209.

Johnson DE (1974). Development of theory: A requisite for nursing as a primary health profession. *Nursing Research 23*, 372–377.

Johnson DE (1980). The behavioral system model for nursing. In Riehl JP, Roy C, eds. *Conceptual Models for Nursing Practice* (2nd ed.). New York: Appleton-Century-Crofts, pp. 207–215.

King IM (1971). *Toward a Theory for Nursing: General Concepts of Human Behavior*. New York: John Wiley & Sons.

King IM (1975). A process for developing concepts for nursing through research. In Verhonick PJ (Ed.), *Nursing Research*, Vol. I. Boston: Little, Brown.

King IM (1981). *A Theory for Nursing: Systems Concepts Process*. New York: John Wiley & Sons.

Lazlo E (1972). *The Systems View of the World*. New York: George Braziller.

Leininger M (1978). *Transcultural Nursing: Concepts, Theories and Practices*. New York: John Wiley & Sons.

Leininger M (Ed.) (1984). *Care: The Essence of Nursing and Health*. Thorofare, NJ: Charles B. Slack.

Levine ME (1967). The four conservation principles of nursing. *Nursing Forum 6*, 45–69.

Levine ME (1973). *Introduction to Clinical Nursing* (2nd ed.). Philadelphia: FA Davis.

Linton R (1936). *The Study of Man*. New York: Appleton-Century-Crofts.

Maslow A (1954). *Motivation and Personality*. New York: Harper & Row.

Mead GH (1934). *Mind, Self and Society*. Chicago: University of Chicago Press.

Miller JG (1978). *Living Systems*. New York: McGraw-Hill.

Moreno JL (1945). *Psychodrama*. New York: Beacon House.

Neuman BM (1980). The Betty Neuman health care systems model: A total person approach to patient problems. In Riehl JP, Roy C (Eds.) *Conceptual Models of Nursing Practice*. New York: Appleton-Century-Crofts.

Nightingale F (1859). *Notes on Nursing: What It Is and What It Is Not*. Harrison and Sons; facsimile edition, 1946. Philadelphia: JB Lippincott.

Orlando IJ (1961). *The Dynamic Nurse–Patient Relationship*. New York: GP Putnam's Sons.

Peplau H (1952). *Interpersonal Relations in Nursing: A Conceptual Frame of Reference for Psychodynamic Nursing*. New York: GP Putnam's Sons (reprinted in 1988 by Macmillan and in 1991 by Springer).

Piaget J (1926). *The Language and Thought of the Child*. New York: Harcourt-Brace.

Piaget J (1969). *The Psychology of the Child*. New York: Basic Books.

Rogers M (1970). *An Introduction to the Theoretical Basis of Nursing*. Philadelphia: FA Davis.

Rogers M (1972). Nursing: To be or not to be. *Nursing Outlook 20*, 42–45.

Rogers M (1980). Nursing: A science of unitary man. In Reihl JP, Roy C (Eds.) *Conceptual Models for Nursing Practice* (2nd ed.). New York: Appleton-Century-Crofts.

Roy C (1970). Adaptation: A conceptual framework for nursing. *Nursing Outlook 18*, 42–45.

Roy C (1976). *Introduction to Nursing: An Adaptational Model.* Englewood Cliffs, NJ: Prentice-Hall.

Roy C (1980). The Roy adaptation model. In Riehl JP, Roy C (Eds.) *Conceptual Models for Nursing Practice* (2nd ed.). New York: Appleton-Century-Crofts.

Roy C (1984). *Introduction to Nursing: An Adaptation Model* (2nd ed.). Englewood Cliffs, NJ: Prentice-Hall.

Selye H (1976). *The Stress of Life.* New York: McGraw-Hill.

Wald F, Leonard N (1964). Toward development of nursing practice theory. *Nursing Research 13*, 309–313.

Watson J (1979). *Nursing: The Philosophy and Science of Caring.* Boston: Little, Brown.

RECOMMENDED READINGS

Allan H (1996). Developing nursing knowledge and language. *Nursing Standard 10*, 42–44.

Boettcher JH (1996). Nurse practice centers in academia: An emerging subsystem. *J Nursing Education 35*, 63–68.

Bradley SF (1996). Processes in the creation and diffusion of nursing knowledge: An examination of the developing concept of family-centered care. *J Adv Nursing 23*, 722–727.

Bream TL, Brams AL, Krenz KD (1992). Beyond the ordinary image of nursing. *Nursing Management 23*, 44–47.

Carper BA (1978). Fundamental patterns of knowing in nursing. *Adv Nursing Science 1*, 13–23.

Castledine G (1994). A definition of nursing based on nurturing. *Br J Nursing 3*, 134–135.

Cooley CH (1902). *Human Nature and the Social Order.* New York: Scribner's.

Day RA, Field PA, Campbell IE, Reutter L (1995). Students' evolving beliefs about nursing: From entry to graduation in a four-year baccalaureate program. *Nurse Education Today 15*, 357–364.

Durkheim E (1947). *Division of Labor in Society*, G. Simpson, trans. Glencoe, IL: The Free Press. Originally published in French, 1893.

Gortner S (1983). The history and philosophy of nursing science and research. *Advances in Nursing Science 5*(7), 1–8.

Henderson V (1964). The nature of nursing. *AJN 64*, 62–68.

Henderson V, Nite G (1978). *The Principles and Practice of Nursing.* New York: Macmillan.

Hughes L (1980). The public image of the nurse. *Advances in Nursing Science, 2*(3), 55–72.

James W (1908). *Pragmatism and the Meaning of Truth.* Cambridge, MA: Harvard University Press.

Johnson DE (1965). Today's actions will determine tomorrow's nursing. *Nursing Outlook 13*, 38–41.

Kritek P (1983). Five nurse leaders discuss social policy statement. *American Nurse 15*(2), 4.

Lilley LL, Guanci R (1995). Applying systems theory. *AJN 95*, 14–15.

Porter EJ (1995). Non-equilibrium systems theory: Some applications for gerontological nursing practice. *J Gerontological Nursing 21*(6), 24–31.

Putt A (1978). *General Systems Theory Applied to Nursing*. Boston: Little, Brown.

Rafferty AM (1996). The theory/practice gap: Taking issue with the issue. *J Adv Nursing 23*, 685–691.

Roper N (1994). Definition of nursing: 1. *Br J Nursing 3*, 355–357.

Roper N (1994). Definition of nursing: 2. *Br J Nursing 3*, 460–462.

Schlotfeldt R (1974). On the professional status of nursing. *Nursing Forum 13*, 16–31.

Steele J (1984). Statement moves us to focus on what nurses fix. *American Nurse 16*(1), 4–21.

Sumner WG (1896, 1906). *Folkways*. Boston: Ginn.

vonBertalanffy L (1956). General systems theory. In Ruben BD, Kim J (Eds.) *General Systems Theory and Human Communication*. Rochelle Park, NJ: Hayden, pp. 7–16.

3

Nursing Research: An Action Path to Professionalization

CHAPTER OUTLINE

Development and Progress of
   Nursing Research
Types of Research Contributing to
   Nursing Science
Chapter Summary

Key Points
References
Classic References
Recommended Readings

LEARNING OBJECTIVES

▶ **1** Discuss Florence Nightingale's monumental contributions to the discipline of nursing and to nursing research.

▶ **2** Explain two reasons for the lack of nursing research development from Nightingale's time until the 1950s.

▶ **3** Discuss the reasons for the acceleration of nursing research since the 1950s.

▶ **4** Describe the role of the National Institute of Nursing Research in relation to the development of nursing research.

▶ **5** Compare and contrast the two methods of nursing research (quantitative and qualitative).

KEY TERMS

American Journal of Nursing (AJN)
correlational study
Crimean War
descriptive study
Florence Nightingale

ethnography
experimental study
Goldmark report
National Institute of Nursing Research (NINR)

nursing research
phenomenology
qualitative methods
quantitative methods
training versus education

Nursing research is an integral aspect of the nursing discipline and is crucial to the development of nursing as a profession. The development of nursing research spans more than 100 years—from the time of Florence Nightingale to the present. Incredible progress in research development has occurred during this period, especially since the mid-20th century. To grasp the significance of these achievements, it is helpful to view the developments in nursing research in the context of four time periods—the Nightingale period, Nightingale to 1950, 1950 to 1980, and 1980 to the present. Nurses have performed a broad range of research studies that have contributed greatly to the development of research science. These research studies fall into two methods of research—quantitative and qualitative. Important examples of both quantitative and qualitative nursing research studies are provided.

Development and Progress of Nursing Research

As an occupation moves toward full professional status, it increases its research productivity. The research is focused mainly on problems dealing with the phenomenon around which the profession develops. For physician researchers, this means research focused on discovering the cause, diagnosis, treatment, and cure for diseases. For the nurse researcher, this means research focused on the whole range of preventive and curative matters related to patient care. With nursing, research has aimed at increasing nursing's scientific knowledge base (empirics) as well as the ethical and esthetic knowledge bases for its practice. Nursing research has not been limited to studies of the delivery of nursing care; it has also focused on the patient as a biopsychosocial being, on self (as in the performance of duties and tasks), and on nursing students as potential professionals and future colleagues. Today, nursing research is increasingly informed by developments in nursing theory. However, as nursing research begins to replicate and validate nursing knowledge in the practice setting and relies on this knowledge to direct nursing practice, nursing will increasingly become recognized as an independent, legitimately autonomous profession.

Foundations of Nursing Research: Florence Nightingale

The foundations of nursing research—like the foundations of modern nursing—were established in the mid-19th century by **Florence Nightingale**. Nightingale was a remarkable person in many ways. She was a highly educated, professionally productive woman in a period in which women—particularly those from wealthy, influential families—were not expected to be highly educated and certainly were not expected to be professionally productive. The role of women during this period was that of household manager, mother, and emotional provider to husband and children. Instead of adhering to this established role, Nightingale broke all tradition and established a lifelong pattern of independence of thought and action early in life when she chose to become a nurse. Furthermore, she used her high social position and her own financial resources to bring about a revolution in the medical and nursing care of soldiers in the British Army.

Nightingale studied medicine on her own and performed hospital apprenticeships in Germany and France. In 1853, she became the supervisor of nurses at a

London hospital whose patients were mainly upper- and middle-class women—work for which she received no pay (Curry, Jiobu, & Schwirian, 1997). Nightingale's opportunity to become an influential player in the health care of her time came with her appointment, at age 33, as Superintendent of the Female Nursing Establishment of the English General Hospitals in Turkey. Kalisch and Kalisch (1995) point out that this elegant title was something of a misnomer because as yet there still was not a nursing establishment for her to superintend. However, she was not to be deterred; shortly after her appointment, she and 38 other women set out for the British military hospital at Scutari, a suburb of Constantinople, to nurse British soldiers wounded in the **Crimean War**.

This hospital was infamous for its wretched conditions, and Nightingale was determined to change them. Her achievements during the Crimean War were unprecedented. When she arrived at Scutari, the mortality rate in the hospital was near 60%. When she left, the mortality rate was less than 2%. After the Crimean War ended in 1856, Nightingale returned to England, where she pursued the two goals that were most important to her: (1) reforming Army sanitary practices and (2) establishing a school for nursing (Kalisch & Kalisch, 1995, p. 36).

Nightingale made extremely important contributions to the dramatic improvement in 19th-century health care and nursing education and also contributed greatly to the development of health statistics. A highly educated woman, she studied abroad with Adolphe Quetelet, a Belgian mathematician and astronomer who conducted research on population, probability theory, anthropometry, and criminology. She found his work fascinating and became a convert and ardent admirer of him and his work (Thomlinson, 1965, p. 30). She became known to a small circle of followers as the "passionate statistician" and was the most vigorous and influential exponent of his new science (Cook, 1913). From Quetelet she learned a good deal about the science and art that describes human society in terms of numbers. She also learned the methods, general aims, and results of inquiry into social facts and forces (Knopf, 1916, p. 44).

■■■ ▶▶▶ CRITICALLY THINKING ABOUT . . .

Should undergraduate nursing students be required to take a research methods course or a statistics course? Why or why not?

During her personal crusade against the unsanitary conditions facing the British army in the Crimean War (seven times as many British soldiers fell from disease as from the enemy before Sebastopol) and, later, in her efforts to improve the health and hygiene of the British army in general, she marshaled an enormous amount of empirical data. Through careful analysis of the data and the development of ingenious ways of graphically summarizing and presenting distributions of results, she persuaded key politicians and decision makers—prime ministers, viceroys, secretaries, parliamentary commissions—to initiate needed health reforms (Cohen, 1984; Nightingale, 1858). Indeed, hers are the first recorded efforts to bring systematically analyzed data to bear on major health policy matters. Her success in using statistical methods in army sanitation reform led to her election to the Royal Statistical Society in 1858. In 1874, she was elected an honorary member of the American Statistical Association.

Nightingale's research and programmatic concerns extended beyond army health matters. In England, she found hospital statistics in a chaotic state: the available statistics gave very little useful information on the proportion of deaths and recoveries and the average duration of hospital treatment for different diseases. There was little information on age and sex differences on disease and recovery. With the assistance of Dr. William Farr (1807–1883), she drew up a standard list of diseases and developed the prototype of a uniform disease reporting system for London hospitals. She and Farr studied the tabulated distributions, and the results of their hospital research were reported in a paper at the 1860 meeting of the International Statistical Congress. As a result, the reporting system they devised was adopted in several parts of England and also spread to the hospitals in Paris (Eyler, 1979).

Beyond her hospital efforts, Nightingale applied statistical analysis to a wide variety of questions, including the health of the aboriginal peoples of Australia, of the British army in India, and of the Bengal native army and the army contingents in northern India. She broadened her inquiries to include the general health of the peoples of India, including such topics as famine, irrigation, education, and usury in the Bombay Deccan (the plateau region of south central India).

In all of her work, she had a flair for compiling and presenting facts convincingly. She was also aware of the problems of accurate interpretation. For example, she argued that mortality statistics should be age-specific and that the crude death rate can be misleading (Nightingale, 1859). Her work—together with that of Quetelet, Galton, Pearson, and Fisher—laid the foundation for contemporary statistical data analysis. In her work, she stood head and shoulders with others of her time, particularly John Snow, William Farr, and Ignaz Semmelweis, who are widely recognized as the founders of modern epidemiology (Rockett, 1994).

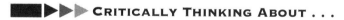 **CRITICALLY THINKING ABOUT . . .**

Was Florence Nightingale's work nursing research or health research? Does it make a difference? Why or why not?

Nightingale to 1950

Nightingale laid the foundations for nursing research, but a tradition of research did not immediately follow. It was almost 100 years later that the nursing research enterprise, as we know it today, really became an established and viable knowledge-building activity to assist nursing in achieving full professional status. How did the pattern of research and scholarship established by Florence Nightingale become disrupted for so long? Two primary factors contributed to the loss of the nursing research ethic in the latter half of the 19th century and into the early 20th century: social norms and education patterns.

Social Norms

The social norms of the time were dictated by the predominant Victorian image of women as weak, dependent creatures, and the vast majority of nurses were women. Even more harmful was the idea that women were the intellectual inferiors of men and that the pursuit of science was entirely too rigorous a task for them to master (Shea, 1997). Although those norms were dying out as the 19th century ended, few women were encouraged to seek a university education—especially not in the sciences required of a competent researcher—in the period from 1900 to 1940.

Education Patterns

The second primary factor contributing to the hiatus in nursing research was the growth pattern of nursing education in the United States. That pattern, which was intact from 1870 until the beginnings of baccalaureate education for nurses in 1909, was the training of nurses in hospital schools of nursing (Dolan, 1973; Shea, 1997). As Mildred Hogstel and Nancy Sayner pointed out:

> The location of these schools in large hospitals with medical schools where (nursing) students were taught by physicians influenced the organization, management, and control under which they functioned. Instead of using many of Nightingale's ideas as a model, these schools fell quickly under the control and supervision of the hospital boards of directors, managers, and physicians. . . . Thus, some of the ideas and functions Florence Nightingale envisioned for nursing were lost. (Hogstel & Sayner, 1986)

It is useful here to differentiate between **training** and **education**, because this difference has significant implications for the place of research in nursing and why nursing research developed so slowly. Training is task-oriented; there is little room for questioning or challenging, activities that are inherent in the research process. In education, by contrast, acquisition of knowledge and development of cognitive skills, fresh ideas, and unique perspectives are encouraged. For well over 50 years, the vast majority of nurses were trained in hospital schools, which resulted in

> trained nurses who were taught, disciplined, or drilled to be fit, qualified, or proficient in their narrowly defined, somewhat static role, which was subservient to male-dominant medicine. The few educated nurses, however, were expected to acquire new knowledge and to use their cognitive abilities to create and evaluate new nursing roles that would evolve in response to societal needs. (Shea, 1997, p. 232)

The likelihood that research progress would occur remained slim until a sufficiently large cadre of nurses received education rather than training.

 CRITICALLY THINKING ABOUT . . .

Should nurses be educated or trained? Does it make a difference? Why or why not?

Early Improvements in Nursing Research

Despite these rather dismal post-Nightingale origins, some leaders in nursing research began to emerge in the early 20th century. There was some attention to patient- and technique-oriented research, but most nursing research in the first half of the 20th century focused on nursing education. Leaders in these early education research efforts are presented in Table 3-1. The initial practice-related research that emerged in the early 20th century focused primarily on morbidity and mortality rates associated with public health problems such as pneumonia and contaminated milk (Carnegie, 1976). For example, Lavinia Dock and Lillian Wald conducted a study in 1902 showing the positive effects of having nurses in schools, and school nurses

TABLE 3-1	EARLY LEADERS IN NURSING RESEARCH	

Year	Researcher	Field
1900	Lavinia Dock	Nursing reformer and staunch advocate for the rights of nursing students in hospital training schools
1906	Isabelle Hampton Robb	First superintendent of the Johns Hopkins Training School for Nurses
1915	Lillian Wald	Pioneer in establishing home health nursing
1912, 1926	Adelaide Nutting	Nursing reformer committed to improving nursing education
1932	Annie Goodrich	Helped establish the Army School of Nursing in World War I and served as its first dean
1923	Goldmark Report (discussed at length in Chap. 1)	One of the most prominent of the studies aimed at improving the education of nurses. Josephine Goldmark, a social secretary whose name the report bears, Adelaide Nutting, Annie Goodrich, and Lillian Wald were members of the committee whose survey yielded the data for the report.

were subsequently employed in New York City and other cities (Roberts, 1954). Another example is the Committee on Public Health Nursing of the National League of Nursing Education, which studied concerns such as infant mortality, blindness, and midwifery in 1913. This group also stated that nursing should bring to bear the scientific approach in distinguishing its role in the prevention of disease and promotion of health.

The first course in nursing research was developed and taught in the 1920s due to the influence of Isabel Stewart, assistant professor in the Department of Nursing and Health at Teachers College, Columbia University. She was also an avowed supporter of removing nursing schools from the control of hospitals (Kalisch & Kalisch, 1995). Also in the 1920s, the *American Journal of Nursing* (**AJN**) started publishing case studies in which scientific criteria were applied to evaluate the appropriateness of the methods applied in each case. These case studies were used as teaching tools (Gortner & Nahm, 1977).

Wars affected the development of research throughout the 19th and early 20th century (Hogstel & Sayner, 1986). For example, the social changes prompted by World War II affected all aspects of nursing, including nursing research. Increased hospital admissions and the needs of the military prompted a serious need for more and better-educated nurses. The nursing research conducted during World War II dealt with hospital environments, the status of nurses, nursing education, and the nursing shortage.

Shortly after the war, the Carnegie Foundation funded Esther Lucille Notter's three-year study of nurses' educational preparation and nursing practices. She echoed the call to move nursing preparation from the training environment of the hospital schools into the academic environment of the university. Notter's work, in turn, prompted many states to carry out their own studies of nursing needs and resources in the immediate postwar period (Simmons & Henderson, 1964).

The research of this period, although slow to develop, formed a foundation of knowledge about patient care and about nurses and nursing students that to this day informs more recent, extensive, and comprehensive studies. It is a heritage of which nurses should be proud, for it clearly told society, and other health care professionals as well, that nursing contained within it a powerful research potential.

1950 to 1980

After more than 25 years of repeated recommendations that nurses should be educated in colleges and universities rather than trained in hospitals, the transition finally began in earnest. This transition had a powerful impact on all aspects of nursing, especially on the nursing research enterprise. The transition of nursing into the academic environment required the discipline to have legitimate academic credentials in educational circles. This requirement meant that nursing had to have a scientifically sound knowledge base and that nurses must demonstrate the capability of generating new, cutting-edge knowledge using established, state-of-the-art, rigorous research methods. The academic environment made it imperative that research become one of the tools of the nursing trade. The groundwork for nursing's current level of research expertise was laid in the 1950s.

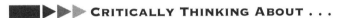 **CRITICALLY THINKING ABOUT . . .**

> As a student in a collegiate program of nursing, do you feel a part of the university or part of the college or school of nursing? Do you identify yourself as a nursing student or as a college student? Does this make a difference to you?

Educating Nurses for University Faculty Roles

One critical aspect of preparing nurses to perform according to the standards and expectations of fellow educators in the universities was the level of educational preparation of prospective nursing teachers. Until the 1950s, nurses with baccalaureate preparation were not plentiful, and nurses holding graduate degrees—especially a doctoral degree—were rare. In 1953, Columbia University opened the door to nurses in their quest for the academic credentials and skills that were so desperately needed if nursing were to progress in its science and as a profession. The Institute for Research and Service in Nursing Education was established at Teacher's College, Columbia University, and provided learning experiences for research for doctoral students (Gortner & Nahm, 1977). Although the focus of this program was nursing education—it granted the EdD degree (Doctor of Education) rather than the PhD degree (Doctor of Philosophy and the highest academic degree granted by universities)—it provided strong emphasis on and support for the academic enrichment of nurses and the appropriate level of education for nurses to function as educators in university settings all over the United States.

Despite these advances, there were few nurses who were qualified to do, or teach, research beyond the baccalaureate level throughout the 1950s. Therefore, as nurses increasingly sought graduate preparation at the master's degree level, most received their education in research methods outside of nursing, usually in departments such as sociology, psychology, education, and biology (Hogstel & Sayner, 1986). As the ranks of doctorally prepared nurses have increased in number (from only about 300 in the 1960s to 11,000 in 1992) (Moses, 1992), more research content has been added to nursing curricula at all levels. Therefore, for the most part, research courses are now taught by nursing faculty rather than by professional colleagues in other disciplines and departments.

The doctoral preparation of hundreds of nurses was greatly facilitated by the Division of Nursing within the Bureau of Health Professions in the Health Resources and Services Administration of the U.S. Public Health Service. In 1955, this agency made funding available for grants, the goal of which was to provide resources for faculty development. This financial support allowed unprecedented numbers of nurse to pursue doctoral study and preparation for research.

The Changing Focus of Nursing Research

The focus of nursing research has changed over time due to three factors:

1. How nurses have been educated to perform research
2. Nursing information needs of the various time periods
3. Broadening and deepening research skills of nurses.

As stated previously, the first graduate programs available for nurses were in the fields of education and social and behavioral sciences. Thus, nurses developed research skills primarily in these areas, and early nursing research was focused on nurses themselves—that is, they began studying nurses and nursing. These early researchers performed studies of nursing education, nursing status, working conditions, and personality characteristics and motivation of nurses. This focus was of concern to some nurse leaders, including Virginia Henderson, who observed that in most occupations, the research focus is on the practice of the discipline rather than on the practitioner. She asked, "Why is it, then, that in our field, studies on the nurse outnumber studies on the practice of nursing more than ten to one?" (Henderson, 1956, p. 99). The most logical answer to her question is that nurse researchers of that period were best equipped to perform research on themselves and their characteristics and behaviors, given their doctoral preparation in education and the social and behavioral sciences. Although some nursing scholars have been critical of this early research focus on nurses rather than on nursing, others view it as a necessary and logical phase of the nursing research progression and of nursing's entry to and emerging importance in academia.

By the late 1950s, nursing research studies focusing on clinical problems started appearing. The first research institute to emphasize nursing research was established in 1957—the Department of Nursing Research in the Walter Reed Army Institute of Research (Stevenson, 1986). Nursing leaders began establishing priorities for the kinds of nursing research that should be supported, and practice-oriented research was targeted as the highest priority. By the end of the 1960s, a wide variety of clinical studies were appearing in the nursing research literature. For example, at Yale University, Rhetaugh Dumas and Robert Leonard (1963) studied nurse–patient teaching and communication. Also in 1963, Lydia Hall published the results of a five-year study that examined alternatives to hospitalization for elderly clients. Hall's findings prompted the founding of the Loeb Center in New York City, a nurse-run care facility that is still providing care for older adults today. It was also during the 1960s that the pioneer nursing theorists began to share their ideas (see Chap. 2).

Clinically focused research continued to develop throughout the 1970s, and by 1976 Elizabeth Carnegie (then editor of *Nursing Outlook*) observed that most of the research published in the nursing journals was clinically oriented. The expanding clinical focus was supported considerably by the expanding number of PhD programs in schools and colleges of nursing nationwide. This expansion continued at a near-explosive rate during the 1980s and into the 1990s. In 1979, there were 22 doctoral programs in nursing; by 1995, there were 62 such programs, from which more than 250 doctorally prepared nurses graduated each year. New programs for doctoral preparation of nursing continue to be developed and implemented; at the heart of these programs is the preparation of nursing scholars who can further the science and profession of nursing through sustained programs of focused, clinically relevant research.

American Nurses Association's Continuing Support for Nursing Research

The American Nurses Association (ANA) has consistently supported the nursing research enterprise as a means of furthering the professionalization of nursing. In 1950, the ANA initiated a five-year study of nursing functions and activities, which culminated in the report *Twenty Thousand Nurses Tell Their Story* (Hughes, Hughes, & Deutscher, 1958). This report was the basis for the ANA's 1959 statements on the functions, standards, and qualifications for professional nurses. At the same time, specialty nursing groups such as community health, psychiatric–mental health, pediatrics, and obstetrics were also developing standards of care. Gortner and Nahm (1977) contend that the research conducted by the ANA and the specialty groups at this juncture provided the basis for the nursing practice standards that guide current nursing practice.

In 1954, the ANA formed the Standing Committee on Research, and in 1955, the American Nurses Foundation (ANF) was chartered. The committee's purpose was to plan, promote, and guide research and studies relating to the functions of the ANA (See, 1977). The purpose of the ANF was to serve as a center for research by raising and distributing funds to support beginning nurse scientists. From 1955 to 1993, the ANF awarded 459 nursing research grants. The first nursing research conference sponsored by the ANA was held in 1965. The 55 researchers attending presented and critiqued studies related to nursing education, nursing students, and hospital personnel (The first American Nurses Association nursing research conference, 1965).

The ANA has made it clear in publications since 1981 that research is a regular part of nursing practice, and that there is an appropriate role for nurses at all levels of preparation in the nursing research enterprise (ANA, 1981, 1985, 1989, 1993). Baccalaureate nurses, although not generally expected to initiate research studies, can often provide the impetus for conceiving and initiating studies through their own observations, ideas, problems, and possible solutions they encounter in their regular clinical practice. The study of head shape distortion among preterm infants (Schwirian, Eesley, & Cuellar, 1986) discussed in Chapter 2 is a perfect example of this kind of study. Baccalaureate (and even associate degree) nurses should be prepared to assist in nursing research by providing support through data collection and pertinent clinical observations they share with the investigators. Baccalaureate nurses should also be knowledgeable consumers of nursing research, critiquing publications responsibly and applying new findings as appropriate.

Nurses who have obtained a master's degree should be prepared to do all of the above and may or may not be prepared to initiate nursing research studies, depending on the nature of their graduate study. Those whose focus in graduate study was highly clinical in nature are best suited to working collaboratively with investigators who have more formal research methods and statistics in their background. However, doctorally prepared nurses have the primary responsibility for initiating and conducting nursing research that is of high quality, is firmly grounded in science, and has significance in nursing practice.

 CRITICALLY THINKING ABOUT . . .

How can you deliver nursing care and do research at the same time? How do you see that happening in the settings where you obtain your clinical education?

The Literature of Nursing Research

One of the requirements of a growing, vital research enterprise (also one of the indicators of its development) is the establishment of peer-reviewed journals dedicated to the dissemination of knowledge gained through research. From the first publication of *Nursing Research* in 1952, there has been steady growth in the number of high-quality journals dedicated to research in nursing (Table 3-2). These journals serve as a rich source of information to practicing nurses and nurse researchers alike.

TABLE 3-2 JOURNALS RELATED TO NURSING RESEARCH

First Published	Journal	General Purpose(s)
1900	*American Journal of Nursing*	General information about nursing practice. Started publishing case studies in 1920s.
1952	*Nursing Research*	Promotion of research in nursing
1953	*Nursing Outlook*	Unsolicited manuscripts on nursing subjects
1962	*Nursing Forum*	Implications of research on nursing professionalization
1963	*International Journal of Nursing Studies*	Promotion of research in nursing
1967	*IMAGE: Journal of Nursing Scholarship*	Research articles and summaries of research on selected topics
1978	*Research in Nursing and Health*	Peer-reviewed journal. Promotion of wide range of research and theory
1978	*Advances in Nursing Science*	Nursing theorists' work and related research
1979	*Western Journal of Nursing*	Analysis of research studies, book reviews, discussions, and debates
1987	*Scholarly Inquiry for Nursing Practice*	Promotion of research crossing disciplinary boundaries in theory and/or methodologies
1987	*Applied Nursing Research*	Promotes research that can be applied to practice
1988	*Nursing Science Quarterly*	Theory-based enhancement of nursing scholarship
1988	*Nursing Scan in Research*	Summaries of research in a "user-friendly" format
1991	*Qualitative Health Research*	Promotion of interdisciplinary qualitative research in health care settings

1980 to the Present

The amount of clinical nursing research increased dramatically in the 1980s and into the 1990s, as did the number of professional journals publishing nursing research (see Table 3-2). In addition, the first volume of a notable publication series, the *Annual Review of Nursing Research*, was published in 1983 (Wesley & Fitzpatrick, 1983). Each year, the editors of this series seek experts in selected areas of nursing research to prepare reviews of research in nursing practice, nursing care delivery, nursing education, and the nursing profession. These annual reviews provide an excellent source of up-to-date information regarding the state of nursing inquiry and research.

One of the most significant factors contributing to the growth of the nursing research enterprise since 1980 was the National Center for Nursing Research (NCNR), established in 1986 under the umbrella of the National Institutes of Health (NIH). Before 1986, limited federal monies had been made available for nursing research through the Division of Nursing; however, the move to NIH added both prestige and financial support to the nursing research enterprise. Dr. Ada Sue Hinshaw was sworn in as the first director of the NCNR in 1986 and served in that capacity until 1994. In 1993, the Center was elevated to full institute status and became the **National Institute of Nursing Research (NINR)**.

The NINR exerts considerable control over the direction of nursing research in this country because it is one of the primary and most prestigious sources of funding for investigators in nursing science. Federal funding for nursing research quadrupled in the first decade of the existence of the NCNR/NINR. The NINR's extramural programs provide grants on a rigorously reviewed and highly competitive basis to researchers in universities, hospitals, and other research centers around the country. However, because the possibilities for research in nursing are almost endless and NINR is the smallest of the NIH institutes, the NINR can fund only a very small proportion of the proposals submitted. Therefore, many important programs (eg, collaborative efforts for clinical trials or consensus conferences) that would benefit the development of nursing science greatly do not receive funding.

The NINR has established priorities for funding that provide a structure within which investigators can develop their programs of research to receive NINR funding. In 1987, the NINR launched the first National Nursing Research Agenda (NNRA) to establish the necessary priorities for funding. The first-phase priorities selected in 1988 included:

- Prevention of and care for low-birthweight infants
- Prevention of and care for human immunodeficiency virus (HIV) infection
- Long-term care for older adults
- Symptom management—pain
- Use of nursing informatics in patient care
- Health promotion for older children and adolescents.

The second-phase priorities, established in 1995 to provide guidelines for the last 5 years of the 20th century, include:

- Community-based nursing models (1995)
- Health-promoting behaviors and HIV/acquired immunodeficiency syndrome (AIDS) (1996)

☒ Remediation of cognitive impairment (1997)
☒ Living with chronic illness (1998)
☒ Biobehavioral factors and immunocompetence (1999).

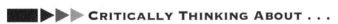 **CRITICALLY THINKING ABOUT . . .**

How often do you read articles about nursing research? How often should you read articles about nursing research?

Significant developments have occurred in nursing research since the time of Florence Nightingale. A timeline of these developments is shown in Figure 3-1. Each development is important and vital to nursing's quest of achieving full professional status. Nursing research is still progressing: developments occur every day in this exciting field, and the possibilities for nursing research development are endless.

Types of Research Contributing to Nursing Science

The nursing research enterprise has grown dramatically in both volume and level of sophistication since its inception with Florence Nightingale, particularly since the mid-20th century. This section explores the range of research that nurses perform in support of the growth of their science and the continuing progress toward the knowledge base required by a fully recognized profession.

Research usually is classified in two ways, by the research method used in the study and by the topic that is studied. The research studies presented in this chapter are classified according to the same schema. Imagine a large two-dimensional mathematical matrix. One axis contains the research methods and strategies used by nurse researchers; the other axis contains the 10 research priority areas defined by the NINR as the foci for the research agenda for the last decade of the 20th century, as well as other research interests pursued by nurse researchers. To provide a better understanding of how nurse researchers have contributed to the development of the nursing science discipline, nursing research studies that fit into selected method-by-topic matrix cells will be highlighted and briefly described. All the studies described below are complete and appear in peer-reviewed professional journals. Some studies were funded by the NINR, some were funded by other sources, and some studies received no funding at all, although the work was judged by the journal reviewers (who are also researchers) to be of sufficient substance and quality to merit publication.

Research Studies Using Quantitative Methods

Quantitative methods are the more traditional approach to research. They rely on using variables that can be quantified, counted, measured, and subjected to rigorous statistical analysis using established models (object and phenomenon) of probability to develop statements about what seems to be true about groups and can be generalized to populations. There is an underlying assumption that reality exists—that there is a real world driven by natural causes. The quantitative investigator must maintain objectivity and distance himself or herself from the subjects of research; objectivity is

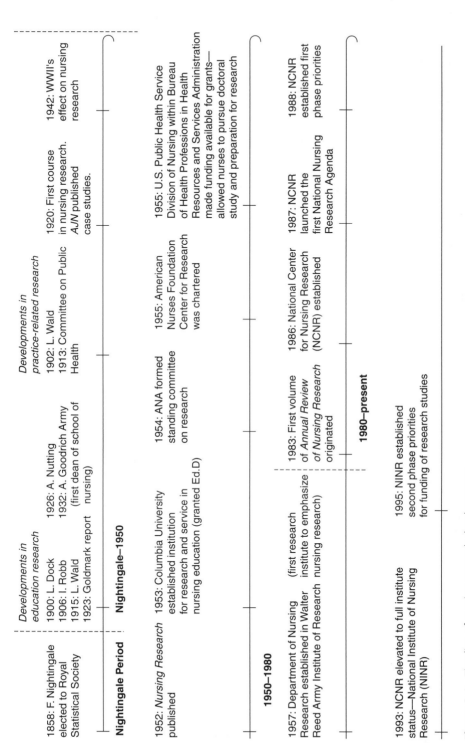

Figure 3-1. Timeline of nursing research developments.

Developments in education research

1900: L. Dock
1906: I. Robb
1915: L. Wald
1923: Goldmark report

1926: A. Nutting
1932: A. Goodrich Army
(first dean of school of nursing)

Nightingale Period

1858: F. Nightingale elected to Royal Statistical Society

Nightingale–1950

Developments in practice-related research

1902: L. Wald
1913: Committee on Public Health

1920: First course in nursing research. *AJN* published case studies.

1942: WWII's effect on nursing research

1952: *Nursing Research* published

1953: Columbia University established institution for research and service in nursing education (granted Ed.D)

1954: ANA formed standing committee on research

1955: American Nurses Foundation Center for Research was chartered

1955: U.S. Public Health Service Division of Nursing within Bureau of Health Professions in Health Resources and Services Administration made funding available for grants—allowed nurses to pursue doctoral study and preparation for research

1950–1980

1957: Department of Nursing Research established in Walter Reed Army Institute of Research

(first research institute to emphasize nursing research)

1983: First volume of *Annual Review of Nursing Research* originated

1986: National Center for Nursing Research (NCNR) established

1987: NCNR launched the first National Nursing Research Agenda

1988: NCNR established first phase priorities

1980–present

1993: NCNR elevated to full institute status—National Institute of Nursing Research (NINR)

1995: NINR established second phase priorities for funding of research studies of great value. The more tightly controlled the study, the better it is (Polit & Hungler, 1997). Typically, four types of studies are considered quantitative (Table 3-3):

1. **Descriptive studies**
2. **Correlational studies**
3. **Experimental studies**
4. Quasi-experimental studies.

Subject selection and experimental treatments are controlled to the greatest extent possible, but an overriding consideration must be the protection of human subjects. These research method terms will become clearer in the examples that follow.

A Quantitative Descriptive Study

Soon Bok Chang, a professor of nursing in Seoul, Korea, and Martha Hill, an associate professor in the Johns Hopkins School of Nursing, wished to assess HIV/AIDS-related knowledge, attitudes, and preventive behaviors among pregnant Korean women (Chang & Hill, 1996). This survey was completed as part of the process of designing patient and public education programs in Korea. Four hundred nine pregnant women at six prenatal clinics in Seoul completed self-administered questionnaires to determine how much they knew about HIV/AIDS and related risk factors.

TABLE 3-3 FOUR TYPES OF QUANTITATIVE RESEARCH STUDIES	
Type	**Description**
Descriptive	These studies describe a phenomenon or phenomena of interest to the investigator. They are usually performed in areas in which little prior information exists.
Correlational	These studies examine the relations between or among variables, using variables that can be measured and analyzed using statistics.
Experimental	These are closest to the "traditional" sciences such as chemistry, biology, and physiology. These types of studies require rigorous control of the research environment (usually in a laboratory), rigorous control over as many variables as possible in the study, and strict adherence to the research protocol from beginning to end. True experimental studies are not conducted using human subjects for ethical reasons.
Quasi-experimental ("almost experimental")	In a quasi-experimental design, full control is not possible. Quasi-experiments are research designs where the researcher initiates an experimental treatment but where some characteristic of a true experiment is lacking. Control may not be possible because of the nature of the independent variable or the nature of the available subjects. Usually what is lacking in a quasi-experimental design is the element of randomization. In other cases, the control group may be missing. However, like all experiments, quasi-experiments involve the introduction of an experimental treatment (LoBiondo-Wood G, Haber J, 1994, p. 221).

The investigators also asked the women about their attitudes about HIV/AIDS, what should be done about the problem, and what types of preventive behaviors they practiced. Chang and Hill also gathered demographic data about the survey respondents (age, marital status, education, socioeconomic status, and length of gestation).

More than 88% of the survey respondents correctly identified four of the six major risk factors for HIV infection (contaminated blood transfusions, multiple sex partners, contaminated needles, and homosexual contact). The group was moderately knowledgeable (55% answered correctly) about intravenous drug use as a risk factor. The women had less knowledge about transmission of the virus via heterosexual contact: only 28% of the respondents knew that the virus can be transmitted by heterosexual vaginal contact. This was of concern because of the high prevalence of Korean husbands who participate in extramarital sex. The lack of knowledge concerning heterosexual transmission of the virus was considered the major finding of this study.

In determining the women's attitudes, Chang and Hill asked questions that fell into two categories: risk appraisal, by assessing risk behaviors, and feelings of discrimination against people who have HIV/AIDS. In terms of preventive behaviors, half the women reported that they engaged in at least one behavior to prevent HIV/AIDS:

- ▪ Avoiding the use of intravenous drugs
- ▪ Encouraging their husbands not to have extramarital sex
- ▪ Not having extramarital sex themselves
- ▪ Making sure any needles that are used on them are sterile
- ▪ Learning more about AIDS
- ▪ Encouraging their husbands to learn more about AIDS.

In addition, 16% of the respondents indicated that they gave condoms to their husbands when the men went away from home. Chang and Hill found that higher rates of preventive behavior were reported among urban residents and among those with higher levels of education. However, they cautioned against overinterpreting this observation, because the numbers of nonurban women and higher-educated women were quite small. A common finding was that the level of measured knowledge was only weakly related to self-reported preventive behavior.

The answers to questions related to feelings of discrimination against people with HIV/AIDS revealed generally negative attitudes toward persons outside the family who had HIV/AIDS. However, many indicated they would continue to associate with, and even care for, a family member with HIV/AIDS.

Based on their research findings, Chang and Hill concluded that the most important aspect of a program of education for Korean women in HIV/AIDS prevention would be to increase the women's appraisal of risk to themselves and others.

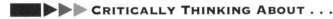 **CRITICALLY THINKING ABOUT . . .**

How could or should information from this quantitative descriptive study affect nursing practice?

A Quantitative Correlational Study

Hamner's study (1996) represents the type of research that is important to nursing science in that it tests a proposition from one of the most prominent theories put forth in nursing, Sister Callista Roy's adaptation model. Although this study was not within an NINR priority area, it was important research. In fact, more studies of this kind are needed to authenticate the utility of extant nursing theories or to provide substantive information for their update and modification.

Jenny Hamner, an associate professor at the Auburn University School of Nursing when the study was published, wanted to test a conceptual framework based on a proposition from the Roy adaptation model. For a group of 60 patients treated in a medical-surgical intensive care unit (ICU), she chose to predict the relations of five variables:

1. Severity of illness
2. Perceived control over visitation (PCV)
3. Hardiness
4. State of anxiety
5. Length of stay (LOS).

She presented four hypotheses regarding the relations among the five variables, which she based on a model elicited from part of Roy's adaptation model. The major variable of interest, to which all variables were compared in the hypotheses, was LOS in the ICU. Her four hypotheses were:

1. Severity of illness would be positively associated with LOS (the sicker one is, the longer the stay).
2. PCV would have a negative effect on LOS (the more control one has, the shorter the stay).
3. Hardiness would have a negative effect on LOS (the hardier one is, the shorter the stay).
4. Anxiety would have a positive effect (the more anxious one feels, the longer the stay).

At least 20 hours after admission to the ICU, the patient–respondents—all of whom were physiologically stable at the time of data collection—completed three surveys: a 15-item Perceived Control Over Visitation Role (an instrument devised by Hamner), Spielberger's State-Trait Anxiety Inventory (a commonly used measure of anxiety), and a Health Hardiness Scale developed by Susan Pollock. Data regarding severity of illness was obtained by using the Acute Physiologic and Chronic Health Evaluation II (APACHE II) score. LOS was obtained from patient records.

Hamner used path analysis, a correlational technique allowing the examination of several variables at once, to examine the relations among the five variables and to test the hypothesized model. Her analysis revealed that 18% of the variance in LOS could be accounted for by the combination of the other four variables. Although that is a statistically significant value, it is still a very small amount of variance. Thus, in general, the data did not provide support for the model Hamner proposed.

One might wonder why research that produced nonsignificant findings and no substantial support for the hypothesized model merits publication. Hamner argued, "Even nonsignificant results in preliminary model testing can inform others about approaches to model testing and are important to report" (Hamner, 1996, p. 219). She also described some factors that may have contributed to her nonsignificant findings. These included measurement problems with the APACHE (which in actuality is a clinical rather than a research tool) and the fact that the PCV scale was newly developed. She also acknowledged that the sample size was small, a factor that works against generating statistically significant findings in analyses such as this. Hamner concluded her report with the following comment: "As nurse researchers move forward in the testing of nursing theory, it is important to understand methodologic imperfections, especially those that are inherent in social science research" (Hamner, 1996, p. 219).

 CRITICALLY THINKING ABOUT . . .

How could or should information from this quantitative correlational study affect nursing practice?

A Quantitative Experimental Study

Gayle Page, a nurse researcher whose background includes the care of pediatric patients, based her program of basic research on her concerns that pain is not managed in children as well as it should be (Page, Ben-Eliyahu, Yirmiya, & Liebeskind, 1993). This led her to initiate her research as her dissertation work while a doctoral student at the University of California, Los Angeles.

Page and her coinvestigators noted in the introduction of the research report that painful stressors such as surgery have been shown to suppress immune function and to enhance tumor development. The purpose of the research was twofold: to study the role of immune mediation in the tumor-enhancing effects of surgery and to explore the role of postsurgical pain in surgery-induced enhancement of tumor development. To arrive at conclusions for the overall study, a separate experiment was conducted for each purpose.

The first experiment, performed to study the role of immune mediation in the tumor-enhancing effects of surgery, consisted of two studies. In the first study, 120 Fisher 344 rats (an inbred strain used for research) were assigned to three groups. One group received anesthesia and abdominal surgery; one group received anesthesia only; and one group served as controls, receiving neither surgery nor anesthesia. Five hours after surgery, all the rats were lightly anesthetized and injected with cells that caused the type of lung tumors known to be sensitive to natural killer (NK) cell activity. Twenty-one days after injection with the cells, the rats were killed using halothane gas, their lungs were removed, and the number of lung metastases was counted.

In the second study, 120 Fisher 344 rats were assigned to three groups—a surgical group, an anesthesia-only group, and an untreated control group. The surgical group was then divided into five smaller groups and injected with tumor cells at different times—24 hours before surgery and 5 hours, 24 hours, 8 days, or 21 days after surgery. The rats in the anesthesia-only group were injected with tumor cells 5 hours after surgery. The rats in this second group were killed 21 days after tumor injection and the number of lung metastases was counted.

The first study revealed that the number of surface lung metastases in animals undergoing surgery was twice that of the other two groups. In the second study, rats injected at the time intervals of 5 and 24 hours after surgery showed significantly more metastases than the rats injected with tumor cells 24 hours before, 8 days after, and 21 days after surgery, as well as the rats in the anesthesia-only group.

These findings, in combination with results from a considerable body of previous research described in the paper, led the researchers to conclude that surgery results in enhanced growth in a tumor sensitive to NK cells "and that this metastatic-enhancing effect occurs only during the time in which this tumor is known to be sensitive to NK cell control" (Page, Ben-Eliyahu, Yirmiya, & Liebeskind, 1993, p. 25). Thus, Page and her coinvestigators met the first goal of this study: further understanding of the role of immune mediation in the tumor-enhancing effects of surgery.

In the second experiment, to determine the impact of an analgesic dose of morphine on surgery-induced enhancement of tumor growth, rats were assigned to one of four treatment groups. The first group had abdominal surgery and received morphine postoperatively. The second group had surgery but received an injection of a vehicle that contained no morphine. The third group received anesthesia and morphine. The last group received anesthesia and an injection of the vehicle without the morphine. The investigators introduced varied amounts and patterns of morphine administration, both preoperatively and postoperatively. They used the same methods for injection of tumor-inducing cells and subsequent assessment of tumor metastases as in the first experiment.

The data from the second experiment showed that "surgery animals receiving morphine manifested significantly fewer metastases than did surgery animals not receiving morphine. Morphine had no effect on the anesthesia-only animals. While surgery animals were less active, ate less and were less responsive to their environment, . . . morphine treatment abolished or shortened the duration of these effects" (Page, Ben-Eliyahu, Yirmiya, & Liebeskind, 1993, p. 24). They stated that the most significant finding of the second experiment was that administration of morphine blocked surgery-induced enhancement of metastatic colonization. This indicates that the experience of postoperative pain is a critical factor in promoting metastatic spread. Their report ended, "If a similar relationship between pain and metastasis occurs in humans, then pain control must be considered a vital component of postoperative care" (Page, Ben-Eliyahu, Yirmiya, & Liebeskind, 1993, pp. 26–27).

An important component of Page's article is the amount of background detail it contained, including the literature review preceding the study, how the experiments were conducted, and how these findings compare to others in the same area of scientific inquiry. This is entirely in keeping with the scientific tradition of one study building on those that have preceded it. Those who would wish to replicate (or challenge) the findings of this study can do so by careful attention to the content of the paper. Such attention to detail may make for tedious and difficult reading, but it also makes for excellent science.

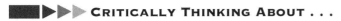 **CRITICALLY THINKING ABOUT . . .**

How could or should information from this quantitative experimental study affect nursing practice?

Research Studies Using Qualitative Methods

Researchers using **qualitative** (also referred to as naturalistic) **methods** take a different approach to research and tend to hold very different underlying assumptions than do quantitative researchers. Qualitative research is growing rapidly in popularity within the nursing research community. There are several reasons for the appeal of a qualitative approach to developing knowledge in nursing, most of which are related to the nature of nursing and those who are drawn to the practice of nursing.

- ☑ Nursing is a holistic discipline, and one feature of any of the qualitative approaches is an emphasis on the entirety of a phenomenon. The phenomenon does not have to be dissected or taken apart to be studied.
- ☑ In nursing, the emphasis is always on the client system and its values and unique perspective. In naturalistic research, subjectivity and values are considered inevitable and even desirable on the part of the researcher.
- ☑ Nursing is highly interactive. The qualitative researcher, rather than being a separated observer, is a participant with the subject in the knowledge development process.
- ☑ The researcher's view of reality is different. Rather than there being just one reality—a fundamental assumption of quantitative researchers—there are multiple realities, each of which is constructed by the individual. One person's reality is not necessarily another person's reality, but both are valid.
- ☑ Naturalistic inquiry takes place in the field, and neither the environment nor the subject of study is controlled. Compared to quantitative studies, relatively few subjects are studied, but each one is studied in great depth.

Some qualitative methods often used by nurse researchers include **ethnography**, grounded theory, ethology, and **phenomenology** (Table 3-4).

A Qualitative Ethnographic Study

Barbara Resnick, a geriatric nurse practitioner in Maryland, conducted a study to explore the factors that increase and decrease motivation in people in a geriatric rehabilitation unit (Resnick, 1996). Resnick used critical ethnography to pursue her research question and interviewed five women who were patients in a 15-bed geriatric rehabilitation unit. All the women were white; the average age was 87. These women were selected because they had been identified by the rehabilitation team as being "unmotivated." Each woman was interviewed at least three times; one woman was interviewed eight times. The repeated interviews achieved two purposes. First, they explored in depth the themes identified by patients as they progressed through the program. Second, they clarified and validated the findings gained in earlier interviews.

In addition to the interviews, Resnick observed each of the women in at least one session of physical therapy, focusing on the interaction of the staff with the patient and her willingness to participate in the program. To strengthen the credibility of the data, Resnick used the rehabilitation team as an expert panel to review her findings and to determine if those findings matched the rehabilitation team's observations. Resnick identified nine themes that recurred in the interviews, themes that either increased or decreased the women's motivation to participate in rehabilitation. Factors that improved motivation were:

- ☑ Having personal goals. These goals included getting better, getting home, and being able to walk independently.
- ☑ Use of humor by the staff. One woman said that humor helped relieve the tension involved with rehabilitation.
- ☑ Caring and kindness on the part of the rehabilitation staff. This showed the women that the staff really cared about them; the women, in turn, were willing to participate in rehabilitation to pay the staff back.
- ☑ Believing in the competence of the staff and in the rehabilitation process. This included positive prior rehabilitation and believing that rehabilitation would help them.

TABLE 3-4	FOUR TYPES OF QUALITATIVE RESEARCH STUDIES

Type	Description
Ethnography	This type of study has its academic roots in anthropology; its focus is culture, with the goal of developing a holistic view of a culture, thereby gaining insights into the behaviors and motivations of members of that culture.
Grounded theory	This theory was developed in the 1960s by Barney Glaser and Anselm Strauss, two sociologists at the University of Chicago. The foci of grounded theory are social processes and social structures. The purpose is to generate broad explanations of phenomena that are grounded in reality. When using grounded theory, one does not start with a highly focused research question; rather, the question emerges as the data are collected. According to Polit and Hungler, "the majority of qualitative nursing studies that identify a research tradition claim grounded theory as the tradition to which they are linked" (1997, p. 205).
Ethology	The roots of ethology are in psychology; its focus is behavior observed over time in a natural, unmanipulated context. It is sometimes called the biology of human behavior, and it "attempts to identify principles that explain the interdependence of humans and their environmental contexts" (Polit & Hungler, 1997, p. 201).
Phenomenology	This type of qualitative study is the most distant from the "hard" quantitative science and does not have its roots in a science at all—its roots are in philosophy. The focus of phenomenologic study is people's lived experience. Phenomenologists believe that essential truths about reality are grounded in those experiences, and their goal is to describe that experience as fully as possible. In-depth conversations are the common sources of data in phenomenologic inquiry; both investigator and informant are seen as full coparticipants. Often, more than one interview is needed.

◘ Getting encouragement from the staff and family.
◘ Basic personality. Some of the women said they had always worked hard and did whatever they had to do to keep going. Therefore, their approach to rehabilitation would be no different.
◘ "Power-with" relationships between the staff and patients. This involves the development of individual capabilities through the interactions and influence of other persons. Power-with interactions were described as occurring "when the staff listened to what the patients said, and understood them" (Resnick, 1996, p. 43).

Factors that decreased the women's motivation were:

◘ Domination (and the patients' response to domination). This will be discussed in detail below.
◘ Belief that rehabilitation was unnecessary.

The major theme that emerged in the interviews with the women was domination in rehabilitation. To be dominated is to be ruled or controlled by a superior power. Resnick determined that the women experienced domination in five general ways:

1. Domination by physical force. They were physically weak and slow and the staff members were able to push and pull them around.
2. Domination by their own bodies. Pain interfered with what they wanted to do, or they simply became too tired.
3. Domination by brainwashing—seemingly endless lectures about what they should or should not do.
4. Domination by the rules and regulations—having to sit up longer than they wanted, or having to go to the dining room even though it was an upsetting experience.
5. Domination by family. Their loved ones did not understand what it was like to be in rehabilitation, but continued to tell them what to do, and they felt pressure to comply.

Several women described hopelessness, valuelessness, and voicelessness in response to domination. Some adjusted to the rules and regulations of the program to fit in or to avoid being disliked. Some resisted the domination by refusing to cooperate. Domination is a "power-over" relationship; although it may produce compliance, it is not a motivating factor. Patients may comply while they are in the rehabilitation setting, but when they go home they will have little or no motivation to perform the activities necessary to continue their improvement or prevent further decline.

Resnick concluded by describing how she used these findings in discussions with the rehabilitation team in an effort to improve the rehabilitation environment by reinforcing the positive motivating behaviors and diminishing the experiences of domination by developing more "power-with" relationships for their patients.

 CRITICALLY THINKING ABOUT . . .

How could or should information from this qualitative ethnographic study affect nursing practice?

A Qualitative Phenomenologic Study

Eileen Jones Porter was a doctorally prepared nurse on the faculty at the College of Nursing, University of Wisconsin–Oshkosh, when she wrote this research paper (Porter, 1995). Her clinical area of interest was the care and well-being of older adults; her specific interest had to do with how older adults maintain independence, a condition highly prized by most older adults. To assess the functioning of older adults, researchers, clinicians, and those who determine eligibility for services commonly use tools measuring activities of daily living (ADLs). Porter felt that the ADL research tradition might not be the best methodologic choice and might not work in the best interest of older adults who are assessed using only an ADL-measuring tool. Porter believed that the focus of ADL research tradition has been on the independent performance of standardized tests and was, therefore, much too limited. Accordingly, she applied the techniques of phenomenology to conduct a study that would provide an alternative approach to assess the functioning of older adults.

Porter set about studying older persons' experiences in the realm of personal independence. Bahr (1986) identified the primary goal of older adults as attaining or maintaining functional independence. Therefore, Porter initiated her study by asking two older widows if anything was more important to them than maintaining independence. Both of the women said that being able to continue to live alone in their own home was more important than being independent. Based on this finding, Porter shifted her focus somewhat, to older widows' experience of living alone at home.

Porter interviewed seven widows who lived in a community of 50,000. There were four criteria for selection into the study:

1. The woman had been a widow for at least 1 year.
2. The woman lived alone in her own home.
3. The woman had at least one child.
4. The woman had not moved to a different community after her husband's death.

All the study participants were white and ranged in age from 75 to 83 years old. Each woman had one or more children living within 30 miles. Two women seemed to be financially comfortable, three were of moderate means, and two appeared to have limited incomes. One woman had a housekeeper provided by a government program; none received any help with personal care.

Porter based the interviews on an open-ended question: "As a person who lives alone, please describe how you do this." She also used probes throughout the interview, such as, "Explain how you decide when you need help with a task" and "Tell me about a situation when you felt successful living at home alone." The interviews were held in the women's homes; this allowed them to demonstrate activities and point out objects that were pertinent to their experience. Interviews were tape-recorded, and the tapes were transcribed; this copy served as the data to which phenomenologic analysis techniques were applied. Porter developed four phenomena that were general structures of the older widows' experiences of living at home alone:

1. Making aloneness acceptable
2. Going my own way
3. Reducing my risks
4. Sustaining myself.

Porter considered the last three as products of a phenomenologic alternative to the ADL research tradition.

GOING MY OWN WAY

Porter described this phenomenon as the ability of the women to fulfill the responsibilities required to live alone: attending to business matters, taking care of one's property, and taking care of oneself. Within each of these general activity areas were subareas of activity; those of particular relevance were "monitoring my performance," "doing what has to be done," and "proving that I am still capable." The women were aware that they experienced deterioration in terms of strength, stamina, balance, and memory. However, by continuously monitoring their own performance, they could assess any deterioration of the tasks they knew they needed to perform to continue to live alone. They used various strategies to maintain their property and themselves. Sometimes they performed the tasks themselves; sometimes they obtained assistance from others, particularly tasks related to property maintenance.

REDUCING MY RISKS

The women monitored their performance and realized that although they were capable of doing a certain task themselves, it might not be safe, smart, or necessary to do so. Porter explained: "the risks involved [in the tasks] were paramount, and the women were trying to reduce these risks" (p. 36). The women reduced their risks by exercising caution, accepting reliance, and bringing their world closer to home. The women knew they had more difficulty in controlling their movements and maintaining their balance than when they were younger, and continually were aware of the need to exercise caution, particularly when they were not at home. They took their time performing tasks and stayed aware of their surroundings as they walked. They also reduced their risk by relying on assistive devices (eg, canes, handrails) as well as modest assistance from other people (eg, holding a daughter's arm when walking to help maintain balance). By spending more time in their own homes (bringing their world closer to home), the women could better reduce risks; they also tried to ensure that someone would come when they needed help.

SUSTAINING MYSELF

Porter stated: "*Sustaining myself* was considered the most fundamental phenomenon of the lived experience. As the women sustained themselves, they acted intentionally in ways that related to the other phenomena such as *reducing my risks* or *going my own way*" (Porter, 1965, p. 37). By sustaining themselves, they kept themselves going so they could continue to live at home alone. They could do this by taking it easy, keeping active but intentionally avoiding excess activity, and using a cane.

Porter noted that some of the women she interviewed would not, by the standards of ADL tools, have been classified as independent. But for these women, independence did not mean performing specific physical tasks; rather, independence meant creating their own schedules, deciding how tasks would be done (even if someone else did it), and getting out into the community. Porter concluded that practitioners working with older adults could do better than simply assessing performance of activities on a five-point scale. She believed it would be more useful to determine how an older adult evaluates the risks of various activities, how that person chooses to minimize those risks, and whether the person's environment provides the opportunity to reduce risks. She went on to suggest that a more individualized assessment method should be adopted that "focuses more on an older person's unique circumstances and less on ADL" (Porter, 1965, p. 41).

◤▶▶▶ CRITICALLY THINKING ABOUT . . .

How could or should information from this qualitative phenomenologic study affect nursing practice?

It is easy to observe from the sampling of quantitative and qualitative method research studies that quantitative and qualitative researchers differ considerably in the questions they ask, the strategies they use to gather and analyze data, and even in the kinds of findings they generate. Some nurse researchers are committed to a quantitative approach to knowledge development; others are equally committed to qualitative approaches. Doctoral programs in nursing routinely include in-depth instruction in both quantitative and qualitative methods, and nursing faculties usually represent a mix of quantitative and qualitative researchers. Increasing numbers of investigators are beginning to incorporate both quantitative and qualitative strategies in their work to explicate and understand the phenomenon of interest more fully.

▶ CHAPTER SUMMARY

As we have seen, the development of nursing research has spanned many years and many important milestones, stretching from the work of Florence Nightingale to the activities of the National Institute of Nursing Research. Indeed, it could be said that nursing research is a growth industry, with an army of bright, dedicated scholars pursuing important research agendas that seem to have unlimited potentials as they stretch into the 21st century. Continued growth in both the quantity and sophistication of nursing research using the broad spectrum of available methods is imperative. It would be counterproductive to limit ourselves to one approach for the sake of uniformity. The richness of nursing lies partly in its commitment to and respect for diversity. The nursing research enterprise deserves the same commitment to maximize the development of a broad scholarly knowledge base for the discipline.

KEY POINTS

▶ 1 Florence Nightingale made many important contributions to nursing practice and research. Her work in military hospitals during the Crimean War helped decrease the mortality rate from 60% to 2%. Her work in England focused on reform of army sanitation practices and establishment of a school for nursing. Using statistics, she persuaded key politicians and decision makers in England to initiate needed health reforms in military and civilian hospitals. Nightingale's work helped improve the health care of her time and helped establish the traditions of nursing research and health care statistics.

▶ 2 Two reasons for the lack of development of nursing research from Nightingale's time until the 1950s were the social norms of the period and the educational preparation of nurses. The view of women during this period was that they were weak, dependent creatures with no aptitude for science and no need to study. Therefore, because only women became nurses, they were not expected, or educated, to perform research. In addition, the educational preparation of nurses occurred, for the most part, in hospital schools, which were controlled by physicians.

▶ 3 Between 1950 and 1980, nursing research developed rapidly as baccalaureate nursing education became a regular part of colleges and universities. In addition, universities established doctoral programs for nurses. This enabled nurses to have the appropriate level of education to function as educators in university settings across the United States. The ANA supported nursing research by forming the Standing Committee on Research and the ANF, which distributed funds to support beginning nurse scientists. Finally, since the first publication of *Nursing Research* in 1952, there has been steady growth in the number of high-quality journals dedicated to research in nursing.

▶ 4 Since the 1980s, the NINR, under the umbrella of the National Institutes of Health, has provided direction and support for the development of clinical nursing research. The amount of clinical nursing research has increased dramatically and has become increasingly focused on significant problems in nursing. The NINR developed first-phase (1987) and second-phase (1995) priorities for nursing research funding to provide a structure within which investigators can develop their programs of research to receive NINR funding.

▶ 5 The two methods of nursing research are quantitative and qualitative. Quantitative studies rely on variables that can be counted, measured, and subjected to rigorous statistical analysis. Four types of quantitative studies are descriptive, correlational, experimental, and quasi-experimental. Qualitative studies are characterized by the entirety of a phenomenon, subjectivity and values, interaction with the subject being studied, multiple realities, and the lack of a controlled environment or subject. Four common types of qualitative studies are ethnography, grounded theory, ethology, and phenomenology.

REFERENCES

American Nurses Association (1981). *Guidelines for the Investigative Function of Nurses.* Kansas City, MO: Author.

American Nurses Association (1985). *Code for Nurses With Interpretive Statements.* St. Louis: Author.

American Nurses Association (1989). *Commission on Nursing Research: Education for Preparation in Nursing Research.* Kansas City, MO: Author.

American Nurses Association (1993). *Position Paper: Education for Participation in Nursing Research.* Washington DC: Author.

Bahr RT, Sr. (1986). Professional and public education initiatives addressing health and related needs of elderly persons. *Community-based initiatives in long-term care* (pp. 63–78). New York: National League for Nursing.

Chang SB, Hill MN (1996). HIV/AIDS and pregnant Korean women. *Image: J Nursing Scholarship, 28,* 321–324.

Cohen IB (1984). Florence Nightingale. *Scientific American, 250*(3), 128–137.

Curry T, Jiobu R, Schwirian K (1997). *Sociology for the 21st Century.* Upper Saddle River, NJ: Prentice-Hall.

Hamner JB (1996). Preliminary testing of a proposition from Roy's model. *Image: J Nursing Scholarship, 28,* 215–220.

Hogstel MO, Sayner NC (1986). *Nursing Research: An Introduction.* New York: McGraw-Hill.

Kalisch PA, Kalisch BJ (1995). *The Advance of American Nursing.* Philadelphia: JB Lippincott.

LoBiondo-Wood G, Haber J (1994). *Nursing research: Methods, critical appraisal, and utilization.* (3rd ed.). St. Louis: Mosby.

Moses EB (1992). *The registered nurse population: Findings from the National Sample Survey of Registered Nurses, March, 1992.* Washington, DC: U.S. Department of Health & Human Services, Public Health Service, Health Resources and Services Administration.

Page GG, Ben-Eliyahu S, Yirmiya R, Liebeskind JC (1993). Morphine attenuates surgery-induced enhancement of metastatic colonization in rats. *Pain, 54,* 21–28.

Polit DF, Hungler BP (1997). *Essentials of Nursing Research: Methods, Appraisal and Utilization* (4th ed.). Philadelphia: Lippincott-Raven.

Porter EJ (1995). A phenomenological alternative to the ADL research tradition. *J Aging and Health, 7,* 24–45.

Resnick B (1996). Motivation in geriatric rehabilitation. *Image: J Nursing Scholarship, 28,* 41–45.

Rockett IRH (1994). Population and health: An introduction to epidemiology. *Population Bulletin, 49,* 1–47.

Schwirian PM, Eesley T, Cuellar L (1986). Use of water pillows in reducing head shape distortion in preterm infants. *Research in Nursing and Health, 9,* 203–207.

Shea FP (1997). Nursing research and its relationship to practice. In Oermann M (Ed.), *Professional Nursing Practice.* Stamford, CT: Appleton-Lange.

Stevenson JS (1986). Forging a research discipline. *Nursing Research, 36,* 60–64.

Werley HH, Fitzpatrick JJ (1983). *Ann Rev Nursing Research, 1.* New York: Springer.

Classic References

Carnegie E (1976). *Historical Perspectives of Nursing Research.* Boston: Boston University Nursing Archives Special Collections.

Cook E (1913). *The Life of Florence Nightingale.* London: McMillan.

Dock LL (1900). What we may expect from the law. *AJN, 1,* 8–12.

Dolan JA (1973). *Nursing in Society.* Philadelphia: WB Saunders.

Dumas RG, Leonard RC (1963). The effect of nursing on the incidence of postoperative vomiting. *Nursing Research, 12,* 12–15.

Goldmark J (1923). *Nursing and Nursing Education in the United States.* New York: Macmillan.

Goodrich A (1932). *The Social and Ethical Significance of Nursing: A Series of Addresses.* New York: Macmillan.

Eyler JM (1979). *Victorian Social Medicine: The Ideas and Methods of William Farr.* Baltimore: The Johns Hopkins Press.

Gortner SR, Nahm H (1977). An overview of nursing research in the United States. *Nursing Research, 26,* 10–33.

Hall LE (1963). A center for nursing. *Nursing Outlook, 11,* 805–806.

Henderson V (1956). Research in nursing practice—when? [editorial] *Nursing Research, 4,* 99.

Hughes E, Hughes H, Deutscher D (1958). *Twenty Thousand Nurses Tell Their Story.* Philadelphia: JB Lippincott.

Knopf EW (1916). Nightingale as statistician. Journal of American Statistical Association, 15, 388–404.

Nightingale F (1858). *Notes on Matters Affecting the Health Efficiency and Hospital Administration of the British Army Founded Chiefly on the Experience of the Late War.* London: Harrison.

Nightingale F (1859). *Notes on Nursing: What It Is and What It Is Not.* London: Harrison.

Nutting MA (1912). *Educational Status of Nursing* (Bulletin No. 7). Washington DC: U.S Bureau of Education.

Nutting MA (1926). *A Second Economic Base for Schools of Nursing and Other Addresses.* New York: Putnam's Sons.

Robb IH (1906). *Nursing: Its Principles and Practices for Hospitals and Private Use* (3rd ed.). Cleveland: E.C Koeckert.

Roberts MM (1954). *American Nursing: History and Interpretation.* New York: Macmillan.

See EM (1977). The ANA and research in nursing. *Nursing Research, 26,* 165–176.

Simmons LW, Henderson V (1964). *Nursing Research: A Survey and Assessment.* New York: Appleton-Century-Crofts.

The first American Nurses Association nursing research conference [editorial] (1965). *Nursing Research, 14,* 99.

Thomlinson R (1965). *Population Dynamics: Causes and Consequences of World Demographic Change.* New York: Random House.

Wald LD (1915). *House on Henry Street.* New York: Henry Holt & Co.

RECOMMENDED READINGS

Abrams KR, Scragg AM (1996). Quantitative methods in nursing research. *J Advanced Nursing, 23,* 1008–1013.

Brandiet LM (1994). Gerontological nursing: Application of ethnography and grounded theory. *J Gerontological Nursing, July,* pp. 33–40.

Bunkers SS, Petardi LA, Pilkington FB, Walls PA (1996). Challenging myths surrounding qualitative research in nursing. *Nursing Science Quarterly, 9,* 33–37.

Freshwater D (1996). Complementary therapies and research in nursing practice. *Nursing Standard, 12*(38), 43–45.

Madjar I, Higgins I (1996). Of ethics committees protocols and behaving ethically in the field: A case study of research with elderly residents in a nursing home. *Nursing Inquiry: J Nursing Scholarship, 3,* 130–137.

Meerabeau L (1996). Managing policy research in nursing. *J Advanced Nursing, 24,* 633–639.

Michel Y, Sneed NV (1995). Dissemination and use of research findings in nursing practice. *J Professional Nursing, 11,* 306–311.

Nolan M, Behi R (1995). Measurement in research. *Br J Nursing, 4,* 402–405.

4

Current Issues in the Evolution of the Knowledge Base for Nursing

CHAPTER OUTLINE

Development and Use of Nursing
   Knowledge
Fostering the Development of
   Nursing Knowledge: Nursing
   Information Classification
   Systems

Chapter Summary
Key Points
References
Classic References
Recommended Readings

LEARNING OBJECTIVES

▶ **1** Understand what is meant by the trifurcation of nursing knowledge and how it affects the development and use of nursing knowledge.

▶ **2** Discuss three barriers to the unification of nursing knowledge.

▶ **3** Describe three strategies for the unification of nursing knowledge.

▶ **4** Discuss the development of nursing information classification systems.

▶ **5** List four common nursing taxonomies.

KEY TERMS

boundary-spanning roles

collaborative research

home health care
   classification (HHCC)
   taxonomy

middle-range theory

North American
   Nursing Diagnosis
   Association
   (NANDA) taxonomy

nursing
   interventions
   classification
   (NIC) taxonomy

(continued)

KEY TERMS (CONTINUED)

nursing information
   classification systems
Nursing Minimum Data
   Set (NMDS)

nursing taxonomies
Omaha problem
   classification
   system (OCS)

research utilization
   (RU) program

In a fully developed profession, practice is based on a knowledge base that is comprehensive, rigorously developed, scientifically sound, and unique to the discipline. Chapter 2 described the important efforts of nursing scholars in the last half of the 20th century to move nursing knowledge to a significantly higher level through the development and promulgation of nursing theories. Chapter 3 discussed the promotion and participation among nursing scientists in the expanding, evolving nursing research enterprise. This chapter will address two salient questions that have arisen from the material in the previous two chapters:

1. What is the current state of the knowledge base for nursing?
2. What should nurses and other players in the health care scene be doing to facilitate further development?

To answer these questions, we will examine one primary issue and two promising trends in the evolution of the knowledge base most appropriate for nursing. The primary issue is that the development of a knowledge base has been hindered by the trifurcation of nursing into theory, research, and practice. This trifurcation will be discussed in depth, and its causes will be explored. Although this issue is still a problem, there are promising trends in the development of nursing's knowledge base. Significant strategies for overcoming this trifurcation have been developed over the past several years that serve as bridges between the three nursing camps. These bridges include research utilization (RU), collaborative research, and the possible utility of using three different approaches to theory incorporation, development, and testing. The second promising trend is the use of computer-based **nursing information classification systems (NICS)**. Use of NICS has significantly moved nursing along in its knowledge base development. The nature and utility of NICS, the criteria for using NICS, and the development of NICS will be discussed in detail.

Development and Use of Nursing Knowledge

The very essence of nursing is practice, the delivery of nursing care, and nursing theory and nursing research exist to serve and improve that practice. The purpose of nursing theory is to provide a logical, holistic conceptual framework for nursing knowledge that guides the practice of nursing. The purpose of nursing research is to provide a sound, dependable, scientific knowledge base that, when embedded within the framework of a nursing theory, is the foundation for consistently effective delivery of nursing care. Nursing theory should shape nursing practice, and the knowledge base from nursing research should inform nursing practice.

There have been significant advances in both nursing theory development and the conduct of nursing research. The delivery of nursing care has improved greatly, largely due to significant technological advances. However, for the most part, nursing practice is still not informed by nursing research, nor is it usually structured by nursing theory. More than 30 years ago, Martha Rogers wrote that nursing is a learned profession and that there is an organized body of knowledge that comprises nursing. She emphasized that the person is at the center of nursing and that nursing science is concerned with understanding the human life process:

> The uniqueness of nursing science lies in the unification of knowledge that constitutes the theoretical basis of nursing practice. The nature of the knowledge determines the scope and limitations of nursing practice. The vision and creativity, the energy and imagination, that are invested in its ongoing elaboration further define the expansion and clarification of nursing's substantive base. (Rogers, 1964, p. 39)

This positive, elegant assertion regarding the state of nursing knowledge has a great deal of appeal to those of us who want to believe the best about nurses and nursing. However, not all nursing scholars or scientists agree that an adequate theory-driven knowledge base exists that will finally propel nursing toward full professional stature. One reason for this is the lack of cooperation and communication between nurses in theory, research, and practice. This trifurcation of nurses (and thus nursing knowledge), the barriers that exist to the functional melding of nursing theory, research, and practice, and strategies for linking these three groups to achieve full professionalization of nursing will be discussed below.

"Trifurcation" of Nursing Theory, Research, and Practice

In the nursing literature, as well as in programs of nursing education, it is common to refer to nursing theory, nursing research, and nursing practice as three distinct and separate entities that are often unrelated and often noncommunicating. A glance at the curricula of most baccalaureate nursing programs would validate the existence of this separation. Nursing research commonly is offered as a separate course in undergraduate nursing programs. Courses relating to practice often are separated into two portions, one dealing with the didactic theory or content and the other dedicated to learning the practice of nursing in clinical settings. This sends a message to students that theory, research, and practice are separate enterprises. Most nursing faculty probably do not intend to convey this message, but unfortunately this is all too often the case.

For at least 30 years, nursing scholars have recognized this mixed message and have repeatedly pointed out that the situation is dysfunctional and will not promote the professionalization of nursing and further the development of comprehensive, functional nursing knowledge (Benoliel, 1977; Fawcett, 1978; Fawcett & Downs, 1992; Henry & Constantino, 1997; Jacobs & Huether, 1978; Levine, 1995; Walker, 1973).

 CRITICALLY THINKING ABOUT . . .

In your clinical courses, was the knowledge you gained based on nursing theory?

Barriers to Unification

Although nursing scholars have consistently called for the narrowing of the gap between practicing nurses and nurse researchers and theorists, nurses in practice are all too often distant from both theory and research. Once they complete their schooling, they do not maintain contact with their nursing scholar teachers. In addition, they typically do not read the journals that contain up-to-date developments in theory and research. Significant barriers persist that keep nursing theory, nursing research, and nursing practice apart and opposed to each other. These barriers include perceived obscurity and irrelevance, isolation of practice from academia, and a theory–research split.

Perception of Obscurity and Irrelevance

Practicing nurses claim that the grand theories of nursing are, for the most part, obscure. As a result of this obscurity, nurses have difficulty incorporating theory into their day-to-day practice. Obviously, theories that are perceived as such will have minimal effect on both the student preparing for practice and the practicing nurse caring for patients. Although many scholars decry the lack of connection between theory and practice, they also recognize why the problem persists. Myra Levine, a noted nursing theorist, is a champion of the necessity for a functional bond between nursing practice and nursing theory but recognizes the mismatch that exists:

> The traditions of nursing leave us poorly prepared to deal with the verbal demands of theory building. Nurses have spoken with their hands, their skills, their ability to observe and respond with appropriate action. . . . The inherent difficulties of communication that characterize nursing practice compromise introducing theory into practice and education because too often the language of theory introduces another set of terms that have little relevance in the workplace. . . . Theoretical language cannot be simply superimposed on the clinical environment. (Levine, 1995, p 12)

The same kind of perceptions of separateness and irrelevance in reference to nursing research exist in the practice community. Formally written nursing research reports often seem as obscure to practicing nurses as do nursing theories.

Isolation of Practice from Academia

In addition to the perception that theory and research are obscure and far removed from practice is the actual physical separation of nurses who do the work of theory and research and nurses who do the work of practice. The world of the theorist or researcher is very different from the world of the practicing nurse. Theorists and researchers typically do their work in university settings; practicing nurses provide services in hospital or community settings. In addition, different standards and norms apply to each group of nurses. The practicing nurse must perform patient-focused activities in the most efficient manner possible; the nurse in academia must focus on teaching and scholarly productivity, which may or may not be delivered efficiently. Accordingly, different types of activities gain rewards in the two settings. To maintain a position or to obtain promotion and salary rewards, the nurse in academia must teach using state-of-the-art knowledge, conduct research, and produce scholarly publications on a regular basis. Hospitals and other health care institutions rarely incorporate such expectations in the reward structure for practicing nurses (Funk, Champagne, Wiese, & Tornquist, 1991).

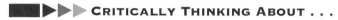 **CRITICALLY THINKING ABOUT . . .**

In your nursing education, have you felt that the world of practice and the work of academic nursing are greatly separated? Explain.

Marian Pettingill, Dee An Gillies, and Carolyn Clark (1994) sent questionnaires regarding factors that encouraged and discouraged research to 404 nurses in the Midwest. Of the respondents, 182 were educators and 222 worked in service settings. The most discouraging factor cited by both academicians and practitioners was the lack of time to devote to research. Half the educators and just over half the practicing nurses expressed this opinion. The second strongest discouraging factor cited by educators was lack of support from nursing administration; practicing nurses cited the lack of nursing staff support. However, these respondents may not represent nurses in general due to the selection process the investigators used. The respondents were selected from membership lists of the Midwest Alliance in Nursing and the Midwest Nursing Research Society. The fact that the nurses were members of these types of organizations demonstrates that they already had an interest in and commitment to nursing research. Thus, the sample of nurses may not be very representative of the two groups in general, particularly of nurses in clinical practice.

Practitioners and scholars also may be isolated from each other because they perceive themselves as being different types of people, they do not expect to share the same perspectives, and they do not care about the same things. Carolyn Hicks, an English psychologist, conducted a study to determine whether nurses would perceive a nurse described as a "good clinician" differently from a nurse described as a "good researcher" (1996). Two groups of practicing nurses were given questionnaires that contained a description of a theoretical job candidate and 15 pairs of bipolar adjectives the respondents could use to describe the applicant. The descriptions of the hypothetical applicants were identical except that one was described as a "good clinician," the other as a "good researcher." The practicing nurses' evaluations of the two hypothetical nurses differed significantly. The "good researcher" was evaluated as being more ambitious, a poorer communicator, less kind, stronger, more logical, more controlled, more confident, less popular, more ruthless, and more rational and analytical compared to the "good clinician." These findings supported Hicks' hypothesis that practicing nurses stay

> shy of research because their constructs of themselves as nurses are incompatible with the prerequisite characteristics of a good researcher. In the simplest terms, they may not conduct research because of assumptions of role inappropriateness, between the nurse as carer and the nurse as researcher. (Hicks, 1996, p. 358)

 CRITICALLY THINKING ABOUT . . .

Have you sensed that nursing clinicians and nursing scholars perceive themselves as being different kinds of people? Explain.

Theory–Research Split

The gulf between nursing practice and nursing theory and research is the most obvious and may be the most problematic in blocking further professionalization of nursing. However, there also is a gulf between nursing theory and nursing research because most of the early nursing theory simply cannot be used in a research framework. As noted in Chapter 2, it is becoming more common to refer to the grand theories developed in the 1960s and 1970s as conceptual frameworks because they do not possess qualities inherent to a theory. In other words, they cannot be logically broken down into propositions, hypotheses, or operational definitions, all the tools required to test the validity of a true theory. Researchers need testable theories to work with, not conceptual frameworks.

Theorizing and researching traditionally have been carried out in universities, and scholars commonly communicate through publications in scholarly journals. Thus, it may be puzzling that such a gulf exists between nursing theories and research. Mary Blegen and Toni Tripp-Reimer (1994, 1997) believe that this gulf exists because of how the early nursing theorists went about their work and the nature of the "theories" they developed. They contend that the conceptual models that emerged in the 1960s and 1970s and into the 1980s were important to nursing because they helped define the discipline of nursing and fostered reform in nursing curricula. Until that time, nursing curricula were largely based on the medical model inherited from the hospital training school tradition. Thus, the development of conceptual models was essential in articulating nursing's own curriculum and identity.

However, the problem with the models was that they developed parallel to, rather than integral to, research efforts. These conceptual models were statements of nursing philosophy and ideology and were eagerly seized on by educators as frameworks to guide curriculum development. However, the models did not present knowledge that could be applied directly in practice, nor could the models be tested through research. Therefore, the nursing theory developed as a type of knowledge during these years has come to be considered by both practitioners and researchers to be too abstract to be useful (Blegen & Tripp-Reimer, 1994, 1997).

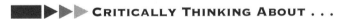 Critically Thinking About . . .

Can nursing curricula ever be independent of the medical model? Why or why not?

Strategies for Unification: Linking Nursing Scholarship to Nursing Practice

Although trifurcation of nursing knowledge is still a significant problem and there are several barriers present that work against unification, significant strategies have been developed to overcome these barriers and unite all three aspects of nursing knowledge. RU and collaborative research have been suggested as bridges to join nursing scholarship and nursing practice. Blegen and Tripp-Reimer (1994, 1997) posited three alternative methods of how theory could be incorporated more fully into nursing research and practice.

Research Utilization

The findings of nursing research are not making their way into nursing practice at an acceptable rate. Marita Titler (1997) noted that the use of research findings in nursing practice originated with Florence Nightingale, but research and practice became separated when the preparation of nurses in hospital training schools did not produce practitioners with sufficient qualifications to conduct research. However, the educational qualification of nurses has increased. In addition, the scientific body of nursing knowledge has increased, and this knowledge must be translated into improved practice.

Establishing RU programs is one strategy for achieving this goal. A **research utilization program** means that there is a specific plan and mechanism for finding, assessing, evaluating, and possibly implementing up-to-date research findings into clinical practice. Although RU is a topic of great interest and holds much promise, it is still not the norm in most nursing care environments. Incorporating RU as a regular facet of nursing care should be a goal for all nurses who wish to engage in the highest quality of practice. Polit and Hungler (1997) have provided general guidelines regarding the scope of responsibility for facilitating RU and have outlined general strategies for researchers, clinicians, and administrators. They believe that much of the responsibility for facilitating RU lies with researchers and call on researchers to focus on six activities:

1. Perform high-quality research.
2. Replicate research and publish the results.
3. Collaborate with practitioners.
4. Disseminate findings aggressively and far beyond the traditional scientific journals that practicing nurses rarely read.
5. Communicate clearly, leaving the jargon of research behind when communicating with clinicians and administrators.
6. Suggest clinical implications of findings clearly and succinctly.

Polit and Hungler also suggest several activities from which practicing nurses could benefit and that could further RU in their practice settings:

1. Read widely and critically.
2. Attend professional conferences.
3. Learn to expect evidence that a procedure is effective; accepting on the basis of simple tradition simply will not do.
4. Seek work environments that are supportive of RU in terms of policies, practices, and rewards.
5. Join or establish a journal club.
6. Collaborate with nurse researchers whenever the opportunity arises.
7. Pursue and participate in any institutional RU projects, as well as appropriate RU projects on a personal or unit level (Polit & Hungler, 1997, pp. 437–438).

Polit and Hungler also acknowledge that there must be institutional support if RU is to become a regular part of nursing practice and patient care. They encourage administrators to:

◪ Foster a climate of intellectual curiosity among nurses rather than unquestioning compliance.
◪ Offer emotional and moral support for nurses who initiate or participate in RU efforts.
◪ Offer financial or resource support for proposed projects.
◪ Reward nurses' efforts in RU activities (Polit & Hungler, 1997, p. 439).

Although these suggestions for administrators seem to be addressed primarily to the administrators in practice settings, they also should be considerations for administrators in the academic units where nursing scholars work. When nurse scholars use their research skills to foster RU in clinical settings, they face challenges that do not exist within the more protected walls of academia. Moreover, when a nursing scholar assists practicing nurses in RU, the outcome may not be the typical product of scholarly research (eg, publication in a respected research journal). Administrators in nursing education should take these factors into consideration when they evaluate the scholarly output of nursing faculty.

Research Utilization in Action

One institution where RU has been put to use and has been effective in improving the quality of nursing care is the University of Iowa Hospitals and Clinics (UIHC). The Iowa model for RU, "Research-Based Practice to Promote Quality Care," is presented in Figure 4-1. This elegant, ambitious model could exist and thrive only in an environment where there is strong support from nursing executives and other leaders in the hospital organization. In an article describing the Iowa model, Marita Titler and colleagues (1994) describe the administrative environment at UIHC as very supportive. The value of research is communicated in many ways:

- ▶ Through staff orientation and leadership programs devoted to nursing research
- ▶ By providing clinical release time for doing research
- ▶ By providing recognition for participating in research and tuition reimbursement for completing research courses
- ▶ By funding nurses for attendance or presentation at local, regional, and national meetings.

■■■ ▶▶▶ CRITICALLY THINKING ABOUT . . .

If you worked at a hospital that had an RU program in place, how would that affect your job and your practice?

Titler explained that there is an established organizational structure at UIHC that facilitates the conduct and use of research. First, there is a department of nursing research headed by a PhD-prepared nurse. There also is broad participation by clinical nurse specialists and staff nurses on committees that support, plan, implement, and evaluate nursing research. These include the department of nursing research committee and seven divisional nursing research committees, one in each of the clinical nursing divisions. Divisional research projects are shared at meetings of the professional nursing council. This provides a forum for discussing the applicability of the project to other departments.

Despite the structural support and administrative amenities, Titler and colleagues still give much of the credit for the success of the UIHC program (in infusing research into practice) to the staff nurses for two reasons. First, the staff nurses are the ones who identify relevant clinical issues that start the process described in the model. Also, any research-based changes are made by staff nurses at the bedside with the support of administrators, rather than being initiated by top-level administrators.

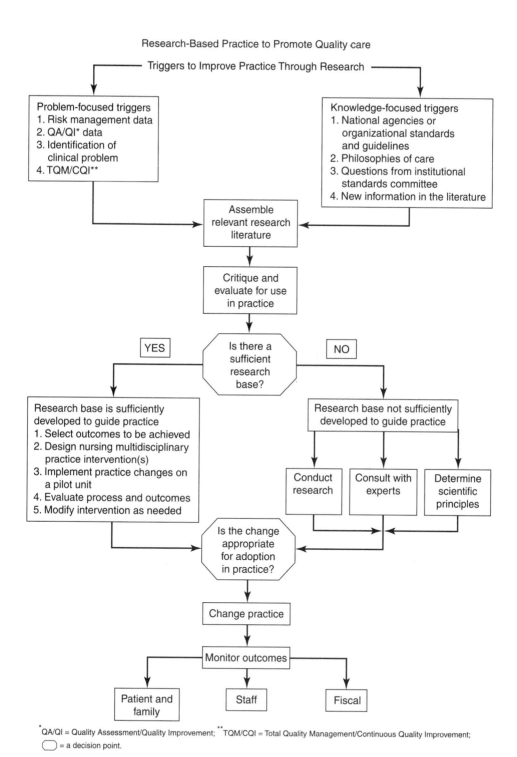

Research-Based Practice to Promote Quality care

Triggers to Improve Practice Through Research

Problem-focused triggers
1. Risk management data
2. QA/QI* data
3. Identification of clinical problem
4. TQM/CQI**

Knowledge-focused triggers
1. National agencies or organizational standards and guidelines
2. Philosophies of care
3. Questions from institutional standards committee
4. New information in the literature

Assemble relevant research literature

Critique and evaluate for use in practice

Is there a sufficient research base?

YES

NO

Research base is sufficiently developed to guide practice
1. Select outcomes to be achieved
2. Design nursing multidisciplinary practice intervention(s)
3. Implement practice changes on a pilot unit
4. Evaluate process and outcomes
5. Modify intervention as needed

Research base not sufficiently developed to guide practice

Conduct research

Consult with experts

Determine scientific principles

Is the change appropriate for adoption in practice?

Change practice

Monitor outcomes

Patient and family

Staff

Fiscal

*QA/QI = Quality Assessment/Quality Improvement; **TQM/CQI = Total Quality Management/Continuous Quality Improvement; ◯ = a decision point.

Figure 4-1. The Iowa model. (Courtesy of the University of Iowa Hospitals and Clinics, Iowa City. Used by permission).

Challenges Facing Research Utilization

Titler (1997) recently raised the question as to whether, in the current climate of stringent cost-containment measures, downsizing, and wide-scale implementation of managed care, RU is a necessity or a luxury. She succinctly identified barriers to RU, current organizational strategies for overcoming those barriers, and future strategies to streamline RU to enhance its viability in a much leaner care delivery environment.

RU efforts may face organizational barriers, such as nurses' lack of authority to change practice and possible lack of cooperation from physicians. Current strategies for managing such problems include hiring a doctorally prepared nurse researcher in the practice environment and incorporating the value of research into job descriptions and merit structures. Future streamlining strategies could include combining RU and quality improvement committees and creating partnerships with nearby organizations or universities.

Another barrier to RU is that most of the federal funding to support nursing research goes to universities, not to practice institutions. Thus, obtaining necessary funding is more difficult in the practice environment. A strategy to counteract such limitations could be to conduct RU projects on a multisite basis and gain assistance from the practice specialty organizations in identifying content areas ready for RU rather than having to conduct one's own research.

Another challenge to establishing and maintaining an RU program is the limitations of knowledge and skills of nurses and their isolation from research-savvy university colleagues. Educators could help eliminate this barrier by preparing their graduates more fully for participation in RU programs—for instance, requirements for participation in journal clubs could be included in regular baccalaureate and graduate programs. Educators also should integrate RU skills into the course of study and could require participation in RU projects as part of the educational experience (Titler, 1997).

Titler also pointed out that another significant barrier to RU lies within research itself. There are not enough replication studies to provide nurses with data to warrant instituting a change in care. There are also barriers surrounding the process of communicating research information so that it can be used knowledgeably and effectively in practice. Statistical reporting can be particularly daunting to practicing nurses, who may not have a sufficient background in statistics to understand complex statistical analysis and what it means. If one does not have access to a comprehensive university-level library, the relevant literature can be difficult to find. Too often researchers tend to write their findings in reports aimed at other researchers; practice implications often are not a part of research reports. Thus, practitioners are given the outcomes, but they receive little direction regarding how the findings could help improve their practice.

A useful trend in solving the communication problem is developing. The number of research columns appearing in practice journals and the number of new journals that emphasize application of research findings (eg, *Applied Nursing Research*) are increasing, and the number of research conferences with a practice focus is growing. To continue to enhance communication of research to practitioners, Titler suggests:

- ◪ A journal dedicated to reporting RU projects
- ◪ More federal funds for RU conferences
- ◪ Increased use of the Internet to share RU protocols. (Titler, 1997, pp. 108–109)

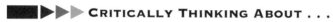 CRITICALLY THINKING ABOUT . . .

How should nursing educators be integrating RU skills into under-graduate nursing curricula?

Collaborative Research

Another bridge for joining nursing scholarship to nursing practice is **collaborative research**, which consists of nurse researchers going into the practice environment and working with nurse clinicians in defining, developing, and implementing research projects focused on improving care delivery. One such collaborative research effort between university researchers and public health department clinicians was described by Pamela Salsberry, Jennie Nickel, and Muriel O'Connell (1991). They reported on the effectiveness of collaborative research during a federally funded project, the Collaborative Home Care Project, which was designed to test the effectiveness of case-management strategies with patients infected with human immuno-deficiency virus (HIV) who were receiving home care. They describe six stages in the collaboration process and the challenges researchers faced at each stage. The first stage was to initiate the contact between the academic nurse researchers and the community clinicians. The university called for nurses in all areas of the community to come together to discuss the epidemic of acquired immunodeficiency syndrome (AIDS) and some possible projects to help deal with it.

Active collaboration between the nurse researchers from the university and nurse clinicians from the health department began with the second stage, which consisted of generating ideas and reaching a consensus about what would constitute a researchable problem. The authors gave the following advice about this stage:

> Individuals considering such collaborative projects should not underestimate the importance of this idea-generating phase, nor should they rush it. Time is necessary for merging the two perspectives, developing open and sharing relationships, and generating ideas. This must be a joint process and not a subtle superimposing of an academically developed research plan onto an existing practice system. (Salsberry, Nickel, & O'Connell, 1991, p. 203)

The authors emphasized the critical role of the contribution of both academicians and clinicians to the quality of the research problem. If the researchers had allowed the research to be formulated without adequate knowledge of design and methods, it may have been difficult or impossible to answer the questions well. This, in turn, might have resulted in findings that were not sufficiently convincing for analysts and policy makers. Conversely, if the clinical insights had not been taken into account in formulating the problem, it may have not have had any significance for the community agency and its patients.

The third stage in the collaborative process was generating a proposal to seek funds for the project. Initially, the work of proposal writing was divided evenly between the researchers and clinicians, but because this did not work out well, they decided together that the primary responsibility for writing the proposal would go to the researchers. However, close contact was maintained with the clinicians, who carefully examined and criticized each draft. In this phase, the differences in the primary orientations of the researchers and clinicians provided significant challenges. The clinicians focused primarily on hands-on daily care; the researchers tended to focus

on theoretical and design integrity of the proposed project. Three content areas required serious discussion and joint development: structure of the protocols, setting
up experimental and control groups, and determining outcome criteria. Two competing needs arose: the project had to be theoretically sound but relatively simple to
implement. Setting up experimental and control groups provoked some tension between the groups. The researchers believed that an experimental group versus control group design was the strongest, most convincing research design. The clinicians
felt that if the experimental intervention was good enough to investigate, then it was
good enough to offer to all patients. The experimental design was ultimately used.

Once the project had been reviewed, approved, and funded, the fourth stage,
implementation, could begin. Once again, different operating styles became apparent. Nurses working in the practice environment must take a high-efficiency approach to delivery of care. Therefore, documentation in patient records was often
minimal and geared toward meeting federal or state requirements, but it was not of
the quality required for a well-documented research project. The health department
staff was especially frustrated by time spent in recruiting subjects, especially when the
recruits decided not to participate or decided later to drop out of the study. From
the staff's point of view, this was simply valuable time lost. From the researchers'
perspective, attrition is simply one of the things that happens in studies involving
people.

The remaining two phases of the project, data analysis and dissemination of findings, had yet to be done when the article was written. However, the authors anticipated some of the issues that might arise. One of the issues would likely be that the
two groups would have differing needs for using the data. Thus, the manner in
which the data would be set up, organized, analyzed, and made available would have
to be very comprehensive and flexible. The authors were aware that continuing regular team meetings would be required.

Despite the difficulties inherent in collaborative research of this kind, these authors believed it was well worth the effort. They concluded:

> A successful collaboration requires a high degree of commitment, openness and
> sharing, and accommodation of differences by all involved. The rewards are found
> in the advancement of nursing at both individual and aggregate levels. (Salsberry,
> Nickel, & O'Connell, 1991, p. 207)

Incorporation of Nursing Theory Into Research and Practice
Earlier in this chapter, we referred to a perception common to both researchers and
practitioners that the first-generation nursing theories have not been particularly useful to either group. Blegen and Tripp-Reimer (1997) addressed this issue using an
interesting approach. They proposed three alternatives of how theory, research, and
practice could function together more harmoniously and more fruitfully, thereby
fostering the professionalization of nursing.

The first alternative is to maintain nursing theory, nursing research, and nursing
practice as relatively separate domains, much as they are now. Such action would be
based on the premise that each kind of nursing knowledge will develop best when
tended with full focus on one primary category. Nurses with interests and skills in
each of the three areas have different perspectives and different skills; it is best to let
nurses in each group develop the category in which their expertise lies. This pattern
has served nursing well for a half-century. However, some refinements would be in-

troduced that would help build bridges between nurses whose work is primarily in improving practice, nurses whose skill lies in theory development, and nurses who devote their careers to research. This position, in essence, is that the basic separated structure will continue to work well if communication between the three groups is implemented.

Blegen and Tripp-Reimer went on to describe possible mechanisms that would serve as bridges to communicate theory effectively to both researchers and practitioners. For the separate-but-communicating model to function well, there is a need for nurses who function in **boundary-spanning roles**. These would include nurses who translate theorists' knowledge into a form useful for researchers and practitioners. Nursing faculty members would serve as the first level of boundary spanners because they capture both the knowledge from theory and the knowledge from research and weave it into the preparation of their students for practice. After graduation, practicing nurses could rely on other boundary spanners, such as continuing education and publications containing developments in nursing theory and findings from nursing research that would be targeted specifically to practicing nurses. Several publications have done exactly that—for example, *Applied Nursing Research, Nursing Scan in Research*, and clinically focused specialty journals that carry columns that bring research to the practitioner.

Those who serve as boundary spanners must identify theoretical developments that need testing and must form relevant research questions. Boundary spanners also must communicate research findings back to theoreticians to enhance the further refinement of theory. Often, researchers have assumed the role of boundary spanner, but this practice has not been totally successful because the orientation of nurse researchers leads them to increase the validity of the general knowledge produced by their studies by removing or controlling the influence of unique individual characteristics of each patient or subjects and setting. On the other hand, nurses oriented to practice must focus on the individual patient's unique characteristics to provide care that truly meets each patient's needs. For the separate-but-communicating model to continue to be useful, more (and better) boundary-spanning strategies between theory and practice and theory and research must be found and used.

■■■ ▶▶▶ CRITICALLY THINKING ABOUT . . .

> In your experience in nursing so far, who have you observed in a boundary-spanning role? What did this person do? How effective was the person as a boundary spanner? Why?

The second alternative proposed by Blegen and Tripp-Reimer is that the categories of theory, research, and practice must be closely connected through application of a structural model. This position is based on the premise that "anything less than full connectedness will continue the current pattern of separateness" (Blegen & Tripp-Reimer, 1997, p. 70). The ideal model for achieving a seamless fabric of unique nursing knowledge brings together academic researchers, nurse theorists, and practicing nurses. Several collaborative models have been tested, but no models have been described that incorporate all three knowledge areas.

Although full collaboration among theorists, researchers, and clinicians is an admirable goal, there are significant limitations to the extent of collaboration that can actually occur. These groups have differing perspectives that can be difficult to surmount. Collaboration requires a great deal of time and effort to ensure good communication. Collaborators must consistently work in teams that draw nurses from multiple settings. This requires a great deal of time and other resources.

Finally, Blegen and Tripp-Reimer present a third alternative—keeping nursing theory, nursing research, and nursing practice separate but connected through development and implementation of user-friendly nursing theory. This position is not the same as the first alternative. The necessary connections among theory, research, and practice are not dependent on boundary spanners, as they are in the first alternative. Rather, the connection is forged by a different kind of knowledge developed by the theorists: knowledge that is closer to practice, testable through the application of research, and built around structures intrinsic to the discipline of nursing. Blegen and Tripp-Reimer explain that if this were to occur, nursing would have the best of all worlds—separateness for development and connectedness to practice (Blegen & Tripp-Reimer, 1997, p. 71). They explain that the key to this ideal connection is the generation and use of **middle-range theory** rather than the first-generation grand theories developed in an earlier time.

Sociologist Robert K. Merton (1957, 1967) called to the attention of researchers the value of middle-range theories for pulling together a wide variety of specific empirical observations that, on their own, would seem to have little to do with the first-generation grand theories. Middle-range theories may be thought of as a set of interrelated hypotheses that aim to explain some specific condition or behavior and inspire verification studies (studies with the goal of testing the specific hypotheses). As verification studies accumulate, the hypotheses of the middle-range theories may be:

➤ Accepted
➤ Modified in some way that identifies the conditions under which the proposition holds and does not hold
➤ Expanded in both scope and number
➤ Rejected outright.

Over time, middle-range theory may come to explain an increasing range of phenomena and thus will have broad explanatory powers. In other words, it will be theory that is applicable for nursing care in all situations, for all groups of people, for all health conditions, and for all health care settings.

An example of a middle-range theory used in a study is presented in Box 4-1. However, as with all examples of middle-range theories, additional propositions may be developed to test the theory, other samples may be studied, and measures other than the ones the Schwirians used may be employed. In addition, the propositions themselves may be tested under more specific conditions (eg, men and women separately or people of different social classes separately). Indeed, further studies must be conducted to obtain a better understanding of the validity, generalizability, and predictability of the particular middle-range theory.

Nursing would be positively served, according to Blegen and Tripp-Reimer, if middle-range theories were to form a central place in nursing research: "It is time to refocus from discussing these larger philosophical systems to producing knowledge that explains patient-related phenomena and helps in the choice and evaluation of interventions" (Blegen & Tripp-Reimer, 1997, p. 72).

Use of middle-range theories would also have several advantages from the perspective of practicing nurses. Although they would need some grasp of research, they

Box 4-1

Example of Middle-Range Theory Used in a Research Study

Two Hypotheses (Basis of the middle-range theory)

1. Over a two-year period and excluding other factors such as experience of critical events, the greater the number and frequency of age-specific health behaviors engaged in (e.g., taking medications as directed, eating a balanced diet, and maintaining social contacts with friends and family), the less the likelihood of a health decline.
2. Over a two-year period and excluding other factors such as experience of critical events, the greater the psychological well-being and psychological hardiness (life orientation), the less the likelihood of a health decline.

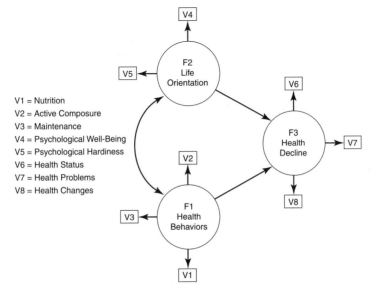

V1 = Nutrition
V2 = Active Composure
V3 = Maintenance
V4 = Psychological Well-Being
V5 = Psychological Hardiness
V6 = Health Status
V7 = Health Problems
V8 = Health Changes

(Schwirian PM, Schwirian KP, Weiss C [1995]. Health behaviors, life orientation, and health decline among older adults. *Journal of Mental Health and Aging* 1[2]:114. New York: Springer; used by permission.)

Study

These hypotheses were tested on a sample of urban older adults using three instruments:

1. Schwirians' Senior Lifestyle Inventory (1993) to measure health behaviors
2. Items from the Philadelphia Geriatric Institute Scale (1984) to measure psychological well-being
3. Younkin and Betz's Psychological Hardiness Scale (1994) Adapted for Older Adults to measure psychological hardiness.

Conclusion

Strong support was found for both propositions. Therefore, support for these propositions lends support for the underlying middle-range theory that engaging in health behaviors and having a positive outlook on life forestalls health decline among the elderly.

*Study—Health Decline Among the Elderly. Schwirian and Schwirian, 1995.

would not be required to read and critique complex research reports. They would not have to try to fit global, highly abstract grand theories into everyday practice. Instead, middle-range theories provide specific descriptions of human responses to illness and detail the nursing interventions applicable to these responses. Nurses still would have to understand the theory, but the task would not seem so difficult. Boundary-spanning activities may still be needed and probably could be provided by nursing educators and RU projects.

 CRITICALLY THINKING ABOUT . . .

> Identify a middle-range theory that you have studied. What was it trying to explain? How could it be tested?

Fostering the Development of Nursing Knowledge: Nursing Information Classification Systems

One alternative to the traditional goal of melding theory, research, and practice to develop and refine a knowledge base for nursing is to generate nursing knowledge using NICS. Before computers were introduced into nursing care settings, nursing information about patients and their care was largely relegated to entries in patient charts and plans of nursing care. These entries were typically idiosyncratic and particularly suited to an individual institution or even an individual department or unit. The nursing record was a transaction log describing what type of care was provided to each patient and when the care was given. Data that were entered had no standardized scheme for coding or classification and thus could rarely be reused for any other purpose. These factors combined kept patient data specific to each patient care event and did not allow for meaningful consolidation of information about groups of patients or patient care events into useful knowledge.

Even when computers were initially introduced into nursing care settings, the systems that were used were still very similar in structure to the precomputer records. Records had simply been moved from a paper storage medium to an electronic storage medium. Retrieving and assembling this unmatched data for important activities such as quality assurance was time-consuming and laborious.

When data were pulled together, findings could be problematic because the information was not necessarily consistent in format, content, or language. It was difficult to generate a clear, generalized picture of actual nursing interventions, the rationale for the interventions, and the resulting outcomes. Although computers did not make a big difference immediately, the technology did permit the rapid assembly of large amounts of data in a way that paper-and-pencil recording never had. This led computer-wise nurses to understand that the computer was a tool that would enable them to develop a knowledge base for nursing based on what nurses actually do when caring for patients. Thus began the development of NICS, a very significant step in the development of a powerful knowledge base for nursing.

Nature and Utility

This approach involves organizing nursing care-based data into NICS using various means of categorization. One purpose of NICS is to define uniformly the realm and language of nursing practice—exactly what nurses do and exactly how they describe it. NICS also can help identify the nursing diagnoses, nursing interventions, and patient outcomes that can be attributed directly to nursing care. The diagnosis identifies the basis and rationale for the nursing intervention; the intervention specifies what the nurse actually did; and the patient outcome provides a measure of the both the appropriateness of the diagnosis and success of the intervention. The development and refinement of computer-based nursing information systems and other computer applications have made this approach to knowledge development possible.

Nurse researchers, nurse educators, nurse clinicians, nurse administrators, and all those who make policy affecting nursing can all benefit from using NICS. Researchers need standardized nursing data to study health problems across populations, settings, and caregivers. Standardized nursing data also enable investigators to link nursing diagnoses with interventions and patient outcomes (McCloskey & Bulechek, 1992; Devine, 1988; Kraegel, 1988; Werley & Zorn, 1989). The development of NICS also can enhance nursing education. A classification system could be used as a basis for generating computer-assisted instruction and curricula that have a nursing focus and could serve as a link between nursing education and clinical practice (McCloskey, 1988). Clinical practice can benefit directly from a classification system that makes documentation of care more effective, supports decision making, and provides a foundation for research-based practice (Werley, Devine, Zorn, Ryan, & Westra, 1991; Werley & Zorn, 1989).

Administrators and policy makers also can benefit from NICS. Administrators will have better information for predicting resource needs and a better understanding of the actual costs involved in nursing care (Leske & Werley, 1992; McCloskey & Bulechek, 1992; Werley & Lang, 1988). Finally, nursing data that document the effect of nursing care can be influential in governmental decisions regarding allocation of health resources and in making health policy decisions (Abdellah, 1988; Kraegel, 1988; Werley, Lang, & Westlake, 1986; Werley & Zorn, 1989).

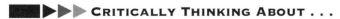 **CRITICALLY THINKING ABOUT . . .**

Which NICS have you studied? What were its elements? How did it help in your nursing practice?

Criteria for Usefulness

If a classification system is to be useful in supporting clinical practice, theory development and testing, and nursing research, it must have certain characteristics and meet certain criteria (Henry & Constantino, 1997). The first criterion is domain completeness—that is, the system must include all the terms necessary to describe the domain or sphere of activity. The second criterion is conceptual clarity and coherence—that is, the system must be consistent with a well-defined conceptual framework but should not be limited to or dependent on a particular model or theory of nursing. This also means that in a good classification system:

1. All definitions are clear and understandable.
2. There is only one way to express each concept.
3. Any term should refer to only one concept.
4. All the terms in a category are in the same class. (Clark & Lang, 1992; McCloskey & Bulechek, 1996; Cimino, Hripsak, Johnson, & Clayton, 1989)

The third criterion is that a classification system should have clear relations between terms and should use commonly understood language to express those relations (eg, "equivalent to," "part of," or "associated with"). Fourth, a classification system should be clinically expressive—that is, it should be the natural language system used in the care environment (Campbell & Munsen, 1992). Finally, a useful classification system must have utility: it must be simple enough for an ordinary practitioner to use; it must work with the family of disease-related and health-related systems common to clinical environments; and it must be based on a central core that can be constantly updated and refined without a great struggle (Henry & Constantino, 1997).

Development of NICS

The development of NICS directed toward establishing a nursing knowledge base has been evolving along four separate but closely related paths over the past 30 years:

1. Nursing Minimum Data Set
2. North American Nursing Diagnosis Association Taxonomy
3. American Nurses Association's leadership and coordination role in NICS development
4. Development of nursing taxonomies that incorporate not only diagnosis, but intervention and outcomes as well.

Nursing Minimum Data Set

As long ago as the 1960s, Harriet Werley, a nursing pioneer of great vision, creativity, and determination in both nursing research and nursing informatics, began to develop the concept of a **Nursing Minimum Data Set** (NMDS) (Werley & Lang, 1988). Early on, Werley understood the importance of having a tool for collecting concise, uniform, standard, comparable nursing data needed by nurses in clinical practice, in administration, in research, and in policy making. The necessary tool also must have utility for nurses in documenting care in any setting. The variables in an NMDS then could be used in computer systems to describe nursing care, measure the quality of care, and determine the cost. Werley's goal for the NMDS was to establish comparability of nursing data across clinical populations, settings, geographic areas, and time. To reach this goal, it was necessary to identify essential data categories and elements and develop uniform definitions for these that were understandable and useful for nurses in practice, research, education, and administration (Werley, Lang, & Westlake, 1986).

By 1985, Werley's longstanding interest in NMDS came to fruition. She had assembled sufficient background information, knowledgeable participants, support from her colleagues at the University of Wisconsin—Milwaukee, and financial backing from the American Hospital Association Foundation to convene an NMDS conference in Milwaukee. She asked Norma Lang, then dean of nursing at the University of Wisconsin—Milwaukee, to serve as cochair of the conference. During the three-day conference, 65 people, including nurse clinicians, administrators, educators, and researchers, discussed the issues involved in the development, implementation, and evaluation of NMDS and generated an initial set (Werley, Lang, & Westlake, 1986).

The nurses attending the conference had expertise in areas of clinical practice, patient classification, nursing diagnosis, quality assurance, nursing information systems, nursing resources allocation, and professional standards. Participants also included public and private health policy experts, information systems experts, a health records specialist, and persons who were knowledgeable about the history of health data systems such as the proposed NMDS.

Thirty of the participants were commissioned to prepare papers in which they provided their perspectives on relevant issues such as conceptual and practical considerations, requirements of various care settings, and systems requirements as viewed by information science and health records professionals. These papers were circulated to all conferees several months before the conference, and seven discussants presented succinct reviews of groups of the papers on the first day. On the second and third days, participants were assigned to one of six task forces to work on developing NMDS content in the following areas: nursing assessment, nursing diagnosis, nursing intervention, nursing outcomes, nursing acuity or intensity, and demographics. Sixteen elements were defined as the appropriate content of an NMDS (Box 4-2).

A full report on the content of the NMDS, including definitions for the categories (nursing care elements, patient demographics, and service) and elements, was prepared by Werley and Lang (1988). This conference and the documents that resulted stand as landmarks in the development of a coherent, unified NICS as a foundation for the necessary knowledge base for the nursing profession. Werley and Zorn (1989) noted that the work on the NMDS was instrumental in encouraging further development of nursing information taxonomies that would include interventions as well as diagnosis, because testing and implementation of the NMDS are impossible without the development and refinement of such classification systems.

 CRITICALLY THINKING ABOUT . . .

If you had been invited to the NMDS conference, what concerns would you have expressed?

Box 4-2
Sixteen Elements of a Nursing Minimum Data Set

- ▸ Nursing diagnosis
- ▸ Nursing intervention
- ▸ Nursing outcome
- ▸ Intensity of nursing care
- ▸ *Five* pieces of patient demographic data
- ▸ Unique facility or service agency number
- ▸ Unique health record number of patient
- ▸ Unique number of principal nurse provided
- ▸ Admission date
- ▸ Discharge date
- ▸ Disposition
- ▸ Expected source of payment

North American Nursing Diagnosis Association

While Harriet Werley was pursuing her interest and setting the stage for the development of the NMDS, another group of nurses dedicated to the development of a logical, coherent system of nursing diagnoses was also moving forward. The development of a standardized nomenclature for nursing diagnosis began in 1973, largely under the leadership of Marjory Gordon, when a group of nurses convened the first national conference on nursing diagnosis. This first conference was followed by several more, and in 1982 the North American Nursing Diagnosis Association (NANDA) was formed. This very dedicated group of nurses has been highly committed to their mission. By the time the NMDS conference was held in 1985, NANDA was in a sufficiently established position to convince the conference participants of the critical importance of including the NANDA diagnoses in the NDMS scheme. The NANDA taxonomy is described later in this chapter.

American Nurses Association

As in most other movements that are instrumental in propelling nursing further toward status as a fully acknowledged profession, the American Nurses Association (ANA) has been instrumental in attending to the development of NICS. In the 1970s, the ANA focused on the development of standards of practice. As part of that process, it identified the elements that must be part of a nursing practice classification: assessment factors, nursing diagnosis, interventions, and outcomes. The later ANA definition of nursing as the "diagnosis and treatment of human responses to actual or potential health problems" reinforced the earlier position (ANA, 1980). The publication in which the definition of nursing was presented also recommended that nurses pursue the development of an NICS. In 1982, the ANA appointed a steering committee on classifications of nursing practice, and in 1991 the steering committee on databases to support clinical nursing practice was formed. This committee was charged with developing clinical nursing practice standards related to nursing classification schemes, uniform nursing data sets, and inclusion of nursing data elements into national databases (Lang et al., 1995).

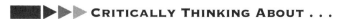 CRITICALLY THINKING ABOUT . . .

What role should the ANA take in the development of standards of practice? Should they make more rules or fewer? Why?

Nursing Taxonomies

One strategy in establishing a useful NICS is the development of **nursing taxonomies**. A taxonomy is an orderly classification of items, ideas, or activities according to their presumed natural relations and according to specific laws or principles (Woolf, 1980; Zielstorff, 1994). Four major nursing taxonomies will be discussed:

1. NANDA taxonomy
2. Nursing interventions classification taxonomy
3. Omaha problem classification system
4. Home health care classification taxonomy.

All four nursing classification systems have been recognized by the ANA database steering committee for use in national and international databases (McCormick, Lang, Zielstorff, Milholland, Saba, & Jacox, 1994). These taxonomies also have been recognized by the National Library of Medicine and incorporated into its metathesaurus to promote easier access to the nursing literature by all health professionals (ANA, 1993; Martin & Norris, 1996).

NANDA TAXONOMY

The **NANDA taxonomy** probably is the most familiar of the classification systems. Since the late 1970s, it has been the predominant classification system for nursing diagnoses (NANDA, 1994; Ozbolt, Abraham, & Schultz, 1990). The NANDA taxonomy is routinely taught in undergraduate nursing programs and used widely in clinical practice in many nursing care settings. The focus of the NANDA taxonomy is nursing diagnoses. A nursing diagnosis is an actual or potential health problem of an individual, group, or community for which a nurses can intervene. The first part of this definition is consistent with the ANA's definition of nursing (see Chap. 1), and the second part makes it clear that a nursing diagnosis is not a medical diagnosis. Nursing diagnoses serve several purposes:

- ☐ They provide nurses with a common language for assessment and identification of and communication about client problems.
- ☐ They provide a mechanism for reimbursement of nursing activities.
- ☐ They are useful in patient and family education, discharge planning, quality assurance, and staffing (Carpenito, 1995).

Since 1982, the list of NANDA-approved nursing diagnoses has grown to almost 130, and more diagnoses continue to be developed and tested. The format has evolved as well. At its most basic, a NANDA nursing diagnosis consists of an actual or potential health problem, along with the etiology or related factors (the probable factors that contribute to the health problem)—for example, Problem: Constipation; Etiology: related to immobility. The health problems are, in turn, grouped into a taxonomy according to nine patterns. The patterns, and an example of a diagnosis for each pattern, are presented in Table 4-1.

NURSING INTERVENTIONS CLASSIFICATION TAXONOMY

The **nursing interventions classification (NIC) taxonomy** was developed at the University of Iowa by a group of academic researchers and clinicians headed by Joan C. McCloskey and Gloria Bulechek. Funding for development and validation of the taxonomy was provided by the National Institute for Nursing Research. The general purpose of the project was to develop a standardized language for nursing treatments to be used in practice, education, and research. The NIC authors believe that the use of this taxonomy will facilitate the inclusion of nursing treatments in health care data sets and ultimately will help determine the effectiveness and costs of nursing interventions (McCloskey & Bulechek, 1995). The NIC taxonomy is designed to be a comprehensive, standardized language descriptive of all interventions nurses do on behalf of patients, including independent nursing interventions as well as collaborative interventions (other health professionals are involved in the intervention). The interventions range from basic to complex, and the entire classification is intended to capture the collective expertise of nurses in all areas of practice.

TABLE 4-1	PATTERNS AND EXAMPLES OF DIAGNOSES FROM THE NORTH AMERICAN NURSING DIAGNOSIS ASSOCIATION (NANDA) TAXONOMY

Pattern	Examples of Diagnoses
Exchanging	Altered Nutrition: More than body requirements
	Urinary retention
Communicating	Impaired Verbal Communication
Relating	Social Isolation
	Altered Family Processes
Valuing	Spiritual distress
	Potential for enhanced spiritual well-being
Choosing	Ineffective Denial
	Noncompliance
Moving	Impaired Physical Mobility
	Activity Intolerance
Perceiving	Body Image Disturbance
	Powerlessness
Knowing	Chronic Confusion
	Impaired Memory
Feelings	Chronic Pain
	Risk for Self-Mutilation.

(NANDA [1994]. *NANDA Nursing Diagnoses.* Philadelphia: Author.)

All the interventions in the NIC are placed within a three-level taxonomy: domains, classes, and interventions. The most global level is the domains level. There are six domains:

1. Basic physiologic—care that supports physical functioning
2. Complex physiologic—care that supports homeostatic regulation
3. Behavioral—care that supports psychosocial functioning
4. Safety—care that supports protection against harm
5. Family—care that supports the family unit
6. Health system—care that supports effective use of the care delivery system.

Each succeeding level of the taxonomy becomes more specific. Level two of the taxonomy consists of classes of interventions. For example, within the basic physiologic domain, there are six intervention classes. The first two are activity and exercise management (interventions to organize or assist with physical activity and energy conservation and expenditure) and elimination management (interventions to establish and maintain regular bowel and urinary elimination patterns and manage complications due to altered patterns).

The third level of the taxonomy, interventions, is the most detailed. Each nursing intervention is spelled out and identified with a four-digit number that can facilitate the entry of the intervention into a computerized health care database for further use and analysis. For example, within the safety domain is the crisis management class, and within this class are interventions such as A6140 (code management), A6200 (emergency care), and A6320 (resuscitation) (McCloskey & Bulechek, 1995). The entire NIC taxonomy consists of 6 domains, 27 classes, and 433 numbered interventions. There are specific steps for placement of a new intervention in the NIC taxonomy, as well as rules for numeric coding of interventions.

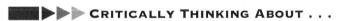 **CRITICALLY THINKING ABOUT . . .**

In your clinical experience, have you seen taxonomies being used? If so, how?

OMAHA PROBLEM CLASSIFICATION SYSTEM

The **Omaha problem classification system (OCS)** originated in the early 1970s when the staff and administrators of the Omaha Visiting Nurses' Association realized it was time for a major revision of the agency's client record system. They realized that this revision would have to incorporate strategies that would generate a clinical database that could be used in a fully integrated, automated management information system. Over a 25-year period, many researchers and clinicians developed the OCS. It was supported by 11 years of funding from the Division of Nursing, U.S. Department of Health and Human Services, and the National Institute of Nursing Research. The goal was to develop a research-based model that could be used in multiple settings, including home care, hospice, public health, school health, prison, and clinic programs.

The OCS consists of three components:

1. Problem classification scheme
2. Intervention scheme
3. Problem rating scale for outcomes.

The problem classification scheme is a taxonomy of nursing diagnoses developed from actual client records. It consists of four levels: domains, problems, modifiers, and signs and symptoms. The domains, the broadest level, are meant to represent the essence of nursing practice. They are environmental, psychological, physiologic, and health-related behaviors. A total of 40 client problems or nursing diagnoses are included within these domains. Each of the patient problems is further elaborated by using modifiers in conjunction with it. A problem may be referenced as health promotion, potential, or actual. It also may be referenced as family or individual. When an actual problem modifier is used, problem-specific signs and symptoms are provided to elaborate the nature of the problem. The developers intended the problem classification scheme to be expandable, rather than exhaustive. Therefore, "other" appears at the end of each domain and each sign and symptom cluster (Martin & Norris, 1996).

The purpose of the intervention scheme is to provide the nurse with a tool that uses standard language and guides both practice and documentation. This scheme was created using data from 275 charts. The intervention scheme is arranged into three levels. The first level is composed of comprehensive categories: health teaching, guidance, and counseling; case management; and surveillance. The second level is an alphabetical listing of 63 targets. A target is the object of a nursing intervention or activity (eg, exercise or safety). Targets help delineate an intervention category that is problem-specific. The third level of the intervention scheme is designed for client-specific information using concise words or short phrases generated by community nurses as they develop plans or document care. This allows a more personalized approach to using a taxonomy than either the NANDA or NIC taxonomy.

The final major component of the OCS is the problem rating scale for outcomes, which consists of three rating scales describing client outcomes in the areas of knowledge, behavior, and status. It was developed to measure progress in relation to the problems specific to the client, to provide a guide to practice, and to be useful in documentation. The scale was designed to be used throughout the entire time of client service. This is particularly relevant in community health settings, where services may not be as intense as in inpatient settings; instead, services may be provided over several weeks, months, or even years.

As independent home care and outpatient services have expanded, so too has interest in OCS. Today this system is in widespread use, although the exact number of users is not known because it exists in the public domain (which means the permission of the developers is not required to use or modify it) (Martin & Norris, 1996).

HOME HEALTH CARE CLASSIFICATION TAXONOMY

Care of clients living in the community also was the focus of the **home health care classification (HHCC) taxonomy**, which was developed at Georgetown University in the late 1980s under the direction of Virginia Saba. Funded by the National Association for Home Care and the Health Care Financing Administration, the Georgetown study was done to develop a method of assessing and classifying home health Medicare patients to predict their need for home care services and to measure the outcomes of their care (Saba, 1994). A national sample of 646 home health agencies participated in the study. Most of the home health Medicare patients (93.8%) whose records formed the basis for the study were 65 or older; of those, more than half were over 75. Sixty percent were females, fewer than half were married, almost a third lived alone, and more than 25% relied on self-care (Saba, 1992b).

The framework for the HHCC consists of 20 home health care components (eg, activity, bowel elimination, cardiac, and urinary elimination). Included within each component is a list of NANDA nursing diagnoses, with coding numbers; a few non-NANDA diagnoses were added to fit the home health care situation more appropriately. The result was a classification scheme of 147 numerically coded nursing diagnoses.

A total of 128 nursing interventions also were categorized under each of the 20 components. Thus, a client who was recovering from a hip fracture at home would be categorized as follows: Activity Component: Nursing Diagnosis—01.5 Physical Mobility Impairment, Intervention—03.1 Ambulation Therapy (included within the Mobility Therapy category of interventions). The intervention outcomes are assessed when the client is discharged from the particular episode of care. An outcome could be 1 = improved, 2 = stabilized, or 3 = deteriorated. As with other classification systems, all diagnoses, interventions, and outcomes for HHCC are assigned numeric codes, and rules are established for the means by which the data are arranged for computer entry (Saba, 1992a).

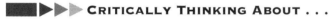 **CRITICALLY THINKING ABOUT . . .**

Should nursing spend more or less time developing taxonomies?

▶ CHAPTER SUMMARY

Science and practice are based on knowledge bases. This chapter has shown that the trifurcation of nursing into theory, research, and practice has made it difficult for a common knowledge base to develop. Nevertheless, over the last several years nurse scientists and clinicians have pursued many activities to bridge the gap among the nursing camps, including such developments as the (RU) approach and the collaborative home care project. In addition to these activities, others have moved nursing toward knowledge base development using nursing information classification systems and nursing taxonomies. The flurry of activity of these information management initiatives over the last 25 years has provided nursing with a strong first generation of information systems that, no doubt, will be refined over the next 25 years and beyond. The current systems will serve as foundations for the next generation of such systems, and the knowledge base for nursing will continue to develop in comprehensiveness, clarity, and utility in support of truly professional nursing practice.

KEY POINTS

▶ 1 The trifurcation of nursing knowledge is the division of nursing theory, research, and practice into three separate areas that are often unrelated and noncommunicating. This trifurcation is dysfunctional and will not promote the development of comprehensive, functional nursing knowledge.

▶ 2 Three barriers to the unification of nursing knowledge are perceptions that theory is obscure and irrelevant, isolation of practice from academia, and a theory–research split.

▶ 3 Many strategies have been developed to bridge the gaps between nurse theorists, nurse researchers, and nurse clinicians and, therefore, unify nursing knowledge. These include (RU), collaborative research, and three alternative methods of incorporating nursing theory into nursing research and practice.

▶ 4 An alternative to the traditional goal of melding theory, research, and practice to develop and refine a knowledge base for nursing is through the development of NICS. This field has evolved along four separate but related paths: the NMDS; development of the NANDA taxonomy of nursing diagnoses; the ANA's leadership and coordination role in nursing information classification systems development; and the development of nursing taxonomies.

▶ 5 Important nursing taxonomies that have been developed and widely recognized are the NANDA's taxonomy, the nursing intervention classification taxonomy, the OCS taxonomy, and the HHCC taxonomy.

REFERENCES

Abdellah F (1988). Future directions: Refining, implementing, testing and evaluating the Nursing Minimum Data Set. In Werley H, Lang N, eds. *Identification of the Nursing Minimum Data Set*. New York: Springer, pp. 416–426.

American Nurses Association (1980). *Nursing: A social policy statement.* Kansas City: Author.

American Nurses Association (1993). Nursing classification recognized by the National Library of Medicine. *American Nurse 25(3),*9.

Blegen MA, Tripp-Reimer T (1994). The nursing theory–nursing research connection. In McCloskey J, Grace HK, eds. *Current Issues in Nursing* (4th ed.). St. Louis: Mosby, pp. 87–91.

Blegen MA, Tripp-Reimer T (1997). Nursing theory nursing research and nursing practice: Connected or separate? In McCloskey J, Grace HK, eds. *Current Issues in Nursing* (5th ed.). St. Louis: Mosby, pp. 68–74.

Campbell KE, Munsen MA (1992). Representation of clinical data using SNOMED III and conceptual graphs. In Frisse M (Ed.), *Proceedings of the 16th Annual Symposium of Computer Applications in Medical Care.* New York: McGraw-Hill, pp. 380–384.

Carpenito LJ (1995). *Nursing Diagnosis: Application to Clinical Practice* (6th ed.). Philadelphia: JB Lippincott.

Cimino JJ, Hripsak G, Johnson SB, Clayton PD (1989). Designing an introspective multipurpose controlled medical vocabulary. In Kingsland L (Ed.), *Proceedings of the 13th Annual Symposium on Computer Applications in Medical Care.* Los Alamitos, CA: IEEE Computer Society Press, pp. 513–518.

Clark J, Lang NM (1992). Nursing's next advance: An international classification for nursing practice. *International Nursing Review, 39,* 109–112.

Devine E (1988). The Nursing Minimum Data Set: Benefits and implications for nurse researchers. In *Perspectives in Nursing.* New York: National League for Nursing, pp. 115–118.

Fawcett J, Downs FS (1992). *The Relationship Between Theory and Research* (2nd ed.). Philadelphia: FA Davis.

Funk SF, Champagne MT, Wiese RA, Tornquist EM (1991). Barriers to using research findings in practice: The clinician's perspective. *Applied Nursing Research, 4,* 90–95.

Henry SB, Constantino M (1997). Classification systems and integrated information systems: Building blocks for transforming data into nursing knowledge. In McCloskey JC, Grace HK (Eds.) *Current Issues in Nursing* (5th ed.). St. Louis: Mosby, pp. 75–87.

Hicks C (1996). Nurse researcher: A study of contradiction in terms? *J Advanced Nursing, 24,* 357–363.

Kraegel J (1988). Potential impact of the Nursing Minimum Data Set on the development of health policy: Public and private. In Werley H, Lang N (Eds.) *Identification of the Nursing Minimum Data Set.* New York: Springer, pp. 370–379.

Lang NM, Hudgings C, Jacox A, et al (1995). Toward a national database for nursing practice. In *An Emerging Framework for the Profession: Data System Advances for Clinical Nursing Practice.* Washington DC: American Nurses Association.

Leske J, Werley H. (1992). Use of the Nursing Minimum Data Set. *Computers in Nursing, 10,* 259–263.

Levine ME (1995). The rhetoric of nursing theory. *Image: Journal of Nursing Scholarship, 27,* 11–14.

Martin KS, Norris J (1996). The Omaha System: A model for describing practice. *Holistic Nursing Practice, 11,* 75–83.

McCloskey J (1988). The Nursing Minimum Data Set: Benefits and implications for nurse educators. In *Perspectives in Nursing 1987–1989.* New York: National League for Nursing, pp. 119–126.

McCloskey JC, Bulechek G, eds. (1992). *Nursing Interventions Classification.* St. Louis: Mosby.

McCloskey JC, Bulechek G (1995). Validation and coding of the NIC taxonomy structure. *Image: Journal of Nursing Scholarship, 27,* 43–49.

McCloskey JC, Bulechek G, eds. (1996). *Nursing Interventions Classification*. St. Louis: Mosby.

McCormick K, Lang N, Zielstorff R, Milholland K, Saba V, Jacox A (1994). Toward standard classification schemes for nursing language: Recommendations of the American Nurses Association steering committee on databases to support clinical nursing practice. *J American Medical Informatics Association, 1(6)*, 421–427.

NANDA (1994). *NANDA Nursing Diagnoses: Definitions and Classification 1995–1996*. Philadelphia: Author.

Ozbolt JG, Abraham IL, Schultz S (1990). Nursing information systems. In Shortliffe EH, Perreault LE, eds. *Medical informatics: Computers in health care*. Menlo Park, CA: Addison-Wesley.

Pettingill MM, Gillies DA, Clark CC (1994). Factors encouraging and discouraging the use of nursing research findings. *Image: Journal of Nursing Scholarship, 26*, 143–147.

Polit DF, Hungler BP (1997). *Essentials of Nursing Research: Methods Appraisal and Utilization* (4th ed.). Philadelphia: Lippincott-Raven.

Saba VK (1992a). The classification of home health care nursing: Diagnoses and interventions. *Caring Magazine, 11(3)*, 50–57.

Saba V.K. (1992b). Home health care classification. *Caring Magazine, 11(5)*, 58–60.

Saba VK (1994). Twenty nursing diagnosis home health care components. In Carroll-Johnson RM, Paquette M, eds. *Classification of Nursing Diagnosis: Proceedings of the 10th Conference*. Philadelphia: JB Lippincott.

Salsberry PJ, Nickel JT, O'Connell M (1991). AIDS research in the community: A case study in collaboration between researchers and clinicians. *Public Health Nursing, 8*, 201–207.

Schwirian PM, Schwirian KP, Weiss C (1995). Health behaviors, life orientation, and health decline among older adults. *Journal of Mental Health and Aging, 1*(2), 111–125.

Titler MG (1997). Research utilization: Necessity or luxury? In McCloskey JC, Grace HK (Eds.) *Current Issues in Nursing* (5th ed.). St. Louis: Mosby, pp. 104–117.

Titler MG, Kleiber C, Steelman V, et al. (1994). Infusing research into practice to promote quality care. *Nursing Research, 43*, 307–313.

Werley H, Devine E, Zorn C, Ryan P, Westra B (1991). The Nursing Minimum Data Set: Abstraction tool for standardized comparable essential data. *Am J Public Health, 81*, 421–426.

Werley H, Lang N, eds. (1988). *Identification of the Nursing Minimum Data Set*. New York: Springer.

Werley H, Lang N, Westlake S (1986). The Nursing Minimum Data Set conference: Executive summary. *J Professional Nursing, 2*, 217–224.

Werley H, Zorn C (1989). The Nursing Minimum Data Set and its relationship to classifications for nursing practice. *Classification systems for describing nursing practice working papers* (American Nurses Association Publications NP-74:50–54).

Woolf HB (Ed.) (1980). *Webster's New Collegiate Dictionary*. Springfield, MA: G & C Merriam Company.

Zielstorff RD (1994). National data bases: Nursing's challenge. In Carroll-Johnson RM, Paquette M (Eds.) *Classification of Nursing Diagnosis: Proceedings of the 10th Conference of the North American Nursing Diagnosis Association*. Philadelphia: JB Lippincott, pp. 34–41.

Classic References

Benoliel JQ (1977). The interaction between theory and research. *Nursing Outlook, 25*, 108–115.

Fawcett J (1978). The relationship between theory and research: A double helix. *Advances in Nursing Science, 1*, 49–62.

Jacobs MK, Huether SE (1978). Nursing science: The theory–practice linkage. *Advances in Nursing Science, 1,* 63–73.

Merton RK (1957). *Social Theory and Social Structure.* Glencoe, IL: Free Press.

Merton RK (1967). *On Theoretical Sociology.* New York: Free Press.

Miller J, Messenger S (1978). Obstacles to applying nursing research findings. *AJN, 78,* 632–634.

Rogers M (1964). *Reveille in Nursing.* Philadelphia: FA Davis.

Walker LO (1973). *Theory, Practice and Research In Perspective.* Paper presented at the American Nurses Association Ninth Annual Nursing Research Conference, San Antonio, TX.

RECOMMENDED READINGS

Barnsteiner JH (1996). Research-based practice. *Nursing Administration Quarterly, 20,* 52–58.

Feldman HR (1996). Teaching research utilization to baccalaureate nursing students. *Western J Nursing Research, 18,* 479–481.

Howell SL, Foster RL, Hester NO, Vojir CP, Miller KL (1996). Evaluating a pediatric pain management research utilization program. *Canadian J Nursing Research, 28,* 37–57.

Jaarsma T, Dasen T (1993). The relationship of nursing theory and research: The state of the art. *J Advanced Nursing, 18,* 783–787.

Lacey EA (1996). Facilitating research-based practice by educational intervention. *Nurse Education Today, 16,* 296–301.

Maeve MK (1994). The "carrier bag" theory of nursing practice. *Advances in Nursing Science, 16,* 9–22.

McSkimming SA (1996). Issues in clinical nursing research: Creating a cultural norm for research and research utilization in a clinical agency. *Western J Nursing Research, 18,* 606–610.

Newman MA (1994). Theory for nursing practice. *Nursing Science Quarterly, 7*(4), 153–157.

Stevens KA (1988). Nursing diagnosis in wellness childbearing settings. *J Obstetrical and Gynecological and Neonatal Nursing,* September-October, pp. 329–335.

Wolgin F (1996). Practice changes through research utilization. *J Nursing Staff Development, 12,* 219–220.

Zwerdling M (1994). The health care delivery system in the year 2000: Nursing care for the societal client. *Nursing and Health Care, 15,* 422–424.

PART III

Nursing Education: At the Heart of Professionalization

5

Basic Nursing Education: An Evolving System

CHAPTER OUTLINE

Development of Nursing Education
Types of Basic Nursing Education Programs
National Nursing Studies: Impact on
   Nursing Education
New Directions in Nursing Education:
   Enhancing Skills for Professional Nursing

Chapter Summary
Key Points
References
Classic References
Recommended Readings

LEARNING OBJECTIVES

▷ **1** Describe the various early traditions that have affected the preparation of nurses.

▷ **2** Understand the impact of Florence Nightingale on nursing education in the United States.

▷ **3** Discuss the development of nursing education in the United States.

▷ **4** Compare and contrast diploma schools, baccalaureate degree programs, and associate degree programs in nursing.

▷ **5** Discuss the importance and impact of selected national nursing studies on the nursing education enterprise.

▷ **6** Discuss the need for critical thinking, leadership and management, and use of nursing informatics in the nursing education curriculum.

KEY TERMS

associate degree
  (AD) programs
baccalaureate
  programs
critical thinking

diploma programs
Institute of Medicine
  (IOM) study
leadership and
  management

National Commis-
  sion on Nursing
  (NCN) study
nursing informatics
Pew Commission
  reports

The history of basic nursing education has roots extending back to the early 19th century. This rich history is filled with significant developments achieved by influential leaders, including Florence Nightingale in England and Linda Richards in America. Out of this history, three types of basic nursing education programs have developed: diploma programs, baccalaureate programs, and associate degree programs, all of which lead to the RN licensure. Several important studies conducted during the 1980s and 1990s have had a significant impact on the development of basic nursing education today and will be used to guide the preparation of nurses in years to come. In addition, new directions for nursing education are being implemented throughout the curriculum of basic nursing education to enhance the skills required for professional nursing. These new directions include critical thinking skills, leadership and management skills, and nursing informatics skills.

Development of Nursing Education

Nursing education has undergone significant developments since its inception more than two centuries ago. This is due to many factors, including key persons, societal needs, and even the crisis of war. Early traditions in nurse training, Florence Nightingale's principles for educating nurses, and the early establishment of nursing education in America all have significantly affected how nurses are educated today in the United States.

Early Traditions in the Preparation of Nurses

People have assumed the caregiving role of nurse for thousands of years. For many people (usually women), caregiving was part of their responsibility in the structure of the family or small group in which they lived. For others, providing nursing care was a calling associated with a religious command to serve others and ease the suffering of humans. In times of war, there has always been a great need for nursing care of those who are wounded, sick, and dying. The preparation of these nurses followed an apprenticeship model—that is, the learner observed a more skilled person in practice. The learner was supervised by that person and modeled his or her behavior accordingly. There was virtually no theory involved; learning was hands-on and pragmatic. If a nurse tried a new technique and it produced positive results, then it became part of his or her practice repertoire and was in turn passed along to apprentices.

Much of the selfless dedication to others that has become part of the cultural expectation for nurses can be traced back to the philosophic underpinnings of medieval religious orders whose members devoted themselves to equal portions of prayer, study, and physical labor, much of which involved caring for the sick. This produced caring, highly skilled nurses in an era when progress in knowledge and the sciences was at a virtual standstill in Western Europe. However, during the Renaissance and after, when great strides were being made in care-related knowledge in the secular world, the rigid nature of religious orders of the time caused them to lag behind in taking advantage of this new knowledge (Catalano, 1996; Kalisch & Kalisch, 1996).

Florence Nightingale: New Principles and Practices in the Education of Nurses

By the time Florence Nightingale came on the scene in the mid-19th century, nursing care in Western Europe had fallen into a state of disrepute. Hospitals were wretched places where poor unfortunates were sent to die among filth and vermin. Nursing was considered a highly undesirable occupation because the religious attendants of earlier times had been replaced by untrained lay people, often women who could find no other means of employment or criminals. Thus, it is not surprising that Florence Nightingale's very proper, very wealthy Victorian family was greatly dismayed when she expressed her desire to become a nurse.

One of the primary tasks to which Nightingale committed herself was the establishment of a school of nursing at St. Thomas' Hospital, London, in 1860. She insisted on six guiding principles that were, to that date, unique in the preparation of nurses (Box 5-1). Nightingale's efforts in establishing the school at St. Thomas' were opposed by most of London's physicians, who considered nurses to be in much the same position as housemaids; nurses, they felt, needed little instruction other than making poultices, enforcing cleanliness, and meeting patients' personal needs (Kalisch & Kalisch, 1996). However, acting with her customary determination, Nightingale succeeded in opening the school, which served as a model for similar schools throughout Europe.

 CRITICALLY THINKING ABOUT . . .

Do you think Nightingale's guiding principles are still important today? Why or why not?

Early Establishment of Nursing Education in the United States

The status of nursing in the United States in the mid-19th century was very much like that in Western Europe: sadly in need of attention and reform. A primary factor that prompted the establishment of the first hospital schools of nursing was the fact

---

Box 5-1

Six Guiding Principles for Preparation of Nurses

1. Nurses should be trained in an educational institution supported by public funds and associated with a medical school.
2. Schools for nurses should be affiliated with a hospital, but not a part of it.
3. Both theory and practice should be included in the curriculum.
4. Administration and instruction in the school should be carried out by paid professional nurses.
5. Students should be selected carefully and be required to live in supervised residences that promote discipline and character.
6. Students should be required to attend lectures, take examinations, and write papers and diaries, and written student records should be maintained.

(Notter L, Spalding E [1976]. *Professional Nursing*. Philadelphia: JB Lippincott.)

that physicians knew there was a dire need for properly trained nurses to care for their patients. At the 1868 meeting of the American Medical Association, its president, Dr. Samuel Gross, recommended the training of nurses and continued to work within the organization to foster that end. A few years later, another physician, Dr. Marie Zakrzewska, was instrumental in starting the first nurse training program in the United States. "Dr. Zak," as she was called, was born in Berlin in 1829 and became interested in medicine at a very early age. She completed study at the school for midwives at the Charité Hospital in Berlin. The knowledge and experience she gained through her education and subsequent practice encouraged her to go even further, but German medical schools refused to admit her because she was a woman. Thus, she decided to come to the United States because it provided more medical educational opportunities for women. In 1854, she met Dr. Elizabeth Blackwell, the first woman to study medicine in America (Baker, 1944). Dr. Blackwell advised the recent immigrant to learn English and also helped Zakrzewska gain admission to Western Reserve University. Zakrzewska earned her MD degree in 1856 and by 1862 had opened her own institution, the New England Hospital for Women and Children in Boston. One of its fundamental missions was the training of nurses. By 1872, the New England Hospital had a new building and had initiated the first American school for the scientific training of nurses. The first diploma was awarded to 32-year-old Linda Richards on October 1, 1873. Thus, Linda Richards was America's first professionally trained nurse (Kalisch & Kalisch, 1996).

In very short order, three American hospitals—Bellevue Hospital in New York City, the New Haven State Hospital in Connecticut, and Massachusetts General in Boston—opened nursing schools modeled after Florence Nightingale's school at St. Thomas' Hospital in London. Linda Richards played a key role in the growth and success of the early training schools affiliated with hospitals. These early hospitals followed the Nightingale model closely: although they were affiliated with a hospital, they were still autonomous organizational entities. However, this organizational differentiation soon changed, as nursing students provided a vast amount of patient care at very little cost to the hospital (Kalisch & Kalisch, 1996).

In the last quarter of the 19th century, the hospital nurse training schools enjoyed great success and experienced unparalleled growth. In 1879, there were 11 training schools in the United States; by 1900, there were 432 hospital-owned-and-operated diploma programs in America (Donahue, 1985). The programs differed in length, from 6 months to 2 years, and each school set its own standards and requirements. Unfortunately, the primary concern was not always the education of the students; the primary concern was staffing the hospital with a continuous, inexpensive source of nurses.

The training school students' work was long, physically demanding, and often demeaning. Lectures and studies were sandwiched into the students' extensive work schedules. Room and board and a small stipend were provided by the hospital. The accommodations tended to be spartan, the food often was of poor quality, and the stipend was meager. During this period, the military and religious heritage of nursing emerged fully, as illustrated in the practice of wearing a uniform, cap, pins (or badges), and sleeve stripes, all of which were symbols of honor and status in the military and in religious orders in which nursing had its roots. Each training school had its own regimented attire; in particular, the nursing cap was an identifying hallmark of each nurse's educational origins. Nurses continued to wear their caps and other parts of their nursing student uniforms with pride long after graduation. Those early nursing uniforms conveyed considerable authority and were highly respected by the public (Kalisch & Kalisch, 1996).

The early hospital nurse training schools in America would have little appeal to nursing students of today, but they accomplished some remarkable achievements. They significantly improved the educational level of, and quality of care provided by, their graduates. Also, the selectivity, discipline, and general aura of confidence that surrounded such schools transformed nursing from an occupation that was reluctantly assumed only by women from the lowest orders of society (criminals and prostitutes) to an honorable, respected occupation.

Types of Basic Nursing Education Programs

As noted above, the first diploma program for nurses in America was established in 1872. The development of nursing education did not stop there. The first baccalaureate program was established in 1909, the first associate degree program in 1952. Therefore, since 1952, there have been three paths that a student may follow to prepare for a career as an RN: a state-accredited hospital-based diploma program, a baccalaureate degree program, or an associate degree program. The programs differ in length, cost, and course of study. When a student has completed the basic program for RNs, he or she is eligible to take the National Council Licensing Examination for Registered Nurses (NCLEX-RN). Having successfully completed the NCLEX-RN, the new graduate may legally practice nursing and may use the initials "RN" after his or her name.

Many nursing leaders have expressed concern regarding the variation in programs by which students can obtain RN licensure. There is no consensus on a nationwide system of nursing education that would standardize preparation for each level of practice, and this variation in preparation for practice is seen as a barrier to the professionalization of nursing. This state of diversity is due, in large part, to the manner in which the various programs of nursing education developed. The development of each type of program will be discussed in detail below. The controversy among nurses in regard to variation in preparation for practice will be discussed in Chapter 7.

 **CRITICALLY THINKING ABOUT . . .**

> What were the most important factors that prompted you to select this type of nursing program? What led you to select this program in particular?

Commonalities Among the Three Types of Nursing Education Programs

Although any discussion of the types of nursing education programs tends to focus on the differences among the programs, Lucy Young Kelly and Lucille Joel (1996) have pointed out that these programs share some characteristics because of changes in society. First, nursing education in all programs is becoming more expensive, and financial support is decreasing for students. One result of this combination of factors is that more and more students are working long hours in addition to pursuing their nursing studies. This puts increasing pressure on students, and faculty are concerned that students simply do not have enough time to devote to their nursing studies.

Second, student populations in all types of programs have become more heterogeneous. In the mid-1970s, a study was conducted of more than 700 recent nursing graduates from all three types of basic programs. At that time, the graduates of associate degree programs looked very different from those who had obtained their basic education in either diploma or baccalaureate programs. Findings from that study, as well as a summary of studies of nursing students from the 1960s and 1970s, revealed that associate degree students tended to be older, married, and studying nursing on a part-time basis due to work and family responsibilities (Schwirian, 1979; Schwirian, 1984). However, these same characteristics are beginning to describe entering classes of baccalaureate students as well. In many cases, students entering nursing study have already earned a baccalaureate degree in another field and may be preparing for a change in career direction.

One area in which diversity has not increased substantially is in the percentages of minority students pursuing study in nursing. The percentage of minority students in all kinds of programs continues to be low.

All three types of educational programs tend to be more flexible, generally in response to these changes in the nature of the student body. Proficiency and equivalence testing, challenge examinations, self-pacing, acceptance of transfer credits, and "fast-tracking" high-ability students to facilitate their progress through the basic program and into graduate work are becoming common practices.

Another commonality among all three types of nursing education programs cited by Kelly and Joel (1996) is that state approval is required for graduates to be eligible to take the RN licensing examination, and national accreditation is available for all basic programs. Accreditation is discussed later in the consideration of ensuring the quality of nursing education programs.

Limited faculty and clinical site resources are two more commonalities among nursing programs. The basic degree expected for obtaining faculty status in the university setting is the PhD Although the number of PhD-prepared nurses continues to increase steadily, there are still insufficient numbers. Therefore, even university programs often must rely on master's-prepared faculty for most clinical teaching and supervision of students. The standard sites for clinical studies of nursing students traditionally have been community and university-affiliated hospitals and clinics. However, hospitals have downsized significantly, so there simply are not as many units and patients to which nursing students may be assigned. Also, the staff mix has changed dramatically in many hospitals, and the amount of informal RN supervision that was once available to students is no longer present. Another difficulty in obtaining sufficient, appropriate sites for clinical study arises from the fact that nursing practice is rapidly moving into the community. Therefore, students should receive increasing amounts of experience in community settings. Although developing the necessary new ties and affiliations is a great challenge, it is one that must be pursued immediately.

Another commonality among programs noted by Kelly and Joel (1996) is that recent social trends and the increasing maturity of students have prompted the faculty and administrators in many nursing programs to include students increasingly in decisions regarding curriculum and policies and procedures used to conduct the business of the school. It is common to have regular student representation on undergraduate and graduate study committees. It also is common to have a student ombudsperson who provides input to faculty and administrators via membership on an executive committee.

Finally, the learning experiences in all three types of programs include experiences in clinical settings and work with a variety of patients and clients.

Diploma School Education

Hospital training schools (diploma schools) for nurses were the first nursing schools and thus the foundation for all future nursing education. These schools were firmly established by 1900 and continued to thrive through the first third of the 20th century. In the 1920s and 1930s, there were approximately 2,000 such programs throughout the country. Until very recently, most practicing nurses in the United States were graduates of diploma schools. Since that peak period of the 1920s and 1930s, the number of diploma programs has decreased steadily: by 1995, only 122 remained in operation, most of which were located in Pennsylvania, New Jersey, and Ohio (National League for Nursing, 1995) (Tables 5-1 and 5-2).

TABLE 5-1	NUMBER OF NURSING PROGRAMS BY TYPE, 1900 TO 1995			
Year	Diploma*	Baccalaureate[†]	Associate (AD)[‡]	Total
1900	432			432
1910		1		
1920	~2000	8		
1930		15		
1940		37		
1950		73		
1958	927	171	38	1136
1960	908	172	57	1137
1967	759	219	276	1254
1970	636	267	437	1340
1975	428	326	608	1362
1980	311	377	697	1385
1985	256	441	776	1473
1990	152	489	829	1470
1995	122	509	868	1499

*Diploma programs data are from many different sources; it was not until 1958 that the National League of Nursing made things "official" and relatively consistent. The number of diploma schools skyrocketed by the 1920s and 1930s, declined through the 1960s, and then declined significantly through the 1970s, 1980s, and 1990s.
[†]Note the slow but steady growth of baccalaureate programs.
[‡]Associate degree programs: there are no data before 1958 because the AD program was not in existence before 1952–57 (when seven "experimental" programs were established and evaluated). Note the phenomenal growth, particularly in the 1960s and 1970s.
Sources:
American Association of Colleges of Nursing (1996). *Peterson's Guide to Nursing Programs,* (2nd ed.). Princeton, NJ: Peterson's.
Educational Preparation for Nursing—1960 (1961). *Nursing Outlook, 9,* 551–553.
Education Preparation for Nursing—1970 (1971). *Nursing Outlook, 19,* 604–607.
National Advisory Council on Nurse Education and Practice (1996). *Report to the Secretary of the Department of Health and Human Services.* Washington DC: U.S. Gov't Printing Office.
National League for Nursing Division of Research (1978). *NLN Nursing Data Book: Statistical Information on Nursing Education and Newly Licensed Nurses.* New York: Author.
National League for Nursing Division of Research (1987). *Nursing Data Review 1987.* New York: Author.
National League for Nursing Division of Research (1994). *Nursing Data Review 1994.* New York: Author.
National League for Nursing Division of Research (1995). *Nursing Data Review 1995.* New York: Author.

TABLE 5-2	NUMBER OF RNs GRADUATING BY PROGRAM TYPE, 1958 TO 2000

Year	Diploma	Baccalaureate	Associate (AD)	Total
1958*	26,143	3,671	425	30,239
1960	24,974	4,132	789	29,895
1967	27,170	6,122	4,639	37,931
1970	22,551	9,069	11,483	43,103
1975	21,562	20,170	32,183	73,915
1980	14,495	24,994	36,034	75,523
1985	11,892	24,975	45,208	82,075
1990	5,199	18,571	42,318	66,088
1993	6,937	24,442	56,770	88,149
2000 projection	5,387	26,492	47,785	79,664

*No systematic records available before the existence of the National League of Nursing. Note the sharp decline in diploma graduates, the steady growth in baccalaureate graduates, and the extraordinary increase in associate degree graduates.

Sources:

American Association of Colleges of Nursing (1996). *Peterson's Guide to Nursing Programs,* (2nd ed.). Princeton, NJ: Peterson's.

Educational Preparation for Nursing—1960 (1961). *Nursing Outlook, 9,* 551–553.

Education Preparation for Nursing—1970 (1971). *Nursing Outlook, 19,* 604–607.

National Advisory Council on Nurse Education and Practice (1996). *Report to the Secretary of the Department of Health and Human Services.* Washington DC: U.S. Gov't Printing Office.

National League for Nursing Division of Research (1978). *NLN Nursing Data Book: Statistical Information on Nursing Education and Newly Licensed Nurses.* New York: Author.

National League for Nursing Division of Research (1987). *Nursing Data Review 1987.* New York: Author.

National League for Nursing Division of Research (1994). *Nursing Data Review 1994.* New York: Author.

National League for Nursing Division of Research (1995). *Nursing Data Review 1995.* New York: Author.

Diploma programs owed their great success to several factors. First, American society was emerging from the Victorian era in which work outside the home was considered unseemly for respectable women. However, due to the nurturing aspect of nursing practice, nursing was one of the occupations considered acceptable and ladylike (the other was school teaching). The second appealing element of diploma nursing programs was the low cost incurred by the students' families. Third, because there were so many of these programs, the student nurse did not need to go very far from home to obtain an education. Finally, many advocates of diploma education cite the advantages of the great deal of direct patient care experience that students received from the very beginning of their program. By the time they had completed their studies and received their diplomas, these nurses were very familiar with hospital practice and routines and could fit into their full nursing responsibilities with very little orientation or extra preparation. In addition, diploma graduates were thoroughly socialized into their roles and usually held fierce loyalties to their own training hospital.

Indeed, in the study of nursing graduates referred to earlier (conducted in the mid-1970s, when there were still more than 600 diploma schools of nursing in the United States), the participants were asked why they chose the type of school they chose (associate degree, diploma, baccalaureate) and why they chose their particular school. The most common answer from the associate and diploma graduates was that it was close to home. The second most common answer for the diploma graduates was that one of their relatives (a mother, an aunt, a sister, a cousin) or one of their friends had attended that school and said it was the very best. Many went on to say that they would give the same advice to girls considering a nursing career (Schwirian, 1979).

Although diploma school graduates were highly prized for their expertise in direct patient care and thorough knowledge of hospital systems, they encountered difficulties if they decided to continue their education by obtaining a baccalaureate degree or a graduate degree, because diploma programs were not certified by the academic accrediting bodies that evaluate and accredit colleges and universities in the United States. Thus, although a diploma nurse may have engaged in 3 years of study in a very rigorous program, he or she could not receive academic credit for courses that would transfer into credits toward a degree in a college or university. In other words, the diploma nurse simply had to start all over again, even to the point of repeating many of the clinical courses he or she had already completed in the diploma program.

One approach to easing this dilemma while still providing the advantages of hospital-based nursing education has been for the hospital school to enter into agreements with nearby colleges to provide instruction in courses that are accredited and carry regular college credit. This practice then allows diploma graduates to transfer part of their credits if they choose to continue their education in an academic setting.

Table 5-1 shows the dramatic decline in the number of diploma programs in the last half of the 20th century. This decline is due to several factors. First, when the diploma schools started, qualifications for the faculty were variable. The teachers usually were nursing and medical staff who were already employed in the hospital; having them teach nursing students added little cost to the program. However, as time went on and more attention was paid to the qualifications of the teachers of nursing, the requirements became more stringent, and the costs of nurse training programs rose as well. Thus, maintaining a high-quality educational program with well-qualified faculty became a costly proposition for hospitals.

Related to the rising cost of diploma programs was a change in reimbursement policies of third-party payers such as insurance companies and the federal government. In earlier times, a hospital's cost of maintaining its nurse training program was passed along into the costs of patient care and services. However, as patient care costs rose and the health care establishment became more cost-conscious, third-party payers no longer were willing to reimburse those "pass-along" costs. Therefore, the rising, nonrecoverable cost of diploma programs changed them from financial assets to financial liabilities.

Another major factor that pulled potential students from diploma schools was the remarkable increase in the availability of associate degree programs that started in the mid-1950s. A final reason that diploma training schools became less popular is that American society in general has increasing expectations regarding higher education. The goal for more and more people is a college education rather than limited technical training. Nurses themselves are increasingly recognizing that a baccalaureate education is the minimum preparation necessary to function successfully in the increasingly complex, competitive, and rapidly changing world of American health care.

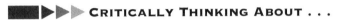 CRITICALLY THINKING ABOUT . . .

Is there a role for diploma schools of nursing today?

Baccalaureate Degree Education

The first program to be considered a **baccalaureate program** in the United States was founded as part of the school of medicine at the University of Minnesota in 1909. This program was modeled closely after the three-year diploma programs that dominated the field at that time. By 1919, 7 more baccalaureate programs had been established (Conley, 1973). An examination of the 1996 edition of *Peterson's Guide to Nursing Programs* (American Association of Colleges of Nursing, 1996) reveals that according to the founding dates given for each of the 625 baccalaureate programs listed, growth remained slow through the first half of the 20th century. The slow growth of baccalaureate programs in the early years can be attributed to several factors:

- ◘ Universities were reluctant to accept nursing as an academic discipline (Chitty, 1997).
- ◘ The number of faculty members who were qualified to teach in university settings was small (Creasia & Parker, 1996).
- ◘ The diploma schools held overwhelming power (Chitty, 1997, p. 38).
- ◘ University education in any field was far more expensive than training in a diploma program.
- ◘ Many of the first generation of baccalaureate programs were 5 years long (3 years of nursing education and 2 years of study devoted to the liberal arts).

Despite initially slow growth in the early 20th century, there has been a steady growth in both numbers of programs and in the programs' influence within the health care environment. The greatest growth in the number of baccalaureate programs has occurred since 1960—nearly a fourfold increase in the number of programs (see Tables 5-1 and 5-2). The quality of the faculties of baccalaureate nursing programs in terms of academic credentials and scholarly productivity also has improved dramatically, especially within the last two decades. Most nursing faculty teaching in baccalaureate programs of nursing today are doctorally prepared members of the academic community. Increasing numbers of nursing faculty provide significant leadership in their universities at large, and many nurses are moving into powerful administrative positions in leading universities all over the country.

The traditional or generic baccalaureate nursing program in nursing is a 4-year program of study in an accredited college or university. Students must meet the same kinds of general education (liberal education) requirements as all the other students to earn their baccalaureate degrees. The nursing program also includes professional education and clinical training for nursing practice. These generic programs are designed primarily for students with no prior nursing experience. Students may be admitted either as freshmen or after the successful completion of 1 or 2 years of "prenursing" requirements (eg, chemistry, nutrition, communications, sociology, psychology, mathematics, history, and humanities). Selection into an upper-division nursing major often is competitive in terms of achievement in the prenursing courses, high-school grade point averages, and ACT and SAT scores. This selectivity allows the school or college of nursing to admit only the academically strongest prenursing students. In addition to theoretical foundations for nursing and clinical nursing practice itself, curricula in baccalaureate programs include nurse leadership, health promotion, mental health, community health, medical and surgical care, psychiatric care, and management. Baccalaureate students typically gain experience in supervised clinical practice in a variety of settings—hospitals, nursing homes, community health agencies, and mental health facilities (Amos, 1996).

Many baccalaureate nursing programs provide "re-entry" programs of study designed for practicing RNs who obtained their basic nursing education at a diploma school or an associate degree program. These are made available to RNs who have determined that the career path they wish to pursue requires a baccalaureate degree as a minimum. Re-entry programs vary widely in terms of requirements and the credits given for students' prior education and experience. Thus, RNs with diploma or associate degree training who wish to continue their education have many choices.

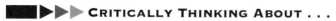 **CRITICALLY THINKING ABOUT . . .**

> Should baccalaureate students be admitted directly into the nursing major, or should they complete most of their liberal studies and then concentrate on nursing as an upper-division major? Why?

Baccalaureate Education: Requirement for Entry Into Practice?

For many years, nursing leaders have identified the importance of requiring baccalaureate preparation for entry into nursing practice. Preparation for nursing, like the preparation for any other profession, belongs in institutions of higher education. Chapter 1 documented study after study (starting as early as 1923) that reiterated that same call. Nevertheless, the American Nurses Association (ANA) created a great furor in 1965 when it published the position paper *Educational Preparation for Nurse Practitioners and Assistants to Nurses.* Some nurses consider this paper the most significant influence on the growth of baccalaureate education in nursing up to that time.

In this position paper, the ANA made it very clear that baccalaureate education must become the basic foundation for professional practice. Moreover, it asserted that students receiving associate degrees were not appropriately prepared for professional nursing practice, but rather were prepared for technical nursing practice. This position elicited strong, vocal opposition on many fronts, including the large number of diploma graduates (who perceived the ANA's position as an insult and a threat) and many physicians (who believed that nurses already were overeducated). However, the ANA maintained its position, and 20 years later it made that position even stronger by adding two additional propositions. First, two levels of nursing practice were to be identified, along with defined competencies for each level, by 1980. Second, by 1985, the minimum preparation for entry into professional practice was to be the baccalaureate degree in nursing (ANA, 1979). Both of these propositions have yet to be implemented well over a decade later. This issue— whether the baccalaureate degree should be the entry into practice—is discussed in detail in Chapter 7.

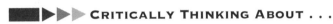 CRITICALLY THINKING ABOUT . . .

Should a baccalaureate degree be required for entry into nursing practice? Why or why not?

Associate Degree Education

Associate degree programs in nursing have taken on a great deal of importance in nursing education and nursing practice during the last half-century. It is unlikely that the current role and function of associate degree programs was either envisioned or intended by the founder of these programs, Mildred Montag. In 1951, Montag completed her doctoral dissertation, in which she described a nursing technician who would be able to perform nursing functions that were much more prescribed and narrower in scope that those of a professional nurse but broader in scope than those of a practical nurse (Montag, 1951). The need for this type of nurse on the nursing care team was seen as very important at that time due to three primary factors:

1. After World War II, there was a tremendous expansion in the hospital industry, including private hospitals, public hospitals, and the Veterans Administration system.
2. The number of diploma programs and graduates had leveled off.
3. The number of baccalaureate nursing programs had not yet begun to climb substantially.

This combination of factors created a great need for more nurses. Therefore, Montag proposed the creation of a new nursing role, the technical nurse. In January 1952, Dr. Louise McManus, director of the Division of Nursing Education at Teachers College, Columbia University, announced a 5-year project aimed at developing and evaluating nursing education programs in junior colleges and community colleges. McManus named Mildred Montag, then an assistant professor of nursing education at Teachers College, as the project coordinator. The purpose of the experiment was to determine if it was feasible to prepare bedside nurses for beginning general-duty positions in a 2-year program (Kalisch & Kalisch, 1996).

Seven community junior colleges were chosen to participate in the experiment. The curriculum of these first programs consisted of about one-third general education and two-thirds nursing education (75% of which was clinical practice). The results of the experiment demonstrated that the associate degree programs were a success: 91.7% of the graduates passed their state board examinations the first time, compared to 90.5% of graduates from all types of nursing programs. Moreover, follow-up evaluation of the program revealed that head nurses described the performance of the associate degree graduates as good as, or better than, recent graduates of other programs in 80% of the cases. It was concluded that a 2-year nursing program could prepare an RN, and it could become an integral part of a community college program (Kalisch & Kalisch, 1996).

This was the beginning of the era of associate degree education for RNs, the first nursing education program to be developed with a systematic plan using carefully controlled experimentation (Kelly & Joel, 1996).

Table 5-1 shows the dramatic growth in the number of associate degree programs, from the 7 experimental schools established in the Columbia project in 1952 to the 868 programs in 1995. Even more dramatic is the increase in the number of graduates from associate degree schools (see Table 5-2). In 1960, associate degree programs produced less than 1,000 graduates; only 10 years later, they were producing well over 11,000 graduates, and that figure continues to climb.

Although the ANA doubtless would have it otherwise, it is clear that the "degree of choice" for entry into nursing practice is the 2-year associate degree program, and it is the fastest-growing segment of nursing education. In its 1996 national sample survey of RNs, the Division of Nursing found that among all employed RNs, 34.6% held the associate degree as their highest degree (Division of Nursing, 1997).

Associate degree programs have grown rapidly since the 1960s for several of the same reasons that diploma programs flourished early in the century:

- ▶ A desperate need for competently trained nurses
- ▶ Low cost to students
- ▶ Geographic accessibility
- ▶ Shorter time required to complete the program than baccalaureate programs

Economic and demographic factors also help explain the rapid growth of associate degree programs. By the early 1960s, the "baby boom" generation reached the age for higher education, and so demand grew. Institutions of higher education grew faster to meet the demand. Moreover, the economy was robust and ready and able to support such expansion in both private and public sectors. It was in the public sector that the associate degree programs benefited hugely. The philosophy spread rapidly that all students who desired higher education should have that opportunity; it should be available in their own community (or a community nearby); and a substantial amount of the support for such education should be public in nature, thereby making education affordable. Two-year community colleges and junior colleges sprung up like mushrooms all over the country, and associate degree nursing programs sprung up with them. Thus, associate degree programs provided preparation for nursing practice that was close to home, was the shortest route to RN licensure, and was low in cost; moreover, none of the cost had to be passed along to patients.

Over time, there have been changes in the philosophy and curricula of associate degree programs. Montag conceived of the program as leading to a terminal degree. Current trends in education, however, include opportunities for associate degree graduates to avail themselves of the higher degree and broader preparation afforded by baccalaureate programs. Some associate degree programs make it clear to students that the associate degree is only the first stepping stone. However, the National Advisory Council on Nurse Education and Practice reported in 1996 that only about 14% of associate degree nurses in practice had gone on for a baccalaureate degree (National Advisory Council on Nurse Education and Practice, 1996).

Montag viewed the job of the associate degree graduate to be technical in nature, free of administrative and leadership responsibilities. In practice, however, associate degree nurses are given the same kinds of responsibilities and leadership assignments as baccalaureate graduates.

Even the name of nurses prepared in associate degree programs has changed. Montag referred to the graduates as "technical nurses," but the use of that term was rejected by the National League of Nursing Council of Associate Degree Programs in 1976 because it implied a status lower than that of a nurse designated as "professional." Since 1976, the term most frequently used is "associate degree" (or AD) nurse.

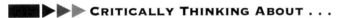 **CRITICALLY THINKING ABOUT . . .**

Today, associate degree programs produce more graduates than any other type of program. What effects does this have on the professionalization of nursing?

National Nursing Studies: Impact on Nursing Education

Important studies on nursing needs, resources, and recommendations for the future of nursing and nursing education were discussed in Chapter 1. These studies are significant, but the recommendations they suggested were not followed and remain buried in the pages of nursing history. However, three nursing studies conducted in the 1980s and 1990s have had a major influence on practices and trends in nursing practice and education and probably will continue to do so:

- ☐ Institute of Medicine study
- ☐ National Commission on Nursing study
- ☐ Pew Health Professions Commission reports.

Institute of Medicine Study

In the late 1970s, there was a shortage of nurses despite both the tremendous growth of associate degree programs and a considerable infusion of federal funds to support nursing education. This created serious debates within the federal government about the need for continued federal aid for nursing education. To bring those debates to an end, Congress mandated in 1979 that a study on nursing and nursing education be conducted by the Institute of Medicine (IOM) of the National Academy of Sciences (IOM, 1983). Congress established four main objectives for the **Institute of Medicine study:**

1. Make recommendations regarding future federal support of nursing education
2. Identify why more nurses do not choose employment in medically underserved areas
3. Determine if and why nurses do not remain in nursing
4. Recommend measures to improve the supply and proper use of nursing resources (U.S. Bureau of Health Manpower, 1979).

In general, the IOM committee determined that the "nursing shortage" was not a shortage at all, but rather a problem of maldistribution of nursing services. The two-year study generated 21 specific recommendations to Congress, most of which had a direct impact on programs of nursing education. These recommendations formed the basis on which nursing policy and funding would be determined throughout the remainder of the 1980s. Some of the most significant recommendations were:

▶ Federal efforts to increase the supply of generalist nurses should be discontinued.

▶ Nurse educators should be encouraged to attract late-entry and minority students in greater numbers.

▶ Opportunities for educational advancement of nurses by facilitating the movement of nurses from one educational level to the next should be improved.

▶ The government should expand its support of fellowships and loans at the graduate level because of continued shortage of RNs prepared for leadership at the graduate level.

One of the most important recommendations in terms of contributing to the continuing professionalization of nursing was recommendation 18: "The federal government should establish an organizational entity to place nursing research in the mainstream of scientific investigation" (IOM, 1983, p. 19). The IOM report is seen as a strong influence on the subsequent establishment of the National Center for Nursing Research in 1986.

 **CRITICALLY THINKING ABOUT . . .**

> The U.S. Congress played a primary role in establishing the objectives for the IOM study it commissioned in the early 1980s. Was this an appropriate action for the government to take?

National Commission on Nursing Study

In 1980, the American Hospital Association appointed the National Commission on Nursing (NCN). The formation of this group was prompted by concern for the "nursing shortage," much like the IOM study. However, the sponsorship (by the American Hospital Association) and composition of this group meant that it would have a different perspective than the IOM study, which was funded by the federal government and was composed heavily of "academic types." The NCN, under the direction of Marjorie Beyers, RN, was established to address nursing-related problems and nursing education issues in the United States and to make recommendations for the future. The committee consisted of 31 members, including nurses and representatives of hospital administration, medicine, business, government, and academia.

The **National Commission on Nursing Study** contained 18 recommendations (NCN, 1983), the most significant of which were:

▶ A need for all three types of nursing programs, with baccalaureate education as an achievable goal

▶ Educational mobility for nurses

▶ Nursing research and strong affiliations between academic institutions and practice settings should be given high priority.

▶ Nurses should regularly be involved in hospital policy making.

▶ Nurses' salaries and benefits should be commensurate with their education, experience, and performance.

One thing the NCN specifically did *not* recommend was that nurses with different educational backgrounds should be used in different ways.

Pew Health Professions Commission Reports

Between 1991 and 1995, the Pew Health Professions Commission produced three reports, which are likely to have more impact on health care education and health care policy than any other series of documents and reports discussed so far. One reason these reports will be so influential is that they span a period in which the health care system in the United States has undergone a complete transformation. The magnitude and speed of change were largely unexpected by most people, including health care professionals. Health care institutions and educators know that changes must be made but are greatly undecided about what those changes must be. The **Pew Commission reports** undoubtedly will provide guidelines to educators, health care institutions, and policy makers for years to come.

In their first report, *Healthy America: Practitioners for 2005* (1991), the Pew Commission set forth "17 competencies describing skills and attitudes needed by the health care providers of the 21st century" (Pew Health Professions Commission, 1995, p. 1). The second report, *Health Professions Education for the Future: Schools in Service to the Nation* (1993), outlined "specific reform strategies for each of the health professions at a time when a national consensus on reforming the health care system seemed imminent" (Pew Health Professions Commission, 1995, p. 1). These first two reports "affirmed that the education and training of health professionals were out of step with the health needs of the American people and offered tools of reform suited to the time and tasks at hand" (Pew Health Professions Commission, 1995, p. 1). In 1993, the commission characterized the emerging health care system as having 10 primary characteristics, the most important of which were:

- ☐ An orientation toward health
- ☐ Intensive use of information and information systems
- ☐ A focus on the consumer
- ☐ A high degree of accountability and interdependence among players in the health care system.

By 1995, the transformations in the health care system that had seemed distant probabilities in the first year of the Pew Commission were well underway, and a clearer image of the reformed health care system had emerged. This system makes dramatically different demands on health care education and health care educators. Accordingly, the 1995 Pew Commission report, *Critical Challenges: Revitalizing the Health Profession for the 21st Century*, provides succinct recommendations for each of the health care professions, including seven general recommendations for nursing (Box 5-2). The commission directed nursing to clarify the practice responsibilities of nurses prepared at different levels. Associate degree nurse preparation should focus on entry-level hospital care and nursing home practice; baccalaureate preparation should focus on hospital-based care management and community-based practice. Nurses prepared at the master's degree level should be prepared for specialty practice in the hospital and independent practice as primary care providers. The commission also recommended reducing the size and number of nursing education programs by 10% to 20%; the programs that should be closed are associate and diploma programs. The number of nurse practitioner programs should be expanded by increasing the level of federal support for students.

Box 5-2

Seven Recommendations of the 1995 Pew Health Commissions Report

1. Recognize the value of the multiple entry points to professional practice available to nurses through preparation in associate, baccalaureate, and master's programs; each is different, and each has important contributions to make in the changing health care system.
2. Consolidate the professional nomenclature so that there is a single title for each level of nursing preparation and service.
3. Distinguish between the practice responsibilities of these different levels of nursing, focusing associate preparation on the entry-level hospital setting and nursing home practice, baccalaureate on hospital-based care management and community-based practice, and master's degree on specialty practice in the hospital and independent practice as a primary care provider. Strengthen existing career ladder programs to make movement through these levels of nursing as easy as possible.
4. Reduce the size and number of nursing education programs (1470 basic nursing programs as of 1990) by 10% to 20%. These closings should come in associate and diploma degree programs. These closings should pay attention to the reality that some areas have a shortage of educational programs and many more have a surplus.
5. Encourage the expansion of the number of master's level nurse practitioner training programs by increasing the level of federal support for students.
6. Develop new models of integration between education and the highly managed and integrated systems of care that can provide nurses with an appropriate training and clinical practice opportunity and that model flexible work rules that encourage continual improvement, innovation, and health care work redesign.
7. Recover the clinical management role of nursing and recognize it as an increasingly important strength of training and professional practice at all levels.

Obviously, these seven recommendations of the 1995 Pew Commission report will have powerful and far-reaching effects on nursing practice, nursing education, and the health care system as a whole.

 CRITICALLY THINKING ABOUT . . .

> The Pew Commission has recommended reducing the number of nursing education programs by 10% to 20%. Does this make sense to you? Explain.

New Directions in Nursing Education: Enhancing Skills for Professional Nursing

As we enter the 21st century, it is clear that the challenges to nursing education and nursing educators have never been greater. This is due primarily to the fact that the practice of nursing in the workplace is changing dramatically. These changes in nursing practice are occurring so rapidly that educators may have absolutely no idea of the nursing practice realities for which they are preparing their students. The old ways with which nursing educators have been comfortable for many years are being sorely challenged. The ways in which students obtain their education and move toward increasing professionalization are changing significantly. Even the colleges and universities in which baccalaureate programs are located are undergoing remarkable organizational and fiscal management changes, often generating challenges so great that the very existence of nursing programs is threatened.

Although this scenario may seem extremely bleak, careful consideration of the myriad of changes and challenges reveals some things that must be addressed in preparing students to practice nursing in today's health care setting. Moreover, there is a body of nursing research that provides some data to help educators make the right decisions and the most productive changes. Three of these new directions in nursing education include:

- ▶ Critical thinking skills
- ▶ Leadership and management skills
- ▶ Use of nursing informatics.

Critical Thinking Skills

Well-developed **critical thinking skills** are essential in making competent clinical decisions. The growing recognition of the importance of developing critical thinking among nursing students is reflected in the recent publication of two books focused specifically on the topic (LeMone & Burke, 1996; Rubenfeld, 1995). We have known for a long time that critical thinking is important. In fact, graduate nurses are expected to hone their critical decision-making skills to a fine edge in a very short time in the practice environment. However, traditional models of curriculum and instruction have obstructed the development of critical thinking. Since 1982, various studies have been performed to evaluate nursing students' critical thinking ability. Some of the findings include:

- ▶ Critical thinking ability is not associated with age or other demographics *per se* (Lynch, 1988; Waite, 1989); instead, critical thinking ability is associated with standard measures of academic achievement (Kokinda, 1989; Lynch, 1988; Waite, 1989).
- ▶ Critical thinking skills were higher among baccalaureate students than among associate degree students (Lynch, 1988), but these critical thinking skills did not change from entry to completion in a baccalaureate program. Therefore, simply spending time in a baccalaureate program does not necessarily make the difference in critical thinking ability (Kintgen-Andrews, 1991; Maynard, 1996; Saucier, 1995).
- ▶ There were no differences in critical thinking skills between groups of students exposed to different nursing curriculum models in baccalaureate programs (Waite, 1989).
- ▶ Critical thinking seems to thrive in learning environments that are not teacher-centered (Newsome, 1989; Sweeney, 1986).
- ▶ Critical thinking is enhanced when students use interactive videodisc technology compared to traditional lectures, the ultimate teacher-centered modality (Klaassens, 1992).

▶ A combination of computer-assisted instruction and a clinical collaboration model in which the student, faculty member, and unit nurse worked as a care team proved effective in developing critical thinking skills (Perciful, 1996).

▶ Critical thinking skills were superior among people who had more actual life experiences (eg, graduates who had entered actual practice [Maynard, 1996] and nontraditional students in a baccalaureate program). These nontraditional students were older, had taken more time between high school and college, and tended to be married and have children. In short, they simply had more direct life experiences (Corder, 1992).

Together, these findings lead one to the conclusion that being actively engaged in the subject matter in some way is the key to fostering critical thinking at any age and in any discipline. Traditional, teacher-centered methods of instruction that rely on learner compliance and passivity must be supplanted by approaches that actively engage the learner if we are to produce nurses who can meet the challenges of nursing practice in today's health care setting.

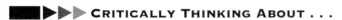 **CRITICALLY THINKING ABOUT . . .**

> Describe the learning activities that enhanced your critical thinking skills during your nursing education.

Leadership and Management Skills

Not very long ago, nursing educators did not need to incorporate significant amounts of content and experience regarding **leadership and management** into undergraduate curricula. Certainly, leadership and management skills were expected of nurses in practice, but those expectations were focused on nurses who had already had extensive experience in practice or nurses who had obtained a graduate degree. This is no longer the case. One of the biggest changes in patient care in hospitals is the use of unlicensed assistive personnel in conjunction with RNs. These patient care teams are under the direct supervision of the RN on the team; thus, the RN is the person accountable for the patient outcomes resulting from any procedures or activities carried out by the unlicensed members of the team.

Unfortunately, little guidance can be obtained from the nursing research literature at this time in terms of preparing undergraduate students for effective leadership roles as they enter nursing practice. Health care systems have changed so fast that this phenomenon is simply too new for data-based information to have accumulated. However, within the last 20 years, a considerable amount of literature regarding the preparation of more experienced, graduate-level nursing students for leadership and management has blossomed. Therefore, the best strategy for nursing educators would be to collect the literature and related research on leadership in nursing practice, adapt it as appropriate, and incorporate it as a regular component of the undergraduate curriculum.

However, incorporating concepts of leadership and management for baccalaureate students must reach farther than the classroom. These concepts must be integrated into the clinical experiences of undergraduate students at all points in their program of study.

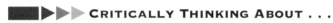 CRITICALLY THINKING ABOUT . . .

How do you feel about assuming leadership and management responsibilities shortly after you have entered nursing practice?

Nursing Informatics Utilization Skills

In **nursing informatics**, nurses use computer technology and management of information to facilitate practice and enhance nursing knowledge (Saba & McCormick, 1996, p. 222). The importance of the ability of practicing nurses to use computers in support of care delivery cannot be emphasized too strongly. Chapter 4 discussed the importance of using nursing information systems in developing the knowledge base for nursing. Nurses who are fortunate enough to be part of that movement must be skilled in the use of computer technology to take full advantage of it and make their own contributions. Almost all nurses will be working in facilities that have some kind of computer-based nursing information system for entry and management of patient and treatment data. New graduates must be ready and willing to put those systems to the best use.

Nursing research data and reports of nursing informatics-related activities suggest that progress is being made in incorporating computer-based activities into undergraduate nursing education. Applications included creating care plans (Doorley, Renner, & Corron, 1994), respiratory assessment (Bratt & Vockell, 1986), and computer-based clinical evaluation tools (Cottrell, Ritchie, Cox, Rumph, Klesey, & Shannahan, 1986). It also has been shown that using computer-assisted instruction materials enhances the effectiveness of student learning (Halloran, 1995; Belfry & Winne, 1988; Boyle & Ahijevych, 1987; Bratt & Vockell, 1986). Nursing faculty members believe that students should have the following computer knowledge:

- How computers work in general
- Ability to use computer-assisted instruction effectively
- Skills in word processing and statistical analysis
- Ability to use hospital information systems effectively (Bryson, 1991).

Various studies evaluating nursing students and computers have shown that simply using computers enhances students' skills (Birx, Castleberry, & Perry, 1996) and that computer applications generally are well received by students (Birx, Castleberry, & Perry, 1996; Jacobson, Holder, & Dearner, 1989; Schwirian, Malone, Stone, Nunley, & Francisco, 1989). Students have shown the strongest preference for learning computer applications for clinical practice and less interest in learning about applications for education and administration (Dover & Boblin, 1991). The consensus of all of the findings is that informatics should be an important part of the undergraduate experience and that students are positive about the field and are benefiting from it.

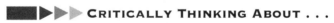 CRITICALLY THINKING ABOUT . . .

Have you had experience with computerized nursing information systems? If so, describe that experience. If not, how are you going to go about getting the experience you will need in practice?

▶ CHAPTER SUMMARY

The growth and development of the nursing education enterprise in the United States in the past century has been nothing less than phenomenal. It has essentially gone through three eras, with a different type of nursing education program being prominent in each era. First came the diploma schools, which laid the foundation for nursing education. Next were the baccalaureate programs, and while they were still developing, the associate degree programs emerged and flourished in the mid-20th century. The diploma schools have been declining since World War II, and now the associate degree programs are the most plentiful, producing 59% of today's nurses. Although only about 25% of the current RN workforce obtained their initial nursing education in baccalaureate programs, these programs provide the broadest background for nursing practice because the study of humanities, science, and the liberal arts are incorporated along with nursing studies (National Advisory Council on Nursing Education and Practice, 1996). In addition, a baccalaureate degree in nursing is a requirement for admission to graduate study in nursing, and we are now entering an era in which preparation for graduate study is becoming recognized as essential to the professionalization of nursing. Thus, a primary challenge to nursing is to give nurses with less than a baccalaureate degree the opportunity to study so that they, too, will be prepared to engage in professional nursing practice in the 21st century.

KEY POINTS

▶ 1 The early traditions that affected nursing preparation included the traditional female role of caregiver, philosophical underpinnings of religious orders, and hands-on, pragmatic apprenticeship roles that occurred during times of war.

▶ 2 Florence Nightingale developed six guiding principles for training nurses that were, to that date, unique. These principles were: nurses should be trained in an educational institution associated with a medical school and supported by public funds; nursing schools should be affiliated with a hospital, but not a part of it; both theory and practice should be part of the curriculum; administration and instruction should be carried out by paid, professional nurses; students should be selected carefully and be required to live in supervised residences that promote discipline and character; and students should attend lectures, take examinations, and write papers and diaries, and written student records should be maintained.

▶ 3 The development of nursing education in the United States is greatly indebted to the insight of Dr. Marie Zakrzewska. "Dr. Zak" opened the first American school for the scientific training of nurses in 1872. In very short order, three more American hospitals opened schools of nursing, modeled closely after Florence Nightingale's school. These hospital-based nurse training schools experienced unparalleled growth in the last quarter of the 19th century, and by 1900 there were 432 such schools in America.

▶ **4** Some of the ways in which the three types of basic nursing programs are similar are that nursing students in all types of programs are generally older, married, and studying nursing on a part-time basis; all educational programs tend to be more flexible; and all educational programs enable the student to take the RN licensure examination. Some of the ways in which they differ is in the length of time it takes to complete the program; the cost of the program; the classes taken; the academic credentials of nursing instructors or professors; admission standards; and the level of skills and knowledge gained.

▶ **5** There have been several significant nursing studies in the 1980s and 1990s regarding the trends in nursing practice and education. These studies include the Institute of Medicine study, the National Commission on Nursing study, and the Pew Health Professions Commission reports.

▶ **6** Nurses in practice are increasingly required to have strong skills in critical thinking, leadership and management, and nursing informatics. Therefore, these skills must be taught in nursing education programs. There is a large and growing body of research directed toward the enhancement of students' skills for truly professional nursing practice.

REFERENCES

American Association of Colleges of Nursing (1996). *Peterson's Guide to Nursing Programs* (2d ed.). Princeton, NJ: Peterson's.

American Nurses Association (1979). *A Case for Baccalaureate Preparation in Nursing.* (Publication No. NE-6 15M). Kansas City, MO: Author.

Amos LK (1996). Baccalaureate programs. In *Peterson's Guide to Nursing Programs,* (2d ed.). Princeton, NJ: Peterson's.

Birx E, Castleberry K, Perry K (1996). Integration of laptop computer technology into an undergraduate nursing course. *Computers in Nursing, 14,* 108–112.

Belfry MJ, Winne PH (1988). A review of the effectiveness of computer assisted instruction in nursing education. *Computers in Nursing, 6,* 77–85.

Boyle KK, Ahijevych K (1987). Using computers to promote health behavior of nursing students. *Nurse Educator, 12*(3), 33–38.

Bratt E, Vockell E (1986). Using computers to teach basic facts in the nursing curriculum. *J Nursing Education, 25,* 247–251.

Bryson DM (1991). The computer-literate nurse. *Computers in Nursing, 9,* 100–107.

Catalano JT (1996). *Contemporary Professional Nursing.* Philadelphia: FA Davis.

Chitty KK (1997). *Professional Nursing: Concepts and Challenges.* Philadelphia: WB Saunders.

Corder JB (1992). The association among critical thinking, clinical decision-making, and selected demographic characteristics of generic baccalaureate students (doctoral dissertation, University of Alabama at Birmingham, 1992). *Dissertation Abstracts International, 53-12,* 6219.

Cottrell BH, Ritchie PJ, Cox BH, Rumph EA, Kelsey SJ, Shannahan MK (1986). A clinical evaluation tool for nursing students based on the nursing process. *J Nursing Education, 25,* 270–274.

Creasia JL, Parker B (1996). *Conceptual Foundations of Professional Nursing Practice* (2nd ed.). St. Louis: Mosby.

Division of Nursing (1997). Advance notes from the national sample survey of registered nurses, March 1996. Rockville, MD: Author.

Donahue MP (1985). *Nursing: The Finest Art.* St. Louis: CV Mosby.

Doorley JE, Renner AL, Corron J (1994). Creating care plans via modems: Using a hospital information system in nursing education. *Computers in Nursing, 13,* 285–288.

Dover LV, Boblin S (1991). Student nurse computer experience and preferences for learning. *Computers in Nursing, 9,* 75–79.

Halloran L (1995). A comparison of two methods of teaching. Computer managed instruction and keypad questions versus traditional classroom lecture. *Computers in Nursing, 13,* 285–288.

Institute of Medicine, Health Care Services Division, Nursing and Nursing Education Committee (1983). *Nursing and Nursing Education: Public Policies and Private Actions.* Washington DC: National Academy Press.

Jacobson SF, Holder ME, Dearner JF (1989). Computer anxiety among nursing students, educators, staff and administrators. *Computers in Nursing, 7,* 266–272.

Kalisch PA, Kalisch BJ (1996). *The Advance of American Nursing* (3rd ed.). Philadelphia: JB Lippincott.

Kelly LY, Joel LA (1996). *The Nursing Experience: Trends, Challenges and Transitions* (3d ed.). New York: McGraw-Hill.

Kintgen-Andrews J (1991). Critical thinking and nursing education: Perplexities and insights. *J Nursing Education, 30*(4), 152–157.

Klaassens EL (1992). Evaluation of interactive videodisc simulations designed for nursing to determine their ability to provide problem-solving practice based on the use of the nursing process (doctoral dissertation, Northern Illinois University, DeKalb, 1992). *Dissertation Abstracts International, 54-01,* 0075.

Kokinda MA (1989). The measurement of critical thinking skills in a selected baccalaureate nursing program (doctoral dissertation, University of Pennsylvania, Philadelphia, 1989). *Dissertation Abstracts International, 50-09,* 2709.

LeMone P, Burke K (1996). *Medical-Surgical Nursing: Critical Thinking in Client Care.* Menlo Park, CA: Addison-Wesley Nursing.

Lynch MH (1989). A measurement of critical thinking in senior baccalaureate nursing students (doctoral dissertation, Marquette University, 1989). *Dissertation Abstracts International, 53-12,* 6219.

Maynard CA (1996). Relationship of critical thinking ability to professional nursing competence. *J Nursing Education, 35*(1), 12–18.

National Advisory Council on Nurse Education and Practice (1996). *Report to the Secretary of the Department of Health and Human Services.* Washington DC: U.S. Government Printing Office.

National Commission on Nursing (1983). *Summary Report and Recommendations.* Chicago: American Hospital Association.

National League for Nursing (1995). *State-Approved Schools of Nursing RN 1995* (Publication No. 19-2689). New York: Author.

Newsome GG (1989). A comparison of the effects of guided design and lecture teaching strategies on the ability of student nurses to solve problems in the clinical setting (doctoral dissertation, University of Georgia, Athens, 1989). *Dissertation Abstracts International, 50-10,* 3144.

Perciful EG (1996). The effect of an innovative clinical teaching method on nursing students' knowledge and critical thinking skills. *J Nursing Education, 35,* 23–28.

Pew Health Professions Commission (1991). *Healthy America: Practitioners for 2005.* San Francisco: UCSF Center for the Health Professions.

Pew Health Professions Commission (1993). *Health Professions Education for the Future: Schools in Service to the Nation.* San Francisco: UCSF Center for the Health Professions.

Pew Health Professions Commission (1995). *Critical Challenges: Revitalizing the Health Professions for the 21st Century.* San Francisco: UCSF Center for the Health Professions.

Rubenfeld MG (1995). *Critical Thinking in Nursing: An Interactive Approach.* Philadelphia: JB Lippincott.

Saba V, McCormick K (1996). *Essentials of computers for nurses.* New York: McGraw-Hill Books.

Saucier BL (1995). Critical thinking skills of baccalaureate nursing students. *J Professional Nursing,* *11,* 351–357.

Schwirian PM (1979). *Prediction of Successful Nursing Performance, Part 3: Evaluation and Prediction of the Performance of Recent Nurse Graduates.* Department of Health, Education and Welfare Publication No. HRA 79-15. Washington DC: U.S. Government Printing Office.

Schwirian PM (1984). Research on nursing students. In Werley HH, Fitzpatrick JJ (Eds.), *Annual Review of Nursing Research, vol. 2.* New York: Springer, pp. 211–237.

Schwirian PM, Malone JA, Stone VJ, Nunley B, Francisco T (1989). Computers in nursing practice: A comparison of the attitudes of nurses and nursing students. *Computers in Nursing, 7,* 168–177.

Sweeney JF (1986). Nurse education: Learner-centered or teacher-centered? *Nurse Education Today, 6,* 257–262.

U.S. Bureau of Health Manpower (1979). *Second Report to the Congress March 15, 1979* [Revised] *Nurse Training Act of 1975.* DHEW Publ. No. HRA 79-45. Hyattsville, MD: The Bureau.

Waite RMI (1989). *A Measurement of Critical Thinking in Senior Baccalaureate Nursing Students.* Unpublished doctoral dissertation, Marquette University, Milwaukee.

Classic References

American Nurses Association (1965). *A Position Paper: Educational Preparation for Nurse Practitioners and Assistants to Nurses.* Kansas City, MO: ANA.

Baker R (1944). *The First Woman Doctor: The Story of Elizabeth Blackwell MD.* New York: Julian Messner Inc.

Conley V (1973). *Curriculum and Instruction in Nursing.* Boston: Little, Brown.

Montag M (1951). *The Education of Nursing Technicians.* New York: GP Putnam's Sons.

Notter L, Spalding E (1976). *Professional Nursing: Foundations, Perspectives and Relationships* (9th ed.). Philadelphia: JB Lippincott.

RECOMMENDED READINGS

Bevis EO, Krulik T (1991). Nationwide faculty development: A model for a shift from diploma to baccalaureate education. *J Advanced Nursing, 16,* 362–370.

Bollenberg R (1991). Differentiated practice: Another threat to the LPN? *J Practical Nursing,* September, pp. 36–37.

Bowles K (1991). Health care trends: A call for advanced knowledge and skills in baccalaureate students. *Focus on Critical Care AACN, 18,* 465–468.

BSN enrollments are falling at a faster rate: AACN finds biggest losses in generic students. *AJN,* April 1987: 529, 542.

Fagin CM, Lynaugh JE (1992). Reaping the rewards of radical change: A new agenda for nursing education. *Nursing Outlook, 40,* 213–220.

Fitzpatrick JM, While AE, Roberts JD (1993). The relationship between nursing and higher education. *J Advanced Nursing, 18,* 1488–1497.

Hegge M (1995). Restructuring registered nurse curricula. *Nurse Educator, 20*(6), 39–44.

Mueller A, Johnston M, Bopp A (1995). Changing associate degree nursing curricula to meet evolving healthcare delivery system needs. *Nurse Educator, 20*(6), 23–28.

Van Meter M (1986). What's happened to diploma education? *R N,* June, p. 86.

Van Ort S, Woodtli A, Williams M (1989). Prospective payment and baccalaureate nursing education: Projections for the future. *J Professional Nursing, 5,* 25–30.

Welcome the thinking nurse! *Nursing Times* 1996;92(26):3.

6

Advanced Education for Nurses: A Hallmark of Professionalism

CHAPTER OUTLINE

The Need for Advanced Education

Master's Degree Preparation for Nurses

Doctoral Degree Preparation for Nurses

Chapter Summary

Key Points

References

Classic References

Recommended Readings

LEARNING OBJECTIVES

▶ **1** Explain the necessity for advanced education in nursing.

▶ **2** Discuss the educational requirements for a master's degree in nursing.

▶ **3** List the four types of advanced practice roles and positions for master's-prepared nurses.

▶ **4** Explain the pathways for pursuing a master's degree.

▶ **5** Discuss the goals of doctoral education in nursing.

▶ **6** Compare and contrast the types of doctoral programs available in nursing.

KEY TERMS

certified nurse-midwife

certified registered nurse anesthetist (CRNA)

clinical nurse specialist (CNS)

doctor of philosophy (PhD)

graduate education

master of science (MS)

nurse practitioner (NP)

postdoctoral training

post-master's degree program

professional doctoral degree

The dramatic changes in the health care marketplace since 1990 are amazing to almost everyone, frightening to many, and paralyzing to some. Nurses fall into each of these categories; most are amazed, many are fearful, and some are simply paralyzed. No group in the health care delivery system will escape the impact of these changes, and things will never go back to the way they once were. One major change that must take place is that advanced education must be examined in a way that was never done before. The need for advanced education in nursing has grown dramatically due to the changes in the health care system. These changes present a threat, but also a challenge. The changes facing nursing will present new opportunities for nurses who have the intelligence, energy, insight, and commitment to take advantage of them. Moreover, meeting these challenges will actually further the professionalization of nursing faster than at any other time in our history. Quite simply, advanced education for a critical mass of practicing nurses is the key to obtaining full professional recognition. This demand for advanced education in nursing will be examined in this chapter.

Some nurses express concern that advanced education in nursing is even more confusing than basic education in nursing. It seems that there are about a million ways to obtain advanced education to meet personal and professional goals. The options are so numerous and diverse that choosing a particular program can be baffling. However, this vast array of options means that nurses have incredible opportunities to establish the career path that is most meaningful and rewarding for them. This chapter will provide a sampling of potential career trajectories involving advanced education.

The two goals for this chapter are:

1. To encourage students who are nearing completion of their basic education for practice to explore the goals they can achieve through advanced education
2. To identify alternative educational pathways available to facilitate goal achievement.

Students should ask themselves four questions before they start reading the rest of this chapter:

1. Where do I see myself in 5 years?
2. Where do I see myself in 10 years?
3. What do I want to achieve in my career as a nurse?
4. What can I do in the course of my career to further the professionalization of nursing?

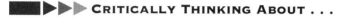 **CRITICALLY THINKING ABOUT . . .**

Have you thought about studying for a master's degree?

The Need for Advanced Education

Advanced education for nurses has expanded greatly in the past 50 years, thereby benefiting the discipline of nursing and enhancing the quality of patient care. However, until now, advanced education was considered largely a means of advancing one's own career and was considered optional on the part of each nurse. Nurses usually made decisions about seeking advanced education in a reactive manner rather than a proactive manner. As most nurses completed their basic nursing education, their plans rarely included graduate or advanced study. Practicing nurses usually decided to pursue advanced education because of some change in the job place, a desire to progress in their position, or a desire to change positions.

However, pursuing advanced education will no longer be optional as we move into the 21st century. Obtaining education, licensure, or certification beyond the basic preparation for practice will be a necessity if one is to continue to practice nursing. The U.S. Department of Health and Human Services (1990) has projected that 200,000 additional master's-prepared and doctorally prepared nurses will be needed by 2005. As discussed in Chapter 5, the third report of the Pew Health Professions Commission (1995) set forth this challenge very clearly in both its projections for needs for health professionals in the 21st century and its recommendations for nursing. The committee projected that up to half of the nation's hospitals will close as patient care moves to ambulatory and community settings. These closings will produce a surplus of 250,000 nurses. Accordingly, the committee recommended reducing the number of basic nursing education programs by 10% to 20% (associate degree and diploma programs). However, the committee also recommended the expansion of master's level programs and an increase in the level of federal support for those students.

The conclusions of the Pew report were strong medicine for all the health professions, but they cannot be ignored; changes must be made. The reactive stance described previously must change. Nurses must establish their career goals early and determine the trajectory that will help them achieve those goals. This, in turn, will help to advance nursing as a profession.

 CRITICALLY THINKING ABOUT . . .

How does advanced nursing education advance nursing as a profession?

Master's Degree Preparation for Nurses

Like baccalaureate nursing education, graduate education for nurses has evolved over time, particularly in the last quarter of the 20th century. **Graduate education—** postbaccalaureate study toward a degree—for nurses began at Teachers College of Columbia University in the early 1920s. This program was designed to prepare nursing educators and administrators. This was the dominant model in 1954 when Rutgers University offered a master's level program to prepare clinical nurse specialists in psychiatric nursing (Redman & Ketefian, 1997). During the 1950s and 1960s, the master's degree was considered a terminal degree, and preparation for teaching and leadership roles was the major emphasis (Jolly & Hart, 1987). In the early 1970s, the importance of graduate-level preparation of nurses to serve as clinical nurse specialists and nurse practitioners emerged and remains the focus in most contemporary master's degree programs in nursing. In 1996, more than 330 National League for Nursing (NLN)-accredited master's degree programs were offered at colleges and universities in the United States (American Association of Colleges of Nursing, 1996). This is 4.5 times as many programs as existed 25 years earlier.

The Basics of a Master's Degree

Assuming the successful completion of a baccalaureate program in nursing and successful completion of the NCLEX licensing examination, the next step on the educational ladder is the master's degree in nursing, usually designated as a **master of science (MS)** degree or a master of science in nursing (MSN) degree. The actual name of the degree is largely a matter of how each college or university designates names for its graduate degrees. Typically, the name attached to the degree makes no difference in terms of professional credentials. In the rest of this discussion, we will use "MS" to signify the generic category of master's degree programs.

MS degree programs vary widely in scope, content, and program goals but have several things in common:

- ▶ MS programs are usually found in senior colleges and universities that also offer a basic baccalaureate degree in nursing.
- ▶ Entrance requirements commonly include graduation from an accredited baccalaureate program in nursing and attainment of a minimum grade-point average of 3.0.
- ▶ Applicants must be licensed RNs.
- ▶ Applicants must complete the Graduate Record Examination, Miller Analogies Test, or some other standardized test.

Many MS programs also require at least 1 year's recent work experience as a RN, but to facilitate more timely progression toward advanced degree preparation, nursing faculties and administrators are considering waiving this requirement (Anderson, 1996). Box 6-1 gives details about the MS process.

MS programs vary from 12 to 18 months of full-time study. Currently, most nurses enrolled in these programs are also employed as RNs, often on a full-time basis, so they pursue their graduate education on a part-time basis. This, of course, means that it takes considerably longer to obtain the degree (see the section Pathways Toward Professional Development below and Fig. 6-1).

The general content of MS programs includes study of nursing theory and constructs of nursing science and their application in practice, as well as study of research methods that can be applied to the development of nursing knowledge and improvement of nursing practice. Physiology and pathophysiology are studied at a more advanced level than in the baccalaureate program. Graduate study in nursing also includes theory and application related to leadership and interpersonal skills that enhance a nurse's ability to improve the health care system (Norbeck, 1996). MS programs also incorporate learning opportunities for advanced clinical study in various settings, depending on the program's objectives and the student's goals.

Advanced Practice Roles and Positions for Master's-Prepared Nurses

Since 1996, nurse practice acts in all 50 states have recognized advanced practice nurses and have promulgated rules and regulations governing their scope of practice. The range of privileges and the extent of autonomy granted to advanced practice nurses vary from state to state.

Nurses in advanced clinical practice fall into four groups: nurse practitioners, clinical nurse specialists, certified nurse-midwives, and certified registered nurse anes-

Box 6-1

The Master's Degree Process

▶ Know your strengths and career desires (the first and most important step).

▶ Start your search by using a publication such as *Peterson's Guide to Nursing Programs: Baccalaureate and Graduate Nursing Education in the U.S. and Canada* (AACN, 1996). This lists all baccalaureate and graduate programs in the U.S. and Canada.

▶ Write for information from each program in which you are interested (addresses are included in Peterson's guide). The school will send you the details about the nature and philosophy of the program, the specialty areas you could expect to study, and often a sample curriculum plan you could expect to follow.
Important Note: If you are pursuing a master's degree as a means of becoming certified in an advanced practice role, make certain that the content and clinical education requirements for completion of the program match the requirements specified by the body from which certification will be sought at the completion of the master's degree.

▶ Determine the quality of the graduate program. Quality depends largely on the composition and qualifications of the faculty; the availability of facilities and state-of-the-art equipment; and opportunities for clinical experience under expert supervision.

▶ Select the program that is rated most highly in the advanced practice specialty you select and that will facilitate the development of those strengths you need to achieve your goals (Norbeck, 1996).

▶ Visit the campus and tour the school or college of nursing.

▶ Complete the application forms.

▶ Take the standardized test(s) that the program requires.

▶ Wait for a decision regarding admission. Decisions regarding admissions usually are made by a committee composed of faculty who teach in the graduate program. Some programs admit graduate students at only one point in the academic year. Others have rolling admissions and admit qualified students as their applications arrive and are processed. On admission, you will be assigned an academic adviser who is a member of the graduate faculty with expertise in your area of interest.

▶ Get started. Full-time study is the most expedient. However, if you must maintain your job while pursuing graduate study, it is possible to study part-time. In fact, most master's degree programs in nursing are accustomed to working with students in that situation. However, as you near the completion of a master's degree program leading to specialty certification, the requirements for clinical study become quite demanding. You may need to change your usual plan of work to meet the clinical practice requirements.

▶ Take final comprehensive examinations devised and evaluated by graduate faculty (students in master's degree programs leading to certification for advanced practice).

▶ Write research thesis (usually only students who are planning to continue on for a PhD).

▶ Follow the procedure stipulated by the body charged with devising and administering the accreditation examination in your chosen advanced practice area and take the necessary examination (only students in programs leading to certification for advanced practice).

▶ Proudly denote your certification status along with the title RN (assuming successful completion of the certification examination).

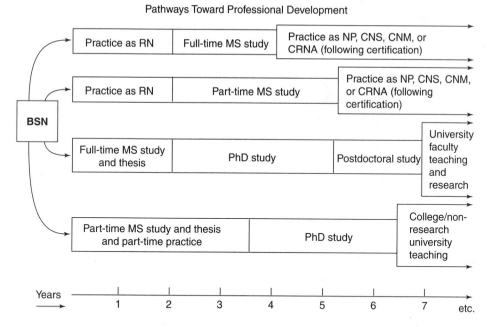

Figure 6-1. There are permutations and combinations of all of these pathways. The important factor is to set a goal and work toward it.

thetists (American Nurses Association, 1993). Table 6-1 lists the number of nurses practicing in each group and the estimated salary for each group.

Nurse Practitioners

The first **nurse practitioner (NP)** program began in 1965 at the University of Colorado. Designed by Dr. Loretta Ford and Dr. Henry Silver, the program was established to prepare nurses to provide primary care services to underserved children. As Carole Anderson (1994, p. 101) pointed out, "initially, there was great resistance to

TABLE 6-1	NUMBER OF NURSES IN EACH CLINICAL PRACTICE CATEGORY AND THEIR ESTIMATED SALARIES	
Title	**Number Practicing in U.S.**	**Estimated Annual Salary**
Nurse practitioner	25,000–30,000	$35,000–$40,000
Clinical nurse specialist	40,000	$30,000–$80,000
Certified nurse-midwife	5,000	$45,000
Nurse anesthetist	25,000	$78,000

(Gillis CL [1996]. Education for advanced practice nursing. In Hickey JV, Ouimette RM, Venegoni SL (Eds.), *Advanced Practice Nursing.* Philadelphia: Lippincott-Raven.)

these programs from graduate faculty in *nursing* schools, and, as a result, the first programs were begun in continuing education divisions. Fortunately, most of these are now graduate programs."

NPs provide basic health care for persons and families, usually in the community rather than in an inpatient setting. NPs perform physical assessments, make nursing diagnoses, and perform nursing interventions. They treat common acute illnesses and injuries, provide immunizations, and assist clients in managing chronic problems such as high blood pressure and diabetes. Depending on the particular state's nurse practice act, NPs may order and interpret x-rays and laboratory tests and prescribe a specified list of medications. One particularly strong element in the practice of NPs is the provision of patient education regarding lifestyles, health care options, and maintenance of optimal function, no matter what the client's objective health status may be.

There are areas of specialization and certification among NPs. Family nurse practitioners are by far the largest group. Many of these NPs are engaged in collaborative practices with physicians and other health care professionals. Many provide health care in community clinics, home health agencies, and well-baby clinics, and an ever-increasing number are establishing independent nursing practices on an entrepreneurial basis. Other areas in which NPs may obtain specialty credentials are pediatrics, adult, gerontology, women's health, psychiatric and mental health, school nursing, and occupational health.

Ted Johnson (1996, p. 23) has called NPs the "in-demand primary care providers." The great need for NPs is a direct outcome of the dramatic overhaul of the health care system in the 1990s. The demand for primary care is escalating rapidly and will continue to do so. Part of the demand stems from the stipulation in increasing numbers of insurance plans and health maintenance organizations (HMOs) that patient care be firmly grounded in, and always initiated by, a primary care provider. Thus, many more primary care providers will be needed. Second, most physicians want to enter specialized practice rather than primary care positions such as family practice or pediatrics. Third, adding to the lack of primary care physicians is the serious maldistribution of their services, leaving many of the nation's inhabitants without access to primary care (Whelan, 1995).

NPs are in an excellent position to fill this serious gap in health care needs, and they are very good at it (Mundinger, 1994). In 1992, the American Nurses Association (ANA) reported that NPs provided more health-promotion activities, such as patient education and exercise prescriptions, than did physicians. NPs also scored higher on diagnostic accuracy and ordered less expensive laboratory tests than their medical counterparts. Moreover, the clients of NPs were more satisfied and demonstrated higher levels of compliance with recommended regimens (ANA, 1992). Other evidence also supports the fact that NPs provide cost-effective primary health care. For example, investigators analyzed the quarterly performance reports from HMOs that had contracted with both physicians and NPs, comparing variables such as the number of emergency room visits by covered patients, the number of hospital admissions, the average length of stay of admitted patients, and the monthly cost of care per patient. The data indicated that the NP practice had 48 fewer admissions per 1000 patients, a shorter length of stay (by 1.5 days), and a monetary savings of more than $1000 per admission (Buppert, 1995).

The discussion of NP preparation in this chapter is focused on MS preparation. However, in the face of the increasing demand for certified NPs, many colleges and universities have instituted **post-master's degree programs**. These programs are designed for the nurse who has already earned an MS in nursing but is not currently certified as an NP. The programs include course work such as advanced pathophysiology, advanced pharmacology, and extensive focused clinical experience under the supervision of a certified NP. These curricula are designed to qualify post-master's nurses to sit for the examinations leading to certification as an NP. This option currently is being pursued by many clinical nurse specialists (CNSs). As hospitals have downsized and reconfigured personnel patterns, many CNSs have found themselves at a disadvantage within the hospitals and are seeking to maintain their advanced practice, possibly in another care environment or in the hospital by serving in a combined NP–CNS role (Hester & White, 1996; Hill, 1996; Chase, Johnson, Laffoon, Jacobs, & Johnson, 1996).

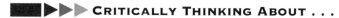 **CRITICALLY THINKING ABOUT . . .**

What do NPs offer in health care that baccalaureate graduates do not?

Clinical Nurse Specialists

The MS preparation of nurses to become **clinical nurse specialists (CNSs)** began in the middle to late 1960s, about the time MS programs for NPs were starting. The CNS role developed within the acute care hospital environment due to a combination of factors. Patient care technology in hospitals had improved at an astronomical rate since the end of World War II, leading to the survival of more acutely ill patients needing increasingly complex care. A high degree of nursing proficiency was required to care for these patients; therefore, it became very important to keep highly skilled, specialized nurses at the bedside.

Before that time, nurses typically moved up in the hospital structure, in terms of both status and income, by moving away from the bedside and into an administrative track. The CNS position afforded clinically expert, highly educated nurses the opportunity to advance within the hospital system without having to leave patient care behind.

> CNS role was conceived as a way of keeping nurses with advanced education in direct patient care. Creation of the role can be likened to the creation of a clinical ladder to be climbed by exemplary and committed bedside nurses who sought both graduate education and a role that allowed them to stay in the clinical nursing arena. (Boyle, 1996, pp. 301–302)

CNSs are expected to be experts in their areas of clinical practice. They have responsibilities for educating nurses and other colleagues in the hospital. They also provide consultation and should take the lead in research utilization efforts. To achieve these goals, CNSs must have completed graduate study in their nursing specialty area. Certification examinations for CNSs in specialty areas such as medical-surgical, maternal-child, psychiatric-mental health, cardiac rehabilitation, and trauma have been available from the American Nurses Credentialing Center (part of ANA) for many years. However, certification is not uniformly required for master's-prepared nurses to function as a CNS. Thus, although CNSs are the largest group of master's-prepared nurses engaging in advanced practice, they are the smallest group of certified advanced practice nurses.

The actual role of a CNS is different in almost every situation, depending on the needs of the health care system and the needs of patients and their families. However, a CNS should be prepared to lead the way in improving care, serve as a clinical leader in terms of skills and knowledge, and be a role model for other nurses. A CNS should also be sufficiently prepared and knowledgeable to act in collaboration with other nurses, physicians, and other members of the health care team. Finally, CNSs have an important role as patient advocates, ensuring that the patient and family members are fully informed about their care and are active participants in decisions regarding that care.

 CRITICALLY THINKING ABOUT . . .

Do CNSs have more responsibility in the health care team than do baccalaureate-prepared nurses?

Nurse-Midwives

Nurse-midwives have been meeting the reproductive health needs of women throughout history. Having women care for other women during pregnancy and childbirth was common centuries before both were moved into the realm of medicine and subsequently treated by physicians as though they were diseases rather than natural processes. Mary Breckenridge influenced the development of nurse-midwifery in the United States in the early 20th century. Breckenridge, an English-trained nurse-midwife who emigrated to the United States in the early 1920s, developed the Frontier Nursing Service in rural Kentucky to meet the nursing and obstetric needs of Scottish, English, and Welsh settlers in the rural Appalachian area. These families often lived many miles from the nearest physician or hospital, so the frontier nurses traveled by horseback to the homes of patients to help those with illnesses or accidents and to assist women in labor.

The practice of nurse-midwifery has changed dramatically. The practice of training nurses in an informal manner has evolved into a formal program of education. Nurse-midwives are educated primarily in MS programs certified by the American College of Nurse-Midwives. Thus, these **certified nurse-midwives** are educated in two disciplines: nursing and midwifery. Certified nurse-midwives have expanded the focus of their practice, which originally centered on pregnancy and childbirth, to provide primary care to women of all ages by establishing a plan of care management with the woman that includes cultural, socioeconomic, and psychological factors that affect a woman's health status (Romaine-Davis, 1997). The definition of nurse-midwifery today is "the independent management of women's health care, focusing particularly on pregnancy, childbirth, the post-partum period, care of the newborn, and the family planning and gynecological needs of women" (Romaine-Davis, 1997).

The American College of Nurse-Midwives has identified central concepts and skills that permeate midwifery practice, including (but not limited to):

- ❏ Promoting family-centered care
- ❏ Communicating and collaborating with other members of the health care team
- ❏ Promoting continuity of care
- ❏ Recognizing pregnancy as a normal physiologic and developmental process
- ❏ Advocating for informed choice and decision making by clients and their families.

Physicians whose practices are in obstetrics and gynecology are routinely incorporating nurse-midwives into their practices. In the increasingly competitive health care marketplace, nurse-midwives are seen as a vital asset in attracting clients who want maximum control over their health and the health of their infants.

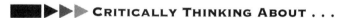 **Critically Thinking About . . .**

Should nurses be engaged in midwifery? Why or why not?

Certified Registered Nurse Anesthetists

Certified registered nurse anesthetists (CRNAs) are the longest-established advanced practice nurses in the United States. CRNA training was established in the late 1800s as the first clinical nursing specialty in response to surgeons' growing needs for experts in anesthesia administration. Sister Mary Bernard of St. Vincent's Hospital in Erie, Pennsylvania, became the first identified nurse anesthetist in 1877. World War I greatly increased the demand for nurse anesthetists in the second decade of this century, and CRNAs have been the principal anesthesia providers in combat areas in every war in which the United States has been engaged since then. The trend to educate CRNAs in MS programs started as recently as the late 1980s, but by 1998 all accredited CRNA programs will be in MS programs (Romaine-Davis, 1997).

CRNAs provide all aspects of anesthesia care. For patients undergoing surgery in hospitals, CRNAs carry out the complete examination and assessment of the patient the evening before the procedure and determine the type of anesthesia to be given on the basis of the patient's physical and psychological status. CRNAs select and order the appropriate preoperative medications and induce anesthesia at the start of the surgical procedure. They monitor the patient continuously throughout the procedure and manage recovery from anesthesia in the postoperative period. Most CRNAs practice in hospital operating rooms, but they also provide service wherever patients require anesthesia (eg, physicians' offices, outpatient surgery centers, labor and delivery, and dentists' offices).

CRNAs could be considered the most highly professionalized group of advanced practice nurses for several reasons:

1. They practice autonomously; no states require medical supervision of CRNAs.
2. Their educational preparation is, in general, the most lengthy and rigorous of the specialty programs. Most advanced practice nurse MS programs require 1 to 2 years of full-time study; CRNA MS programs require 2 to 3 years of full-time study. The educational preparation in the knowledge and clinical skills involved in anesthesia administration are the same as that of anesthesiologists (physicians specialized in anesthesia administration).
3. CRNAs have a strong identity with their professional organization. Ninety-six percent of CRNAs are members of the American Association of Nurse Anesthetists, the highest membership rate in any professional organization within nursing (Romaine-Davis, 1997).

Critically Thinking About . . .

Why do you think CRNAs are more closely aligned with their professional organization than are other nurses and nurse specialists?

Pathways Toward Professional Development

Preparation for advanced practice in nursing, whether it is as an NP with a specialty area, a CNS, a certified nurse-midwife, or a CRNA, follows a relatively common trajectory. However, there are different pathways toward the goal of an MS degree. In addition, the nurse's goals for practice after completing the MS may influence certain components of the MS program. Planning is very important if a nurse is to make the best use of available time, money, and opportunities to achieve satisfying career goals. Figure 6-1 shows the general process of preparation for advanced practice and identifies critical decision points and factors each nurse should consider. The starting point in this model is successful completion of the baccalaureate nursing degree and attaining licensure as an RN.

Practice First Versus Direct Progression

The first decision a nurse needs to make is whether to practice nursing for a specified period of time before entering graduate study. Many nurses favor this option, for several reasons. First, a new baccalaureate graduate rarely has finely honed nursing and clinical decision-making skills. However, this argument does not apply in the case of the new graduate who became an RN through an associate degree program and already has several years of practice experience. Second, supporters of the "work before you go on" school of thought assert that a nurse cannot possibly expect to practice at an advanced level if he or she has not practiced at the basic level. Third (and perhaps most important), unless the new baccalaureate graduate is like the experienced associate degree nurse mentioned above, he or she has experienced only a tiny sample of nursing practice in each of the specialty areas—actually only a few weeks per area. For some new graduates, that tiny sample is enough for them to know they had found the career focus of their dreams. However, the realities of the practice world are very different from the clinical teaching environment and may give them a very different perspective about how they want to pursue their careers. Other new graduates have not developed any specific specialty practice preferences. For them, direct practice would be very helpful in sifting through the remarkable number of career choices nurses have.

Unfortunately, some insist that new graduates must "pay their dues" by practicing before pursuing graduate study. Fortunately, this punitive stance is taken by fewer and fewer contemporary nurse educators.

Although there are good reasons for practicing nursing for several years before entering graduate study, there are also nurses (usually nursing educators) who advocate direct entry into graduate study soon after a nurse completes the baccalaureate degree and obtains RN licensure.

First, it is much easier to continue on in the role of student. When nurses enter practice, they soon become accustomed to a "real income" rather than the customary "student pittance," and they improve their lifestyle considerably. They develop a commitment to their job and often assume responsibilities involved in establishing and maintaining a family. Going back to school can be a very wrenching experience and can create significant personal strain and role conflicts for nurses who have been established in practice for several years.

A second factor related to job and family obligations has to do with mobility in terms of choosing the best graduate program of study. No single graduate program could provide all the possible options. Therefore, if a nurse is "place-bound" by various responsibilities, there is little choice but to enter a program that is geographically accessible, even though it might not be suitable for his or her specific career goals. Alternatively, a nurse may choose not to pursue advanced education at all. This would be a loss to both the nurse and to nursing.

Another factor in support of continuing directly into graduate school is that one's "studenting" skills remain sharp. Many older students who take graduate courses experience a great deal of anxiety, not only because their studenting skills are not as sharp after years of disuse, but also because technology has made the learning environment very different from what they remembered.

A final argument for going directly into advanced nursing study is that the nurse probably will reach his or her career goals much faster. This is especially true for nurses who choose to enter teaching and research in universities. They need to plan for 2 years of master's level study, at least 3 years (usually more) of doctoral study, and 1 or 2 years of postdoctoral experience to obtain a faculty position in a school or college of nursing they consider desirable. For these nurses, it would certainly seem that "the sooner the better" would be their motto. Being prepared for higher positions at a younger age also has implications for the magnitude of a nurse's lifetime earnings, simply because higher positions are associated with higher incomes.

 CRITICALLY THINKING ABOUT . . .

Which would be best for you—going directly to graduate school or practicing for 2 or 3 years before continuing your education?

The Master's Degree as a Stepping Stone to the Doctoral Degree

In addition to obtaining certification for an advanced practice role, another option that master's-prepared nurses may choose is to continue their graduate education toward a doctor of philosophy (PhD) degree. The nature and purpose of this degree are described more fully in the next section. The nurse who is considering obtaining a PhD, either immediately after the MS or sometime in the future, should expect to complete a research thesis as part of the MS program. Because the PhD is considered primarily as preparation for research and teaching in higher education, PhD admissions committees customarily seek evidence that applicants have at least a beginning background in graduate-level research methods and some experience in conducting an independent research project. In fact, although many MS programs are leaning toward providing a course of study that qualifies graduates to take certification examinations, it may be possible to bypass the requirement for extensive clinical study and focus on completing a research thesis instead. Obviously, in that case, the nurse would forgo the opportunity for obtaining certification but could advance directly into PhD study.

Another option is to complete the rigorous clinical requirement *and* write a thesis. This would require more time, but this nurse would be excellently positioned for both clinical certification and advanced practice and admission to a PhD program.

Doctoral Degree Preparation for Nurses

The first doctoral education in nursing was initiated at Teachers College, Columbia University, in 1933 and at New York University in 1934. Both offered the doctor of education (EdD) degree. These programs produced many of nursing's early leaders, who worked for the improvement of nursing education (Parietti, 1990). In 1954, the University of Pittsburgh initiated a PhD program in nursing. Since then, doctoral education for nurses has advanced steadily. The 1996 *Peterson's Guide to Nursing Programs* identified 65 doctoral programs in nursing. This does not take into account the nurses who seek doctoral preparation in other disciplines and sciences related to nursing.

Doctoral programs for nurses have developed in three phases (Grace, 1978; Murphy, 1981):

- ◪ Phase I (inception to 1959) consisted of education for nurses to carry out functional roles in education and leadership
- ◪ In phase II, nurses received doctoral education in a second discipline such as psychology, sociology, or physiology. This was referred to as "nurse scientist" training and was largely supported by the federal government between 1960 and 1969.
- ◪ Since 1970, we have been in phase III, the doctoral education of nurses in and of nursing.

These phases reflect significant growth toward the status of nursing as a true profession.

The general goals of doctoral education are to expand nursing's scientific knowledge base through research and scholarly activities and to prepare nurses to serve in leadership capacities in a variety of spheres within nursing and society (Crowley, 1977). If nursing is to progress as a scholarly, scientific discipline, vast numbers of nurses must be prepared at the doctoral level. They can then exert leadership in influencing nursing's course in the health field. If nurses remain less educated than other players in the health care arena, they cannot expect to be treated with respect or to affect decision making. A doctoral degree is a respected credential in academia and is a source of power for faculty.

Acquiring a doctoral degree does not automatically produce a scholar, but it does provide the research and statistical knowledge and experience required to facilitate the preparation of scholarly work. Many well-known researchers and scholars began their scholarly activities on a small scale. Through experience, they secured a remarkable track record of research and publications, which have greatly influenced nursing's growth as a scientific discipline. Moreover, increasing numbers of these persons consistently publish the results of their research endeavors; others continue to publish new insights into problems plaguing nursing's professional advancement. Doctoral programs in nursing prepare nurses to become faculty members in colleges and universities, deans of schools of nursing, administrators in medical centers, and researchers and theorists in nursing (Chitty, 1997).

There are actually five graduate degree titles offered in nursing:

- ◪ PhD (doctor of philosophy in nursing)
- ◪ DNS (doctor of nursing science)
- ◪ DNSc (doctor of nursing science)
- ◪ DSN (doctor of science in nursing)
- ◪ DN or ND (nursing doctorate).

However, 83% of nursing doctoral programs offer the PhD degree (American Association of Colleges of Nursing, 1997). The doctor of philosophy degree in nursing and the other doctoral programs in nursing are discussed in detail below.

The Doctor of Philosophy Degree in Nursing

The **doctor of philosophy (PhD)** degree is recognized as the research doctorate and is widely accepted in higher education. The major job market for nurses with doctorates is within colleges and universities. At colleges and universities, the PhD degree (in contrast to the so-called "clinical doctorates," which will be discussed later) is considered the most prestigious. Therefore, a nurse whose goal is to teach and do research at the university level would do well to follow a course of action leading to the PhD. Nurses may also earn a PhD in many areas related to nursing, such as physiology, neuroscience, pharmacology, anatomy, education, biologic science, and the social and behavioral sciences. In fact, until the 1970s, that is exactly what nurses seeking doctoral preparation did, simply because there were no doctoral programs in nursing. However, if a nurse's goal is to obtain a faculty position in a university's college of nursing, he or she should know that a PhD in nursing (although not always stated as such in the hiring criteria) is clearly the degree of choice among graduate nursing faculty and college of nursing administrators. Therefore, graduates with nursing degrees are in more favorable positions than applicants whose earned their PhD in another discipline.

 CRITICALLY THINKING ABOUT . . .

Should all nurse PhDs have their degree in nursing, or should some come from other science fields, given the earlier discussion of the knowledge base for nursing?

Success in a nursing faculty position at a university usually entails three activities: teaching, research, and service. The criteria for each of these activities are clearly spelled out in documents and rules relating to gaining advancement in rank and salary within the university. Usually, university faculty members are required to teach at both the undergraduate and graduate levels. They also are expected to serve as academic advisers to students and provide guidance to students who are working on master's theses and doctoral dissertations. Another element of the teaching role is service as faculty adviser to student organizations.

Research is the second major activity in which PhD-prepared nurses engage as university faculty members. Research may be conducted alone or with collaborators who share similar interests. A nursing faculty member may collaborate with other nursing colleagues or with colleagues in other departments throughout the university. Increasingly, the expectation for faculty members, particularly those at research universities, is that they will develop a program of research that they pursue in increasing depth throughout their career. Moreover, faculty members are expected to obtain funding to support their research from sources outside the university. These sources may include the National Institutes of Health, foundations such as W.K. Kellogg and Robert Wood Johnson, organizations that have a particular disease focus (eg, the American Heart Association, the American Lung Association), and private or industrial sources such as pharmaceutical companies and manufacturers of medical equipment.

The range of topics that nursing faculty members study is very broad. Samples of nursing research topics were presented in Chapter 3. When research is completed, the results should be written up and reported in professional journals, clinical practice journals, or books. Publication is a significant expectation for all university faculty members. Research and publication may not be such a high priority for a faculty member at a smaller college. Faculty at smaller colleges tend to have a heavier teaching load, and research and publication are not emphasized to the degree they are at larger, research-oriented universities.

Service has many components and varies greatly from school to school and even within the same system. One form of service is serving on departmental and university committees. In academic systems, faculty governance is highly prized, and faculty participate in decision making to a much greater extent than do employees in most other organizations. Thus, many committees are necessary to accomplish the work of the university, and the service of many faculty members is required. Another form of service is service to a professional organization such as the ANA, the state nursing association, Sigma Theta Tau (the honorary society for nursing), and specialty practice organizations such as American Association of Critical Care Nurses. PhD-prepared nurses are expected to assume leadership at all levels in such organizations as part of their professional service. A third kind of service is leadership in community organizations that are related to a nurse's area of expertise. For example, a faculty member whose expertise is smoking cessation could participate in and provide leadership and service to the local, state, or national lung association. A faculty member whose specialty is cardiology might be active in the American Heart Association.

In some college and university schools of nursing, the faculty role also has a component of nursing practice. This means that in addition to an earned doctorate, a faculty member would be expected to hold certification as an advanced practice nurse and provide nursing care regularly to maintain that certification. Proponents contend that this ensures that faculty members maintain clinical expertise and do not become relegated to the "ivory tower," high above the realities of practice in the real world. Opponents argue that requiring certification and regular faculty practice seriously endangers the research mission of nursing, and that building a sound, scientific knowledge base for nursing should be a higher priority.

Professional Doctoral Degrees in Nursing

Several schools offer doctoral degrees that are generally called "professional" degrees. The intent of **professional doctoral degrees** is not to prepare scholars for research and the development of theory; that is the purpose of the PhD. Rather, professional doctorates were conceived of as an advanced practice degree with an emphasis on clinical practice and clinical research.

Professional doctorates have several degree designations. The doctor of nursing science (DNS) is the most common professional doctorate and is intended to bridge the gap between practice and research (Allen, 1990). Advocates of the DNS (as well as the DNSc, also called doctor of nursing science) contend that because nursing is a practice discipline, "all intellectual endeavors should be connected to the practice concerns of nursing" (Redman & Ketefian, 1997, p. 164). Boston University initiated the first professional nursing doctorate (DNS) in 1960, followed by the University of California—San Francisco in 1964 (Matarazzo & Abdellah, 1971).

Other doctoral programs stressing the clinical rather than the academic nature of nursing since the 1970s (American Association of Colleges of Nursing, 1987) include the doctor of science in nursing (DSN) and the nursing doctorate (DN or ND), which is designed for the person with a baccalaureate or master's degree in a field other than nursing who wants to pursue nursing as a career. The first of these programs was established by Case Western Reserve University in 1979. Unlike the other nursing doctorates, however, the DN is seen as a first professional degree that prepares graduates for basic nursing practice; the DN represents neither an advanced nor an investigative degree. Proponents of the post-baccalaureate DN argue that it should be the degree required for entry into practice, just as the MD and the DDS are required for entry into practice in medicine and dentistry, respectively.

The professional doctoral degrees (with the exception of the DN) would be of greatest interest to nurses who plan careers in clinical rather than academic settings. Graduates of such programs would be qualified to provide clinical leadership in hospitals, community agencies, and local, state, and federal government agencies.

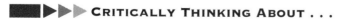 CRITICALLY THINKING ABOUT . . .

Should the DN be the basic degree for entry into practice to put nurses on a more level playing field with other health care practitioners?

Postdoctoral Training in Nursing

Postdoctoral training for nurses who have completed a PhD in nursing consists of 1 to 3 years of focused study under the close supervision and mentorship of an experienced nurse researcher in a research-intensive environment. This guided research experience enables the recent PhD to get focused in research and to get a substantial start on a program of research that will be carried well into his or her career. Postdoctoral training is relatively recent in nursing. Before this time, nurses seeking postdoctoral training obtained it in disciplines other than nursing and usually did so on their own initiative.

The impetus to the growth of postdoctoral training in nursing came after the establishment of the National Institutes of Nursing Research (NINR) within the National Institutes of Health in 1985. Ada Sue Hinshaw, the first director of the NINR, stated that the purpose of postdoctoral training is "to provide time, space, an intellectual and colleague support system, as well as a safe risk-taking environment for becoming an independent researcher" (Hinshaw, 1991, p. 83). The overall goal of NINR support for postdoctoral training is to enable nurses to "position ourselves so that we can shape the cutting edge of science" (Hinshaw, 1991, p. 82).

Currently, 13 universities offer postdoctoral training under funding from the NINR, and 9 postdoctoral fellowships are individually funded through NINR. Other sources of support for postdoctoral study include the National Science Foundation, the Robert Wood Johnson Foundation, the American Nurses Association Minority Fellowship Program, and the W.K. Kellogg Foundation. The postdoctoral level of study is now recommended more and more for nurses who plan to pursue teaching and research careers at research universities. As more opportunities and support become available, postdoctoral training will no doubt become increasingly common among nursing scholars.

▶CHAPTER SUMMARY

Advanced education for nurses has grown dramatically in recent years and offers the best hope for further development in the professionalization of nursing. This fact is becoming widely recognized within the discipline, and faculty members routinely provide strong encouragement for students to pursue advanced study. Other members of the health care system also have come to realize the vital contributions that can and must be made by nurses with educational preparation beyond the baccalaureate degree. Master's degree programs in nursing have grown over the past 30 years, as have doctoral programs in nursing. Still, only 2.2% of registered nurses held master's or doctoral degrees in 1996 (Division of Nursing, 1997). This must change.

One of the most significant factors in the demand for advanced educational preparation for nurses is the current and projected need for dramatically increased numbers of primary care personnel in the redesigned health care delivery system. The economic and social factors that are driving this system are changing forever the manner in which health care will be delivered and managed in the United States. A massive infusion of advanced practice nurses—especially nurse practitioners holding specialty certification and certified registered nurse-midwives—is imperative at least until 2020. This also means that there will be a much greater demand for PhD-prepared nurses to teach in graduate programs of nursing in colleges and universities throughout the United States.

The changes in the health care system have indeed put stresses on nursing, but at the same time they have set the stage for success by providing an unparalleled demand for highly educated, truly professional nurses. We must seize this opportunity.

KEY POINTS

▶ 1 To continue to practice nursing into the next century, education, licensure, or certification beyond the basic preparation for nursing practice will be necessary. In fact, the U.S. Department of Health and Human Services has projected that 200,000 additional master's-prepared and doctorally prepared nurses will be needed by 2005.

▶ 2 To pursue advanced education in nursing (a master's degree), a student must have completed an accredited baccalaureate degree in nursing, passed the NCLEX-RN licensing examination, attained a minimum grade-point average of 3.0 during undergraduate study, and completed a standardized test (eg, Graduate Record Examination, Miller Analogies Test). In addition, some programs require at least 1 year of nursing practice.

▶ 3 Nurses in advanced clinical practice fall into four groups: nurse practitioners, clinical nurse specialists, certified nurse-midwives, and certified registered nurse anesthetists.

▶ 4 There are different pathways a nurse can follow in pursuing a master's degree. The recent baccalaureate graduate can practice before going on to graduate study or go directly into graduate school. Another option available (for both the nurse who practiced and then went to graduate school and the nurse who went directly to graduate study) is to focus their master's degree preparation as a stepping stone for the PhD.

▶ 5 The goals of doctoral preparation for nurses include expanding nursing's scientific knowledge base, performing research, providing leadership within nursing and society, advancing nursing as a scientific discipline, affecting decision making in the health care community, gaining respect and power in the health care community, and advancing nursing as a profession.

▶ 6 The five types of doctoral programs available for nursing are PhD (doctor of philosophy in nursing), DNS (doctor of nursing science), DNSc (doctor of nursing science), DSN (doctor of science in nursing), and DN or ND (nursing doctorate).

REFERENCES

American Association of Colleges of Nursing (1996). *Peterson's Guide to Nursing Programs*, 2d ed. Princeton, NJ: Peterson's.

Allen J, ed. (1990). *Consumer's Guide to Doctoral Degree Programs in Nursing* (Publication No. 15-2293). New York: National League for Nursing.

American Nurses Association (1993). *Nursing Facts From the ANA.* Washington DC: Author.

Anderson CA (1994). Graduate education in primary care: The challenge. *Nursing Outlook, 42,* 101–102.

Anderson CA (1996). The nurse Ph.D.: A vital profession needs leaders. In AACN *Peterson's Guide to Nursing Programs*, 2d ed. Princeton, NJ: Peterson's, pp. 25–26.

Boyle DM (1996). The clinical nurse specialist. In Hamric AB, Spross JA, Hanson CM (Eds.) *Advanced Nursing Practice: An Integrative Approach.* Philadelphia: WB Saunders.

Buppert C (1995). Justifying nurse practitioner existence: Hard facts to hard figures. *Nurse Practitioner, 20*(8), 43–47.

Chase LK, Johnson SK, Laffoon TA, Jacobs RS, Johnson ME (1996). CNS role: An experience in retitling and role clarification. *Clinical Nurse Specialist, 10,* 41–45.

Chitty KK (1997). *Professional Nursing: Concepts and Challenges.* Philadelphia: WB Saunders.

Division of Nursing (1997). *March 25, 1997, Report to American Association of Colleges of Nursing.* Washington DC: U.S. Department of Health & Human Services, Public Health Service Health Resources and Services Administration, Bureau of Health Professions.

Gillis CL (1996). Education for advanced practice nursing. In Hickey JV, Ouimette RM, Venegoni SL (Eds.) *Advanced Practice Nursing: Changing Roles and Clinical Applications.* Philadelphia: Lippincott-Raven.

Grace H (1978). The development of doctoral education in nursing: An historical perspective. *Journal of Nursing Education, 17*(4), 17–27.

Hester LE, White MJ (1996). Perceptions of practicing CNSs about their future role. *Clinical Nurse Specialist, 10,* 190–193.

Hill NC (1996). Advanced practice in nursing: Conceptual issues. *J Professional Nursing, 12,* 141–146.

Hinshaw AS (1991). The federal imperative in funding postdoctoral education: Indices of quality. *Proceedings for the 1991 Forum on Doctoral Education in Nursing. Postdoctoral Education in Nursing Science: Purpose Process Outcome.* Amelia Island, FL: University of Florida, pp. 81–108.

Johnson T (1996). Nurse practitioners: The in-demand primary care providers. In AACN *Peterson's Guide to Nursing Programs* (2nd ed.) Princeton, NJ: Peterson's, pp. 23–24.

Jolly ML, Hart SE (1987). Master's prepared nurses: Societal needs and educational realities. In Hart SE (Ed.), *Issues in Graduate Nursing Education* (Publication No. 18-2196.) New York: National League for Nursing, pp. 25–31.

Mundinger M (1994). Sounding board: Advanced-practice nursing—good medicine for physicians? *N Engl J Med, 330,* 211–213.

Murphy JF (1981). Doctoral education in, of, and for nursing: An historical analysis. *Nursing Outlook, 29*(11), 645–649.

Norbeck JS (1996). Master's programs. In AACN *Peterson's Guide to Nursing Programs 1996.* Princeton, NJ: Peterson's, pp. 20–22.

Parietti E (1990). The development of doctoral education in nursing: A historical overview. In Allen J (Ed.), *Consumer's Guide to Doctoral Degree Programs in Nursing* (Publication No. 15-2293). New York: National League for Nursing, p. 1532.

Pew Health Professions Commission (1995). *Critical Challenges: Revitalizing the Health Professions for the 21st Century.* San Francisco: UCSF Center for the Health Professions.

Redman RW, Ketefian S (1997). The changing face of graduate education. In McCloskey JC, Grace H (Eds.), *Current Issues in Nursing* (5th ed.). St. Louis: Mosby, pp. 161–168.

Romaine-Davis A (1997). *Advanced Practice Nurses: Education, Roles, Trends.* Sudbury, MA: Jones & Bartlett.

U.S. Department of Health and Human Services (1990). *Seventh Report to the President and Congress on the Status of Health Personnel in the United States.* Washington DC: Author.

Whelan E (1995). The health corner: A community-based nursing model to maximize access to primary care. *Public Health Reports, 110*(2), 184–188.

Classic References

Crowley DM (1977). Theoretical and pragmatic issues related to the goals of doctoral education in nursing. *Proceedings of the First National Conference on Doctoral Education in Nursing.* Philadelphia: University of Pennsylvania School of Nursing, pp. 25–29.

Matarazzo J, Abdellah F (1971). Doctoral education for nurses in the United States. *Nursing Research, 20,* 404–414.

RECOMMENDED READINGS

Aroian J, Meservey PM, Crockett JG (1996). Developing nurse leaders for today and tomorrow. *J Nursing Administration, 26*(9), 18–26.

A study comparing characteristics of nurse anesthesia programs with the success rate on the certification examination. *J American Association of Nurse Anesthetists, 64,* 76–80.

Clarke PN, Glick DF, Laffrey SC, Bender K, Emerson SE, Stanhope M (1996). Doctoral education in community health nursing: A national survey. *J Professional Nursing, 12,* 303–310.

Gunn IP (1996). Health educational costs provider mix and healthcare reform: A case in point—nurse anesthetists and anesthesiologists. *J American Association of Nurse Anesthetists, 64,* 48–52.

Harris RB, Sillero G, Corbo J, Cupka P, Lee A, Sinski A (1996). Development and testing of a clinical self-timetable for acute care graduate CNS students. *J Nursing Education, 35,* 419–422.

Kent J (1995). Evaluating preregistration midwifery education. *Nursing Times, 91*(24), 38–40.

Ketefian S, Lenz E (1995). Promoting scientific integrity in nursing research, part II: Strategies. *J Professional Nursing, 11,* 263–269.

Lenz E, Ketefian S (1995). Promoting scientific integrity in nursing research, part I: Current approaches in doctoral programs. *J Professional Nursing, 11,* 213–219.

Lloyd A (1990). Ethics and health. *Nursing Times, 86*(25), 36–37.

Mackintosh C, Bowles S (1997). Evaluation of a nurse-led acute pain service. Can clinical nurse specialists make a difference? *J Advanced Nursing, 25,* 30–37.

Martin SA (1996). Applying nursing theory to the practice of nurse anesthesia. *J American Association of Nurse Anesthetists, 64,* 369–372.

Pickersgill F (1995). A natural extension? *Nursing Times, 91*(30), 24–27.

Reilly L, Carlisle J, Mikan K, Goldsmith M (1996). External review for promotion and tenure in schools of nursing. *Nursing Education Today, 16,* 368–372.

7

Nursing Education: Issues and Challenges

CHAPTER OUTLINE

Entry Into Practice
Accreditation
Diversity
Other Issues

Chapter Summary
Key Points
References
Recommended Readings

LEARNING OBJECTIVES

▶ **1** Explain why the issue of entry into nursing practice has been a problem for nursing for almost a century.

▶ **2** Describe the concept of differentiated practice and why it may be a solution to the entry-into-practice debate.

▶ **3** List the reasons why accreditation of nursing education programs is important.

▶ **4** Discuss the changes in nursing accreditation.

▶ **5** Discuss the reasons why enhancing diversity within nursing education and nursing practice is important.

▶ **6** Describe some strategies that can be used to enhance diversity within nursing education.

KEY TERMS

accreditation
American Association
   of Colleges of
   Nursing (AACN)
certification
competencies
credentialization

differentiated
   nursing practice
diversity
license
National League
   for Nursing
   (NLN)

Minority Academic
   Advising Program
   (MAAP)
pathways model
Pew Health
   Professions
   Commission

The advent of the 21st century offers unparalleled challenges and opportunities to nursing, the nursing education enterprise, and nursing educators. The nursing practice milieu is undergoing a dramatic transformation. Nursing as a discipline, and nursing educators in particular, must recognize the opportunities and respond to the challenges to forward the professionalization of nursing. It is clear that fewer nurses who can function only at the basic level will be needed. However, there is a great need for more nurses who are qualified to engage in advanced practice and provide scholarship and leadership in higher education in nursing. This chapter addresses three primary challenges that nursing leaders and nursing educators must meet: entry into practice, accreditation, and diversity (encouraging and dealing with it in student populations and in the clients for whom nurses care).

Entry Into Practice

Entry into practice has been referred to as the "issue that will not go away" (Moloney, 1992). Earlier chapters made clear that since 1923, nursing leaders have been calling repeatedly for the baccalaureate degree as a requisite for entry into practice. But a person can still qualify to be an entry-level RN by completing a two-year associate degree, a three-year diploma program, a four- or five-year baccalaureate degree, a 2-year post-baccalaureate master's degree, or a two- or three-year nursing doctorate degree, as well as various combinations of these programs (Camilleri, 1997). Is it any wonder that the general public, academic counselors, and professionals in and outside of nursing find it difficult to comprehend why nursing has been unable to put its house in order and offer one form of basic nursing education for professional nursing?

The entry-into-practice issue has even been the subject of an examination from an ethical perspective analyzing the implications of the issue and associated dilemmas for the nursing student and graduate (Hess, 1996). The author stated that the required single nursing licensure examination perpetuates the belief that there is no difference in training and capabilities of nurses who go through the various schooling pathways toward becoming an RN. In other words, the single nursing licensure examination is misleading to the public. This examination led to the author to conclude that "the status quo in nursing practice, licensure, and education is morally unacceptable" (Hess, 1996).

 CRITICALLY THINKING ABOUT . . .

Do you agree with Hess that the status quo in nursing practice, licensure, and education is morally unacceptable? Why or why not?

Impact of Diploma Schools

Moloney, a nurse researcher and an ardent advocate of the baccalaureate degree as the minimum preparation for entry into nursing practice, questioned why the entry dilemma has remained unresolved, even though two levels of practitioners (professional with a baccalaureate degree and technical with an associate degree) were proposed by the American Nurses Association (ANA) as far back as 1965 (Moloney,

1992). The answer lies in the numbers—the numbers of nurses and nurse educators who believed they had something to lose if the 1965 ANA resolution was accepted and implemented nationally. If fact, the ANA probably suffered a membership loss and alienated many diploma-prepared nurses because of its 1965 position paper (Kelly & Joel, 1996).

Until the mid-1980s, more than half the RNs in the United States were prepared in hospital diploma schools of nursing. These nurses perceived the acceptance of the baccalaureate degree as the minimum preparation for entry into practice as an insult and a threat to them in many ways. Many feared disenfranchisement within nursing; others felt that they would be treated as second-class citizens in employment settings. Still others were simply affronted that the nursing skills that they prized so highly, and at which they were so adept, were being replaced with academic standards and study that they felt really did not have anything to do with being a competent, kind, and caring nurse (Camilleri, 1997). Thus, until the mid-1980s, the huge numbers of diploma-prepared nurses, who did not agree with the ANA resolution, presented an effective obstacle to implementing the requirement for baccalaureate preparation for entry into nursing practice.

Impact of Associate Degree Schools

As discussed in Chapter 5, the dominance of diploma schools has been in sharp decline since midcentury, so their numbers are not the same obstacle they once presented. However, as the numbers of diploma school-prepared nurses were declining, another group of RNs prepared in 2-year associate degree programs were increasing in number to assume the numerical dominance the diploma nurses held in the first half of the century.

Mildred Montag, the founder of the associate degree movement, clearly intended that associate degree graduates should be designated as technical nurses and baccalaureate graduates as professional nurses, but this is not what occurred. It was demonstrated in the mid-1950s that graduates of the first experimental associate degree programs could successfully pass the RN licensing examinations. Thus, the associate degree program became an approved path for entry into professional nursing. A person could qualify to become an RN through an associate degree program in half the time and at less than half the cost of a baccalaureate program. Moreover, hospitals—the primary employer of RNs—rarely differentiated between associate degree and baccalaureate degree nurses in either salary or job assignments; this is still the case.

These factors essentially guaranteed the phenomenal growth of these programs and the numbers of nurses graduating from them. As a result, associate degree graduates clearly outnumbered baccalaureate graduates by 1970 and have continued to do so every year since. Thus, the RN workforce is still dominated numerically by nurses holding less than a baccalaureate degree, and the largest single group of nurses are graduates of associate degree programs (Division of Nursing, 1997).

In general, the associate degree contingent of practitioners and educators remains opposed to implementing the requirement of baccalaureate education for entry into practice, for many of the same reasons that diploma graduates were opposed in an earlier time. It is not likely that their opposition will lessen any time soon.

Transforming Entry Into Practice Into a Non-Issue

These numbers and their consequences may seem to establish a grim prognosis for the enhancement of professionalization through increasing basic educational requirements in nursing in the foreseeable future. However, other nursing leaders have reshaped the seemingly endless and fruitless discussion of the entry-into-practice issue by simply making it a non-issue. The National Commission on Nursing Study (1983), described in an earlier chapter as being influential in shaping nursing practice and education in the last part of the 20th century, concluded that there was a need for all types of nursing programs, and that baccalaureate education should be considered an achievable goal if sufficient attention were given to between-program articulation, thereby promoting educational mobility for all nurses. Of course, this study was sponsored by the American Hospital Association, whose members typically did not differentiate among baccalaureate- and nonbaccalaureate-prepared nurses. Another factor that may have influenced the findings was that the study was initiated primarily in response to the nursing shortage of the early 1980s.

 CRITICALLY THINKING ABOUT . . .

Is it important for nursing to have multiple entry points into basic practice?

More recently, and perhaps more importantly, the 1995 report of the **Pew Health Professions Commission** (discussed at length in Chap. 5) stated as its first recommendation to nursing:

Recognize the value of the multiple entry points to professional practice available to nurses through preparation in associate, baccalaureate and masters programs; each is different, and each has important contributions to make in the changing health care system. (Pew Health Professions Commission, 1995, p. vi)

In short, the commission simply directed nursing to set aside the persistent argument about an apparently insolvable issue and get on with the business of improving nursing and the health care system. The Pew Commission also recommended that nursing's professional nomenclature be consolidated so as to have a single title for each of the three levels of nursing preparation and service. Finally, the commission recommended that the practice responsibilities of each of these levels be distinguished (deTornyay, 1996).

Differentiated Practice

To date, the "single title" recommendation from the Pew Commission has not been addressed widely. The reluctance of nursing to pursue this recommendation is understandable, given the history of contention, disagreement, and divisiveness among nurses that was engendered by the proposed introduction of the labels or titles of "professional" and "technical" almost a half-century ago. However, since the 1980s, the ANA, the National League for Nursing, and the American Association of Colleges of Nursing (AACN) have all addressed the need to distinguish levels of practice responsibilities and have identified roles and competencies of nurses prepared at the associate and baccalaureate levels. The specific definition of such roles and competencies lays the foundation for **differentiated nursing practice**.

Differentiated nursing practice means that there is a clearly defined structure of the roles and functions of nurses according to their experience, education, and competence. Implementation of the concept of differentiated practice shifts the focus from a person's ability to obtain RN licensure to his or her actual nursing responsibilities and rewards. Titles are not at issue; rather, the focus in differentiated practice is structuring the roles and responsibilities of nurses according to their educational preparation and clinical competence. Nurses with different education and competencies are qualified to care for different kinds of clients in different settings. By differentiating nursing roles along the continuum of patient care, it is possible to match the knowledge and skills of nurses to the needs of patients (AACN, 1995). A differentiated practice model also defines a structure for determining salaries according to preparation and competencies (McClure, 1991; Forsey, Cleland, & Miller, 1993; Oermann, 1997).

The differentiated practice model presented by AACN defines the nature of the client populations who are best served by associate- and baccalaureate-prepared nurses, along with the appropriate scope of practice and definitions of the most appropriate health care settings in which service should be provided.

The appropriate practice for associate degree nurses is the provision of care to individual clients and families within a specified work period in a manner that is consistent with identified goals of care. The associate degree nurse is prepared to function in structured health care settings in which policies, procedures, and protocols are established and in which there is recourse to assistance and support in terms of a full range of nursing expertise. The associate degree nurse would not be expected or required to make independent nursing decisions.

The practice of the baccalaureate nurse is broader. He or she cares for people, families, aggregates, and communities. His or her responsibility for client care spans the entire care episode. The baccalaureate nurse is prepared to function in both structured and unstructured settings. In unstructured settings, established policies, procedures, and protocols may not exist, so independent nursing decisions may be required.

The AACN also developed a list of **16 competencies** grouped within three general categories:

1. Provision of direct care competencies
2. Communication competencies
3. Management competencies.

Within the first category (provision of direct care), associate degree nurses are deemed competent to provide direct care to clients with common, well-defined nursing diagnoses. In contrast, baccalaureate nurses are competent to provide direct care to clients with complex interactions of nursing diagnoses.

Level of complexity also differentiates associate from baccalaureate nurses in terms of communication competencies. Associate degree nurses are expected to use basic communication skills, such as encouraging clients to express their needs and supporting their coping behaviors. Baccalaureate nurses are described as employing complex communication skills in client care, such as promoting effective coping behaviors and facilitating changes in behavior.

Management competencies also vary between associate and baccalaureate nurses; in general, the management responsibilities of baccalaureate nurses are broader (AACN, 1995).

Models for differentiated practice contain elements other than different levels of educational preparation. These elements will be discussed more fully in Chapter 10.

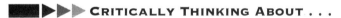 CRITICALLY THINKING ABOUT . . .

What is your response to the concept of differentiated nursing practice?

Resolving the Entry-Into-Practice Issue

The ultimate solution to the entry-into-practice issue—the "issue that will not go away"—actually may not lie only in the actions of well-meaning nursing educators and nursing leaders. It may also lie in the broader societal context and the inexorably changing requirements and demands of the health care marketplace.

First, projected hospital closings will have a great impact on nursing. As noted earlier, the third report from the Pew Health Professions Commission (1995) predicted the closing of as many as half of acute care hospitals and a loss of up to 60% of hospital beds. Therefore, hospital nursing positions will be lost.

Second, there is an increasing emphasis on moving health care into the community. As a result, nursing will move into the community as well, and nurses who practice in the community will find more autonomy, as well as more independent responsibility and decision making—important elements of professionalism. Nurses practicing in the community will also find that the demands on them in terms of their critical thinking skills and independent judgment will increase exponentially compared to their responsibilities in hospital nursing.

Third, there will be a decline in the number of schools that prepare nurses at the associate degree and diploma levels. The Pew Commission recommended eliminating up to 20% of these programs.

A fourth factor promoting change in nursing is the aging of the nursing workforce. The current mean age of practicing nurses is 42.3 years (Division of Nursing, 1996, March). This group is composed primarily of nurses with less than baccalaureate preparation; thus, the proportion of baccalaureate nurses could increase within the nursing workforce. However, it is uncertain whether the positions opened through retirement of nonbaccalaureate nurses will be filled by baccalaureate nurses or by unlicensed personnel.

Sixty-two health executives interviewed in 1995 anticipated that "In the next 5 to 10 years, the number of older RNs who will leave the labor force will exceed the number of entrants" (Buerhaus & Staiger, 1997).

Finally, there is a great demand for advanced practice nurses to serve in primary care practice roles, and rapidly increasing numbers of nurses are responding to those demands by obtaining advanced degrees and certification.

Sometime early in the 21st century, all these factors are bound to intersect. The result may be an entire generation of nurses who are more educated, more skilled, and more professionally oriented than ever before. In short, the societal forces that are driving changes in the American health care system may accomplish, within a decade or two, what 100 years of teaching, preaching, pronouncing, and cajoling within nursing could not.

►►► CRITICALLY THINKING ABOUT . . .

>With the likely closing of hospitals and the shifting of nursing care
>to other settings, is the hospital clinical experience today as impor-
>tant as it was in the past?

Accreditation

Accreditation in nursing education is a major element in maintaining high quality in
nursing programs at all levels. This section discusses the nature and importance of
accreditation, gives a brief history of accreditation in nursing education, and addresses some issues surrounding accreditation.

It is important to understand the terms that are relevant to program accreditation and related issues. The first is the general concept of **credentialization.** Credentials are written proof of a person's qualifications that communicate to others the nature of his or her competence. Credentials also provide evidence of a person's
preparation to practice in a specific occupation. For nurses, credentials may include
diplomas, degrees, licenses, and certificates. Schools and programs award diplomas,
degrees, and sometimes certificates on successful completion of a specified course of
study.

A **license** is a legal credential conferred by an individual state. In nursing, every
state has a board of nursing, the body legally designated to protect the welfare of the
state's citizens by awarding licenses to practice nursing to those who are qualified.

Certification of individual nurses also may be provided by a nongovernmental
authority, usually a specialty practice professional organization such as the Critical
Care Nurses' Association. This kind of credential should not be confused with a legal
license. Certificates are usually granted on completion of an educational program approved by the organization and successful completion of a standardized examination
approved by the organization. Certification of nurse-midwives and nurse anesthetists
was discussed in Chapter 6. The ANA also provides certification in other areas of advanced nursing practice (eg, nurse practitioners).

Accreditation is the certification of organizations. Accreditation provides documented validation of the qualifications of the organization to carry out its stated
goals and objectives. Like other forms of credentialization, accreditation is intended
to protect the public's interest. The public should be assured that the accredited organization can and does deliver the goods and services it promises in a manner that
meets very specific criteria set by the accrediting agency. Accreditation is the process
of granting approval, providing with credentials, or vouching that standards have
been maintained or met (Association of Specialized and Professional Accreditors,
1995).

Accreditation in Nursing Education

All nursing programs must be publicly accredited by their respective state boards of
nursing for their graduates to take the examination for licensure (currently the
NCLEX-RN). Although it is not a requirement, nursing programs also may seek voluntary accreditation. Voluntary accreditation exceeds the minimum standards set for

state board accreditation. It is a voluntary review process of educational programs conducted by a professional accrediting agency. The program desiring accreditation pays to have the accreditation conducted. Accrediting agencies compare the educational quality of the program undergoing review with established standards and criteria. Accrediting agencies are approved by, and gain their authority from, the U.S. Department of Education (Chitty, 1997).

Historically, the accreditation of schools of nursing came about as a result of concerns among nurse practitioners and nursing leaders about the quality and standards for nursing education.

> An accredited program voluntarily adheres to standards that protect the quality of education, public safety, and the profession itself. Accreditation provides both a mechanism and a stimulus for programs to initiate periodic self-examination and self-improvement. (Chitty, 1997, p. 46)

The process of becoming accredited and maintaining accreditation benefits various groups, including students, faculty, administrators, graduates, practicing nurses, and consumers of nursing services. Accreditation entails self-assessment and peer assessment of how well a program is meeting professional standards (Association of Specialized and Professional Accreditors, 1995).

The accreditation status of a nursing program is especially important to its students. First, a basic requirement for admission to almost all graduate programs in nursing is successful completion of an accredited baccalaureate program. Second, eligibility for certain scholarships and loans depends on being enrolled in an accredited nursing program. Finally, most employers of nurses are most interested in hiring graduates of accredited programs, because they too are seeking assurance that their new nurse employees have had an academically and clinically sound educational experience.

National League for Nursing Accreditation

Since 1952, the **National League for Nursing (NLN)** has been the official accrediting agency for most nursing programs in the United States, including practical nursing programs, diploma school programs, associate degree programs, baccalaureate programs, and master's degree programs. Doctoral degree programs in nursing have not been included in the NLN accreditation process because it is generally understood that the right and responsibility for ensuring the quality of any university doctoral program (including doctoral programs in nursing) belongs to the graduate school, which is an integral part of the university (Redman & Ketefian, 1997). The program of accreditation is conducted through four NLN councils:

1. Council of Practical Nursing Programs
2. Council of Associate Degree Programs
3. Council of Diploma Programs
4. Council of Baccalaureate and Higher Degree Programs.

Each council determines its own criteria and updates them periodically.

Criteria and standards in four areas are reviewed during the accreditation process:

1. Administration and governance
2. Finances and budget
3. Faculty, students, and resources
4. Program outcomes.

Since 1991, each type of program has been evaluated against the standards of established outcome criteria. These outcome criteria, also established by each council, are specific to the particular type of school. Outcome criteria used to evaluate associate degree programs include:

- Rates of admission, retention, and graduation
- Scores of graduates on the NCLEX
- Patterns of employment of students after graduation.

The outcome criteria for baccalaureate programs include:

- Evidence of critical thinking
- Communication skills
- Knowledge and skill in therapeutic nursing interventions
- Graduation rates
- Patterns of employment after graduation.

When a program is under review for accreditation, a self-study is conducted by a faculty and administration committee to show how the program meets the established criteria. Then a review team composed of educators from similar types of programs in similar institutions conducts a site visit to review the self-study and to meet with a variety of persons and groups associated with the program, including faculty members, students, and administrators in the school of nursing as well as administrators in the college or university in which the nursing program is housed. Finally, the site visit team prepares a report detailing its findings and recommendations, and these are presented to both the program being reviewed and the appropriate NLN council. The council then makes the decision about accreditation status for the program; it may include recommendations for change or specific conditions with which the program must comply to be accredited.

Changes in Nursing Education Accreditation

In the early 1990s, the general issue of accreditation in higher education came under close scrutiny of the U.S. Congress when its members determined that the default rates on federal student loans were climbing. They determined that a possible cause might be problems with the regional accreditation programs, and that closer federal oversight should be mandated. Accordingly, in 1992, when the Higher Education Act was reauthorized, new criteria were added to ensure appropriate procedures for monitoring student aid and achieving appropriate outcomes (AACN, 1996). This caused a crisis in nursing accreditation when the U.S. Department of Education notified the NLN in 1995 that it did not meet the newly established requirements for accrediting bodies (Tanner, 1996). The more rigid criteria for accreditation were the source of the NLN's problems with obtaining renewal of its recognition to accredit nursing programs. Currently, the NLN has not been disapproved (simply not reapproved), which means it is still accrediting. It is implementing the requirements for accrediting bodies set forth by the Department of Education and is scheduled to go before that department soon to seek reapproval.

The NLN's difficulty in complying with the Department of Education regulations was only one problem in the accreditation processes within nursing education. Concerns over accreditation had been growing since the 1960s, and as a result the following question began to be asked within baccalaureate and master's degree programs: "How many accreditations must nursing programs be expected to endure?" Universities, in general, participate in accreditation by regional accrediting agencies such as the North Central Association to ensure quality of education in the overall university. Many consider NLN accreditation to be a duplicate of regional accrediting agencies and costly in terms of time, resources, and money. Moreover, if a school of nursing wishes to offer a specialty leading to certification for, say, nurse-midwives or nurse anesthetists, it must undergo yet another round of accreditation for each specialty.

Moreover, concerns have been expressed regarding which nursing organization should be accrediting nursing programs. Should it be the NLN, which has been the "accreditor by tradition" for more than 50 years? Should it be the ANA, which serves as the leader in promoting professionalization in nursing? Or should it be the AACN, which was created to provide support and resources for baccalaureate and graduate education in nursing and whose "primary mission is to advance the quality of professional nursing education programs at the baccalaureate and graduate-degree level" (Anderson, quoted in AACN, 1996)? Kelly and Joel noted that although the ANA and the AACN have periodically asserted that the role of accreditation should be theirs, neither one has made any progress in wresting accreditation from the NLN (Kelly & Joel, 1996, p. 451). However, this is likely to change with the developments occurring within the AACN, which are described below.

AACN and Accreditation

The **American Association of Colleges of Nursing (AACN)** represents more than 500 member colleges and universities offering baccalaureate, graduate, or specialty programs in nursing education (Copp, 1997). The deans and directors of each nursing program represent their institutions in the AACN, and from this large group several nursing leaders are elected to the AACN board of directors. For several years, the AACN board of directors has received expressions of concern from nursing educators and policy makers in higher education regarding the processes for nursing accreditation. These concerns were reflected in the actions of the board when, in 1989, it commissioned a special staff report on issues surrounding accreditation. Since then, the board has considered not only matters of specialized accreditation but also more general accreditation of baccalaureate and higher degree programs in nursing.

In 1995, the board adopted the goal to have the AACN assess the feasibility of assuming some role in the accreditation process. This was done "in response to the dynamic state of accreditation in general, and with accreditation bodies in nursing not only proliferating, but also projected to increase" (AACN, 1996, p. 3). In October 1995, the AACN board established the AACN Task Force on Nursing Accreditation, chaired by Linda Amos. The charge to the task force was to explore aspects of specialized accreditation, to present a report of their findings to the membership, and to make their recommendation on what role, if any, the AACN should play in the accreditation of baccalaureate and graduate nursing programs.

The task force surveyed schools who were members of AACN, held open forums to air concerns, interviewed representatives of 25 specialized accrediting agencies, and reviewed the literature on accreditation, certification, credentialing, and licensure. Their data revealed consistent concerns. Member schools reported an average of 3.5 instances of accreditation reviews, not including the school's experience with regional accreditations. They also reported that nursing accreditation costs ranged from $2,000 to $50,000, in addition to the fees charged by the accrediting agencies. These findings prompted the task force to conclude:

> The growing concerns regarding costs of accreditation, the proliferation of specialized accrediting bodies for nursing, the redundant and duplicative processes associated with the various review entities, and the increasing financial pressures in the higher education community have created a need to form a new structure and process for nursing education that will provide for a coordinated and streamlined accreditation process. (AACN, 1996, p. 4)

The task force report was approved by the board of directors and sent to members. At their meeting in October 1996, AACN members passed by a vote of 246 to 59 a proposal that AACN take the lead in creating a new alliance for overseeing accreditation of baccalaureate and higher degree programs in nursing (Brider, 1996). Carole Anderson, then the president of the AACN and the dean of the College of Nursing at Ohio State University, proclaimed that this vote was "nothing less than a resounding mandate to move baccalaureate and graduate nursing education to a new level of readiness for the next millennium" (AACN, 1996).

The AACN plans to assemble a new accreditation alliance (separate from the AACN) that would ensure representation from the various groups involved in setting standards for baccalaureate and graduate programs in nursing, including specialty practice areas and faculty from all programs and types of schools. This new nonprofit accreditation entity will seek recognition as an accrediting authority through the U.S. Department of Education, and it is expected that accreditation services from the AACN-established entity will be operational in 1998. The AACN's receiving approval to accredit baccalaureate and master's degree programs means that for the first time, there is likely to be competition within the nursing accreditation scene.

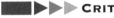 CRITICALLY THINKING ABOUT . . .

Who should the accrediting body be for baccalaureate and higher education programs in nursing? Why?

Diversity

The culture and practice of American nursing during its first century has been directly derived from the fact that the vast majority of nursing students, nursing educators, nursing practitioners, and nursing leaders have been white, female, and of Western European origins. However, demographic trends and changes in health care inform us that this nursing culture, which has served most of us well for the past 100 years, will not continue to do so. For nursing to achieve leadership in American health care in the 21st century, the key words can no longer be similarity, compliance, and conformity. The new key word must be diversity, and inherent in that is self-directedness, responsibility, and culturally competent care.

By **diversity**, we mean the presence in the population of a wide variety of racial, ethnic, and cultural groups with differing value systems, cultural practices, and customs. Increasing diversity provides a challenge to nursing education in two ways. First, diversity offers challenges to nursing educators to make changes within the nursing education institution so that it is more responsive to, and appropriate for, increasingly diverse student populations. One way of doing this is by implementing the Minority Academic Advising Program program, which is discussed later in this chapter. Second, the increasingly diverse client populations in the United States demand that nurses be sensitive to cultural differences among clients and also well prepared and eager to provide care that is culturally competent. For example, in emergency departments of large cities, caregivers and staff members must be prepared to function in a bilingual environment such as English and Spanish.

The changing health care scene puts additional emphasis on the importance of culturally competent care. It used to be that most of the care was provided by hospitals (by caregivers who were often mostly white and Eurocentric), where clients immediately are put in an inferior situation by the fact that the physicians and nurses clearly have the upper hand. Hospitals are alien environments to most people, and many fear that their care may be endangered if they violate the established norms of the hospital system. This is not the case when care moves to the community. If nursing care is going to have any positive impact on client outcomes, it must be framed within the client's cultural environment, norms, and expectations. The nurse is now in the client's world rather than the other way around, and his or her success depends on fitting into the culture of the community, just as the success of the hospitalized client depended on his or her fitting into the culture of the hospital.

Diversity Within Nursing Education

Although there are distinct variations by geographic region, nursing students, like practicing nurses themselves, are primarily female. They also are primarily white (particularly in baccalaureate programs), and they usually enter the nursing program between the ages of 19 and 21. This picture is slowly changing, but to be responsive to the care needs of clients and communities in the 21st century, it must change much more rapidly. This section addresses the issues and trends regarding two groups who are greatly underrepresented among nursing students: members of racial and ethnic minorities and men.

Racial and Ethnic Minorities in Nursing Education

The new century will bring with it a rapidly increasing demand for culturally appropriate nursing care for a population that is increasingly racially and ethnically diverse. Figure 7-1 provides a comparison of the racial and ethnic composition of the 1996 nursing workforce, the racial and ethnic composition of the 1996 U.S. population, and projections for the racial and ethnic composition of the U.S. population into the 21st century. Figure 7-2 shows that the percentage of minority students graduating from basic RN programs actually declined from 1989 to 1993 (when combined with total enrollment figures for all nursing programs in the United States). What may be even more troublesome is the fact that other data in this NLN report show that mi-

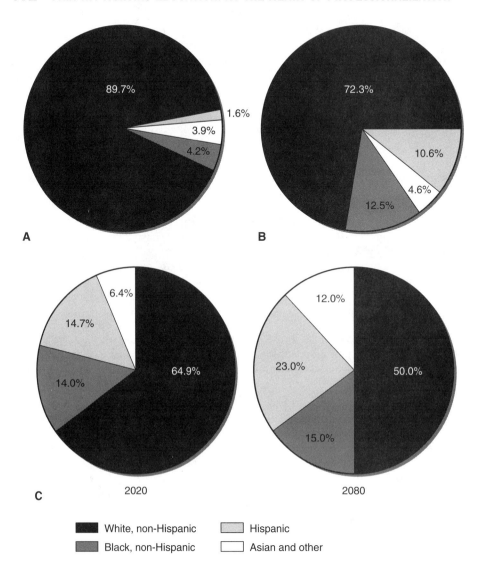

Figure 7-1. (A) Racial and ethnic composition of the 1996 nursing work force. **(B)** Racial and ethnic composition of the 1996 U.S. population. (Sources for **A** and **B:** Division of Nursing [March 25, 1997]. *Report to American Association of College of Nursing.* Washington DC: U.S. Department of Health & Human Services, Public Health Service, Health Resources and Services Administration, Bureau of Health Resources; National Sample Survey of RNs, March 1996, and Bureau of Census, BLS, Current Population Survey, March 1996.) **(C)** Projected changes in U.S. racial and ethnic composition. (Sources for **C:** Brinkerhoff DB, White LK, Riedmann AC [1997]. *Sociology,* 4th ed. Belmont, CA: Wadsworth; Bouvier L, Gardner RW [1986]. Immigration to the U.S.: The unfinished story. *Population Bulletin 41*[Nov]:1–50; Davis C, Haub C, Willette J [1983]. U.S. Hispanics: Changing the face of America. *Population Bulletin 33*[June]:1–43; O'Hare WP [1992]. America's minorities: The demographics of diversity. *Population Bulletin 47*[4].)

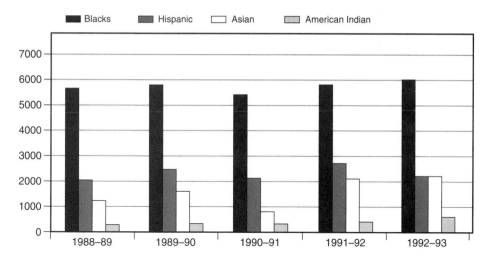

Figure 7-2. Decrease in the number of minority graduates in all basic RN programs, 1988–89 to 1992–93. (Division of Research, National League for Nursing [1995]. *Nursing Data Review 1995.* New York: Author.)

nority students gain admission to and enroll in nursing programs but are the least successful in graduating (Division of Research, National League for Nursing, 1995).

It is clear from these data that there is a significant discrepancy between the racial and ethnic distributions within nursing and nursing education and those within the populations we are preparing students to serve. This was recognized by the National Advisory Council on Nurse Education and Practice in 1996. One of the council's recommendations was that "federal resources should be used to assure that the composition of the basic nurse workforce is reflective of the overall society as an important vehicle for enabling access to, and the delivery of, appropriate nursing services" (National Advisory Council on Nurse Education and Practice, 1996, p. 9). Indeed, culturally diverse practitioners enhance nursing by broadening the perspectives of nurses and clients, and the lack of baccalaureate-prepared minority nurses is bound to have an adverse influence on current health care reform measures and clinical health care issues (Dowell, 1996). Health statistics for ethnic minorities suggest that their health needs differ from the needs of white patients, and the lack of culturally sensitive care by health care providers results in a poorer quality of care. Therefore, the lack of sufficient numbers of minority nurses should be of great concern to nursing practice and to those who educate future practitioners.

Racial and ethnic minority populations traditionally have been greatly underserved in the American health care system. Since the 1960s, the government has increased efforts to provide accessible, cost-effective care to these populations, and the Department of Health and Human Resources plays a major role in that effort. Several fine programs have been launched, such as the National Health Service Corps, the Health Career Opportunity Program, Centers of Excellence in Minority Health, and Student Assistance Programs (U.S. Department of Health and Human Services, 1991).

However, an underlying assumption of such programs is that sufficient minority students will be recruited into the health professions to help meet the health care needs of underserved minority communities. And, as seen in the previous data, that clearly is not happening. According to Patricia Castiglia, "Nursing can no longer sustain itself without incorporating, to a greater extent, diverse minority groups into the profession" (Castiglia, 1997, p. 581).

For the past 25 years, numerous efforts have been made to increase the numbers of ethnic and racial minorities in nursing, but the racial and ethnic composition of both nursing students and practicing nurses has remained virtually the same (Castiglia, 1997). Alternative strategies for recruiting and retaining minority students must be explored, implemented, and evaluated.

 CRITICALLY THINKING ABOUT . . .

> Does the racial and ethnic mix of your nursing education program reflect the racial and ethnic composition of the area that your program serves? What contributes to this situation?

Increasing Racial and Ethnic Diversity in Nursing Education Programs

An entire issue of the *Journal of Nursing Education* in 1996 was devoted to cultural diversity in nursing education. At the beginning of the issue, the editor, Christine Tanner, raised four important questions:

1. What are we doing with regard to minority student recruitment and retention?
2. How culturally competent are we as faculty?
3. How do we help our students become more culturally competent?
4. How Eurocentric is our curriculum? (Tanner, 1996, pp. 291–292)

MINORITY ACADEMIC ADVISING PROGRAM

One article in this issue of the *Journal of Nursing Education* described a supplementary retention program for African-American students in a baccalaureate program in a southern state (Hesser, Pond, Lewis, & Abbott, 1996). This **Minority Academic Advising Program (MAAP)** was provided for 114 African-American students; another 608 students (primarily white) served as a comparison group. MAAP provided a variety of activities focused on enhancing retention of African-American students, the cornerstone of which was a special advising effort provided by one nursing faculty adviser and two senior-level African-American peer advisers. Other activities included consultation and referral assistance from a MAAP coordinator who was an expert in reading and study skills and a special fall orientation program to introduce African-American students to MAAP services and personnel. They also generated a quarterly newsletter and arranged for Black History Month presentations by prominent African-American professionals (role models). The MAAP program spanned the entire university campus, and a campuswide administrative network was established to enhance communication and improve coordination of retention services. Therefore, the group in nursing had a strong support system for its work.

On entry to the program, the MAAP participants had significantly lower grade-point averages and SAT scores; 11 students were at high risk of failing. After participating in the MAAP program, however:

1. Students' retention-to-graduation rate increased 5.3%, to 96.1%.
2. Their nursing grade-point average increased nearly one-quarter of a letter grade.

3. Their time-persisted-in-program increased by 0.7 months.
4. Their nursing board examination pass rate increased by 15 percentage points (Hesser, Pond, Lewis, & Abbott, 1996).

THE PATHWAYS MODEL

Another article in the same issue of the *Journal of Nursing Education* described the **pathways model**. The purpose of this model is to affirm the diversity of background, learning styles, and career aspirations for students in baccalaureate and graduate nursing education. The article focused on the preparation of faculty as mentors for students with disadvantaged backgrounds. The pathways model centers on the interaction between nursing faculty and students who come from diverse and sometimes economically or educationally disadvantaged backgrounds. The goals include the empowerment of both students and faculty, enabling them to work together by focusing on potentials rather than deficits (Rew, 1996).

The pathways model uses a travel analogy based on three major concepts:

- ▶ Students travel a diversity of roads, arriving at the learning environment from a variety of backgrounds.
- ▶ The "learning landscape" contains a wide variety of signs, maps, tour guides, and other resources that students and faculty use to facilitate safe passage of the student through the terrain.
- ▶ Students develop and use unique, self-built pathways to enter the world of nursing practice.

The role of the faculty is critical to the success of the pathways model. Faculty members need three things to manage issues related to cultural diversity of students: awareness of their own social and cultural biases and beliefs, knowledge about other cultures and societies, and skills in adapting teaching strategies to address other ways of learning (Rew, 1996).

Faculty Role

The crucial role of nursing faculty in providing an environment where racially and ethnically diverse student populations can flourish has been emphasized by many writers concerned with increasing diversity within nursing education. In another article in the *Journal of Nursing Education*, Campbell and Davis (1996) pointed out that faculty commitment to enhancing racial and ethnic diversity in nursing is the key ingredient to successful recruitment and retention of minority students. Even without organized programs (eg, MAAP, the pathways model), when faculty are committed to student success, students are more successful. Even without widespread institutional commitment, minority faculty members can assume an activist role in minority student retention and make themselves available to serve as role models and sources of social support (Campbell & Davis, 1996).

Majority faculty also have an important role to play in facilitating the success of minority students. They can serve as models of commitment and sensitivity for colleagues who may have less experience with minorities and less awareness of minority students' needs and learning styles. They also can influence administrators to support the development of programs and services for minority students.

Finally, all faculty must advocate for the incorporation of knowledge of cultural differences into policies, curricula, and instructional practices (Campbell & Davis, 1996).

A qualitative research study conducted by Marilyn Yoder (1996) found that faculty do not always measure up to such standards. She based her conclusions on data obtained from in-depth interviews with 26 nurse educators and 17 minority nurses who were recent graduates. All respondents were, or had been, associated with nursing programs in California. Yoder described five patterns in faculty responses to ethnically diverse nursing students:

1. Generic. These educators tend to have a low level of cultural awareness. Although they identify individual differences among students, they do not consider ethnicity to be an important factor that contributes to these differences. They assume that ethnic students do not have needs that differ from the general student population. They also tend to insulate themselves from student ethnic diversity.
2. Mainstreaming. These educators show a high level of cultural awareness and identify many special needs of ethnic students. They assume that student problems are the result of student deficiencies and lack of knowledge regarding expectations of the majority culture. Therefore, they direct their efforts toward helping students adapt to the mainstream or dominant culture. They feel that if the students understand the expectations and conform to them, they are more likely to succeed.
3. Culturally intolerant. These educators were perceived by recent graduates as unwilling to tolerate cultural differences and were seen as barriers for minority students. Faculty observations supported the students' perceptions.
4. Struggling. Faculty in this category were seen as moving from a lower to a higher cultural awareness and were struggling to adapt their teaching to be responsive to students' diverse cultural needs.
5. Bridging. Faculty in this group possess high cultural awareness and demonstrate high culturally adaptive instructional responses to student diversity. These educators value diversity, respect cultural differences, and encourage students to maintain their ethnic identity and to function biculturally. "The majority of students who were interviewed did not experience a bridging pattern with their educators" (Yoder, 1996, p. 319).

■■■ ▶▶▶ CRITICALLY THINKING ABOUT . . .

Does your nursing institution have a program such as the MAAP program or the pathways model? If not, should it?

Men In Nursing Education

Men are entering nursing education programs at an increasing pace (Fig. 7-3), but they still constitute a minority of nursing students (about 13%) and a distinct minority in practice (about 4%). Figure 7-3 also shows that associate degree programs have been the programs of choice for men since 1985. However, substantial gains have been made in men's enrollment in baccalaureate education as well, especially since 1989 (Division of Research, National League for Nursing, 1995).

REASONS FOR SMALL NUMBERS OF MEN IN NURSING

Men have not always been a minority in a "women's occupation"; the numerical dominance of women in nursing actually did not come about until almost the begin-

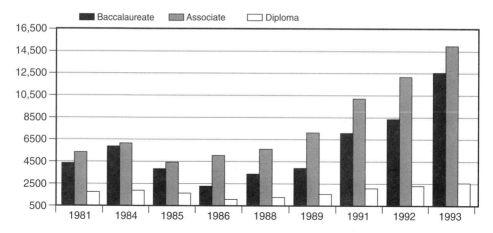

Figure 7-3. Consistent average increase of 12.36% in enrollments of men in all types of programs. (Division of Research, National League for Nursing [1995]. *Nursing Data Review 1995*. New York: Author.)

ning of the 20th century. Women were the traditional caregivers within the home, but in the institutions set up to care for the sick outside the home, caregivers were often men—priests, members of holy orders, physicians' assistants, or members of the military (Bullough, 1997). However, when Florence Nightingale made her dramatic changes in nursing and nursing education, changes that would forever change the occupation, she asserted that nursing was a female discipline. The role of men in caregiving was restricted to supplying physical strength when needed, such as lifting and moving patients (Chitty, 1997).

When a version of the Nightingale training school was imported to the United States in the late 19th and early 20th centuries, students in those schools served as a supply of cheap labor to a rapidly growing number of hospitals. In effect, they staffed the hospitals in return for room and board and a bit of education. The students needed to be available for hospital work at all times, so the hospitals established homes for them. This also fit in with the dominant notion of the time that women needed to be protected. The homes were restricted to women only, placing one more barrier in the way of any men who attempted to gain entry into nursing (Bullough, 1997).

Thus, in the United States, there has been a long history of discrimination against men in nursing. This kind of prejudice was rooted in traditional definitions of the male and female roles in American society: men were expected to perform physically laborious tasks, and women were expected to be caregivers. In 1914, Hornsby and Schmidt observed that the only reason a male would be in nursing was that he was a failure in life's mainstream: "It has become a maxim that a trained male nurse would not be a nurse if he were fit for any other occupation, and that is probably true" (Hornsby & Schmidt, 1914, p. 335).

The military also contributed to the nonstatus of men in nursing, although the military was simply perpetuating a social prejudice that was widespread in American society. In 1901, when the U.S. Army Nurse Corps was organized, it specifically excluded male nurses. When male nurses were drafted into the military in World War I, they did not staff the hospitals; they fought in the trenches. The same thing happened in World War II. However, after World War II, many veterans obtained their college educations through the G.I. Bill, and many of them chose nursing. This started the slow but steady increase of the numbers of men in nursing. Many military corpsmen entered nursing schools after World War II, and they have continued to do so after every subsequent major military conflict (Chitty, 1997; Bullough, 1997).

MEN IN NURSING: MOTIVATION, ATTITUDES, AND EXPERIENCES

A major factor contributing to the attractiveness of nursing as a career for men was the improved salaries and working conditions that occurred in the 1950s and 1960s. Moreover, male nurses generally were, and still are, paid more than female nurses. Part of this disparity is due to the areas in which men chose to work. Much higher proportions of men became nurse anesthetists and nurse administrators, both of which are high-paying positions. However, another part of the salary disparity before the 1960s and 1970s was due simply to the common practice of paying men more than women for doing the same work (Bullough, 1997).

Perkins, Bennett, and Dorman (1993) studied 146 male nursing students, 70% of whom were enrolled in associate degree programs, to determine why they had chosen nursing as a career. More than 80% of the respondents had prior experience in a health-related occupation (eg, military corpsman, emergency medical technician, or nursing assistant). Most of the men had a spouse or female relative who was a nurse, and they received the most support for their decision to become nurses from their wives, mothers, and female friends. Figure 7-4 shows that more than one third of the respondents cited job opportunity and availability, financial incentive, job security, and career flexibility as their reasons for choosing a nursing career. Only 11% of the men students claimed that a desire to contribute to a helping profession was their primary motivation to enter nursing.

These students also were asked what specialty areas they wished to pursue in nursing. The areas of nurse anesthetist, intensive care, and emergency room accounted for almost half of the men's responses (Perkins, Bennett, & Dorman, 1993).

Kelly, Shoemaker, and Steele (1996) studied male students' perceptions of the motivational factors, barriers, and frustrations they encountered in becoming a nurse. The researchers held four focus groups that incorporated 18 male students in

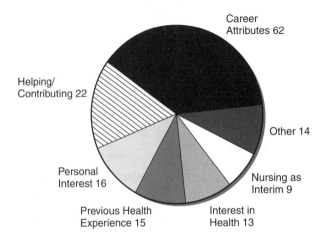

Figure 7-4. Reasons men choose nursing and the number of respondents citing the reasons. (Perkins JL, Bennett D, Dorman RF [1993]. Why men choose nursing. *Nursing and Health Care* 14[1]:36.)

one associate program, two baccalaureate programs, and one diploma program. Five specific interview topics were established:

1. Image of nursing
2. Motivations to enter and persist in nursing school
3. Barriers they encountered in becoming a nurse
4. Problems they may have had after entering nursing school
5. Recruitment of other men into nursing.

All the men felt that the public image of nursing was poor and largely promoted by television's depiction of nurses. However, they also noted that the image is improving. The men cited a variety of practical as well as altruistic motives for entering nursing, including job availability and security, the desire to help people, and the variety of job opportunities open to nurses. Parents, sisters, and wives were their major sources of support in making their career decisions. Like the sample in the Perkins, Bennett, and Dorman study, prior experience in health-related occupations was common for these men (11 of 18 participants).

The male students were asked about barriers they experienced in their quest to become nurses. They cited a lack of information from counselors, a fear of being perceived as unmanly, and changes in their family roles when they had to give up their role as primary income provider to return to school. Indeed, many nontraditional students (which includes men) often must make extensive and difficult arrangements with their spouses, children, elderly parents, and employers to go to nursing school (Copp, 1995). The male students also said they had received little or no guidance from high school counselors (Dowell [1996] also identified poor guidance from high school counselors as a barrier to racially and ethnically diverse students).

In general, male students perceived their nursing schools as being supportive, and explained that the excitement and satisfaction of their clinical experience was their greatest reward. However, many were shocked about how much effort it took to do well in the nursing program, and most said it was much harder than they had anticipated.

The authors concluded their article with some advice to nursing programs interested in recruiting men:

1. Market nursing in an androgynous manner. Do not perpetuate the notion that nursing is a "women's career."
2. Emphasize factors that seem to appeal to men, such as job security and diversity, as well as the concept of helping others.
3. Because family members have been found to be a significant source of support for the career decision, include them in the recruitment process.
4. High school counselors need to be more informed and should be encouraged to promote nursing as a career for men as well as for women.
5. Faculty members must not isolate male students. Men must be provided with learning opportunities equal to those provided to women in terms of laboratory and clinical assignments.

▶▶▶ CRITICALLY THINKING ABOUT . . .

Do the men and women in your nursing program share the same career goals, expectations, and educational experiences? Explain and give examples.

Other Issues

In addition to the three major issues currently facing nursing education, there are other issues that also require attention.

One issue is the proliferation of doctoral titles in nursing. This issue, addressed in Chapter 6, causes almost as much confusion within nursing and outside of nursing as the entry-into-practice issue. Shake Ketefian has argued that nursing would be best served by defining a single doctoral title that contains within it the options to pursue one's professional goals in the most appropriate way.

Another challenge is to establish and affirm an attitude within nursing education that nursing is a career, not simply a job. This attitude alone will contribute substantially to the professionalization of nursing. Choosing and embracing a career carries with it a commitment to lifelong learning and a continuing desire to improve one's skills, knowledge, and understanding. Nursing educators must address this issue with all their students in every course they teach, and nursing school administrators must support these efforts in every way.

Finally, nursing educators must be prepared to change the total configuration of nursing education, probably within the next two decades. There is no way of knowing what the new configuration might be; anything is possible, and no option should summarily be dismissed. The American health care scene is changing rapidly, and if nursing educators do not keep up with the pace, nursing will be left behind, and that would be inexcusable. The changes in the health care system that are likely to come about have the potential for providing opportunities for nurses that have never existed before, and nursing educators must prepare their students to take advantage of these opportunities.

▶ CHAPTER SUMMARY

Three significant issues of concern within nursing education have been addressed in this chapter.

The first issue is the longstanding dilemma surrounding entry into nursing practice. This issue has been a thorn in the side of nursing for most of the century. Calls for making the baccalaureate degree the minimum preparation to enter the practice of nursing have come repeatedly from many and varied sources, but there is still disagreement and dissent within nursing. Unless nurse practice acts all over the country are changed radically, which is highly unlikely, many men and women will continue to choose the shorter, more economical associate degree path to obtain RN licensure and enter basic nursing practice. Thus, it would seem that the best strategy is to follow the directives established by nursing leaders in organizations such as the ANA, the NLN, and the AACN. In other words, the concept of differentiated nursing practice should be further developed and implemented. This concept is based on nurses' qualifications for practice, which in turn are based on education, demonstrated competencies, and nursing experience.

Differentiated practice directives must be implemented within nursing workplaces by nursing leaders in those institutions and systems. Thus, it may be considered more of a nursing practice issue than a nursing education issue. However, nursing education has a pivotal role to play in ensuring the viability of the concept of differentiated practice. The primary challenge within nursing education is to ease the transition from one educational program to the next to encourage the maximum number of nurses to attain the level of education and expertise that will assist them in achieving a satisfying career in nursing and will enable them to provide the best and most appropriate nursing care to their clients.

The second issue is the accreditation of nursing education programs to ensure a quality education to nursing students and quality nursing care to the public. Ensuring the quality of nursing education through rigorous accreditation is extremely important in the continuing professionalization of nursing. There are several problems to be solved, including the multiplicity of accrediting bodies and the escalating costs of accreditation to educational institutions. The accreditation process in nursing is changing. If the AACN's proposal and plan to establish a new accreditation alliance comes to fruition, the course of accreditation in programs of nursing education could be substantially changed and improved. The goal is to standardize, coordinate, and streamline the accreditation of nursing education programs and program elements while maintaining, or even raising, the standards of quality for nursing education and nursing care.

The third issue, and perhaps the one on which we have the most work to do, is related to the lack of diversity in nursing student populations and thus within nursing itself. Student, faculty, and practitioner populations are largely uniform and homogeneous, and such homogeneity can easily produce rigid, stagnant, and inflexible educational environments. To change the nature of the nursing population, nursing programs and schools must change themselves. Schools must become more flexible, must seek and employ more diverse faculty and administrators, and must develop curricula that reflect the growing awareness of culturally sensitive care. Recruiting and retaining students with diverse backgrounds must become a significant focus within nursing research and nursing policy.

The number of men entering nursing education and nursing practice is rising slowly but steadily, unlike the trend among racial and ethnic minorities. Recruitment of minority students is particularly hampered by financial limitations, because many members of racial and ethnic minorities are financially disadvantaged. More full scholarships must be made available to attract minority students and enable them to persist in school to graduation. It is not enough simply to attract students from racial and ethnic minorities; schools also must take steps to increase retention and successful completion of programs. High attrition rates among students in general have been linked to lack of affiliation, lack of sufficient financial aid, lack of faculty contact, lack of faculty commitment, and lack of institutional policies that demonstrate an awareness of and concern for student development (Dowell, 1996). Students who are members of racial and ethnic minorities are at an even higher risk for failure in such barren educational environments. Schools of nursing would do well to conduct careful self-examinations to determine their strengths and weaknesses in meeting the special needs of racial and ethnic minorities and men. They would then be in a position to build on their strengths and fix their weaknesses by curriculum development and enhancement, stronger programs of financial support, role modeling and mentoring, and cultivation of learning environments that celebrate diversity.

KEY POINTS

▶ 1 **The issue of entry into nursing practice has been a problem for almost 100 years. Nursing leaders have called for having the baccalaureate degree as the minimum degree for entry since 1923, but alternative pathways to RN licensure remain. The main reason for the inability to resolve** the issue is the large number of diploma and associate degree nursing graduates throughout the 20th century, who have had a significant negative impact on the implementation of proposals requiring the baccalaureate as the basic degree to enter nursing practice.

▶ 2 Differentiated practice refers to a clearly defined structure of the roles and functions of nurses according to their experience, education, and competence. It offers a possible solution to the entry-into-practice debate because it clearly states what jobs and salaries the different types of nurse graduates should have. The primary responsibility for implementing differentiated practice lies within the realm of practice. However, nursing education would have the responsibility of providing the opportunity for nurses in the lower levels to advance through education.

▶ 3 Voluntary accreditation of nursing education programs (in addition to public accreditation by a state board) is important because it assures students and the public of a high quality of nursing education and care. Although accreditation is voluntary, most nursing programs seek accreditation because it benefits their students.

▶ 4 The general process of voluntary nursing accreditation (accreditation beyond the minimal accreditation by a state board) involves ensuring that the nursing program meets established criteria and standards. This entails a comprehensive self-study by the nursing school desiring accreditation, a site visit conducted by a panel of faculty members from similar schools, and the panel's review and recommendations made to the board of the accrediting agency.

▶ 5 Concerns began to arise as early as the 1960s about the excessive number of accrediting bodies and which nursing organization should be accrediting nursing programs. In 1995, the Department of Education informed the NLN that it did not meet the requirements for an accrediting body (although not disapproved, the League is still awaiting reapproval of its license to accredit). In the late 1980s, after receiving expressions of concern from nursing educators and policy makers about the process of nursing accreditation, the AACN established a task force to explore nursing accreditation and what role the association should play in accreditation. Members of the association voted overwhelmingly for a proposal that the association would take the lead in creating a new alliance for overseeing accreditation of baccalaureate and higher degree nursing programs. Their goal is to be licensed to accredit by 1998.

▶ 6 Enhancing diversity within nursing education and nursing practice is important because racial and ethnic minorities and men have long been sorely underrepresented in nursing. As the U.S. population becomes increasingly diverse, it is vital that nursing care is culturally sensitive and culturally responsive. Thus, part of the responsibility of nursing education is to prepare many more nurses of culturally diverse backgrounds to improve the nursing care to a rapidly expanding segment of the U.S. population.

▶ 7 Some strategies that can be used to enhance diversity within nursing education include setting up formal and informal programs with colleges and universities that support minorities and men. These may include setting up programs such as the MAAP or the pathways model, working with nursing faculty to ensure that they provide an environment where racially and ethnically diverse student populations can flourish, offering more minority scholarships and financial aid, encouraging high school guidance counselors to promote nursing as a career option to men and racial and ethnic minorities, including family in the recruitment process, and emphasizing factors of nursing that appeal to men and minority students.

REFERENCES

American Association of Colleges of Nursing (1995). *A Model for Differentiated Nursing Practice.* Washington DC: Author.

American Association of Colleges of Nursing (1996, November). *Fact Sheet: An Alliance for Accreditation of Nursing Higher Education.* Washington DC: Author.

Anderson CA (1994). Graduate education in primary care: The challenge. *Nursing Outlook, 42,* 101–102.

Association of Specialized and Professional Accreditors (1995). *The Role and Value of Specialized Accreditation.* Chicago: Author.

Brider P (1996). AACN moves to launch new accrediting alliance. *AJN, 96,* 67–72.

Buerhaus PI, Staiger DO (1997). Future of the nurse labor market according to health executives in high managed-care areas of the United States. *Image: Journal of Nursing Scholarship, 29,* 313–318.

Bullough V (1997). Men in nursing: Problems and prospects. In McCloskey JC, Grace HK, eds. *Current Issues in Nursing* (5th ed.). St. Louis: Mosby.

Camilleri DD (1997). Nursing education for the 21st century: Old traditions and new challenges. In McCloskey JC, Grace HK, eds. *Current Issues in Nursing* (5th ed.). St. Louis: Mosby.

Campbell AR, Davis SM (1996). Faculty commitment: Retaining minority nursing students in majority institutions. *J Nursing Education, 35,* 298–303.

Castiglia PT (1997). Minority representation in nursing educational programs: Increasing cultural awareness. In McCloskey JC, Grace HK, eds. *Current Issues in Nursing* (5th ed.). St. Louis: Mosby.

Chitty KK (1997). *Professional Nursing: Concepts and Challenges* (2nd ed.). Philadelphia: WB Saunders.

Copp LA (1995). Respecting the nontraditional student. *J Professional Nursing, 11,* 65–66.

Copp LA (1997). Faculty uninformed in the information age? *J Professional Nursing, 13,* 1–2.

deTornyay R (1996). Critical challenges for nurse educators. *J Nursing Education, 35,* 146–147.

Division of Nursing (1996, March). *Advance notes from the National Sample Survey of Registered Nurses March 1996.* Rockville, MD: Division of Nursing, Bureau of Health Professions, Health Resources and Services Administration.

Division of Nursing (1997). *March 25, 1997, Report to American Association of College of Nursing.* U.S. Department of Health & Human Services, Public Health Service, Health Resources and Services Administration, Bureau of Health Professions. Washington DC: Author.

Dowell MA (1996). Issues in recruitment and retention of minority nursing students. *J Nursing Education, 35,* 293–297.

Division of Research, National League for Nursing. (1995). *Nursing Data Review 1995.* New York: Author.

Forsey LM, Cleland VS, Miller B (1993). Job descriptions for differentiated nursing practice and differentiated pay. *J Nursing Administration, 23,* 33–40.

Hess JD (1996). Education for entry into practice: An ethical perspective. *J Professional Nursing, 12,* 289–296.

Hesser A, Pond E, Lewis L, Abbot B (1996). Evaluation of a supplementary retention program for African-American baccalaureate nursing students. *J Nursing Education, 35,* 304–309.

Kelly LY, Joel LA (1996). *The Nursing Experience: Trends, Challenges, and Transitions.* New York: McGraw-Hill.

Kelly NR, Shoemaker M, Steele T (1996). The experience of being a male student nurse. *J Nursing Education, 35,* 170–174.

McClure ML (1991). Differentiated nursing practice: Concepts and considerations. *Nursing Outlook, 39,* 106–110.

Moloney MM (1992). *Professionalization of Nursing: Current Issues and Trends* (2nd ed.). Philadelphia: JB Lippincott.

National Advisory Council on Nurse Education and Practice (1996). *Report to the Secretary of the Department of Health and Human Services on the Basic Registered Nurse Work Force.* U.S. Department of Health & Human Services, Health Resources & Services Administration, Bureau of Health Professions, Division of Nursing. Washington DC: U.S. Government Printing Office.

National Commission on Nursing (1983). *Summary report and recommendations.* Chicago: American Hospital Association.

Oermann MH (1997). Professional nursing practice. In Oermann MH (Ed.), *Professional Nursing Practice.* Stamford, CT; Appleton & Lange.

Perkins JL, Bennett DN, Dorman RE (1993). Why men choose nursing. *Nursing and Health Care, 14,* 34–38.

Redman RW, Ketefian S (1997). The changing face of graduate education. In H. Grace & J.C. McCloskey (Eds.), *Current Issues in Nursing* (5th ed.). St. Louis: Mosby.

Rew L (1966). Affirming cultural diversity: A pathways model for nursing faculty. *J Nursing Education, 35,* 310–314.

Tanner CA (1996). Accreditation under siege. *J Nursing Education, 35,* 243–244.

Tanner CA (1996). Cultural diversity in nursing education. *J Nursing Education, 35,* 291–292.

U.S. Department of Health and Human Services (1991). *Nursing: Health Personnel in the United States, 1991: Eighth Report to Congress* (Prepublication Report). Washington DC: Author.

Yoder MK (1996). Instructional responses to ethnically diverse nursing students. *J Nursing Education, 35,* 315–321.

Classic Reference

Hornsby JA, Schmidt RE (1914). *The Modern Hospital: Its Inspiration, Its Architecture, Its Equipment, Its Operation.* Philadelphia: WB Saunders.

RECOMMENDED READINGS

Froman RD, Owen SV (1989). Predicting performance on the National Council Licensure Examination. *Western J Nursing Research, 11,* 334–346.

Hess JD (1996). Education for entry into practice: An ethical perspective. *J Professional Nursing, 12,* 289–296.

Hutchens GC (1994). Differentiated interdisciplinary practice. *J Nursing Administration, 24*(6), 52–58.

Marquis B, Lillibridge J, Madison J (1993). Problems and progress as Australia adopts the bachelor's degree as the only entry to nursing practice. *Nursing Outlook, 41*, 135–140.

Raymond MR (1988). The relationship between educational preparation and performance on nursing certification examinations. *J Nursing Education, 27*, 6–9.

Spencer-Cisek P, Sveningson L (1995). Regulation of advanced nursing practice: Part two—certification. *Oncology Nursing Forum, 22*(8), 39–42.

Spicer JG, Ripple HB, Louie E, Baj P, Keating S (1994). Supporting ethnic and cultural diversity in nursing staff. *Nursing Management, 25*, 38–40.

Tanner CA (1996). Cultural diversity in nursing education. *J Nursing Education, 35*, 291–292.

Thomas B, Arseneault A (1993). Accreditation of university schools of nursing: The Canadian experience. *International Nursing Review, 40*(3), 81–94.

Tullman DF (1992). Cultural diversity in nursing education: Does it affect racism in the nursing profession? *J Nursing Education, 31*, 321–324.

PART IV

Nursing Practice and Professionalization

8

Nursing Career Opportunities

CHAPTER OUTLINE

Nursing in Acute Care Hospitals
Nursing in Ambulatory Care Settings
Nursing in the Community
Nursing in Long-Term Care Facilities

Chapter Summary
Key Points
References
Recommended Readings

LEARNING OBJECTIVES

▶ **1** Discuss the factors that contributed to the growth of hospitals in the United States.

▶ **2** List seven elements that make hospitals good environments in which to practice nursing.

▶ **3** Discuss the ways in which nurses contribute to patient care in ambulatory care settings.

▶ **4** Discuss nurses' contributions to care in the community.

▶ **5** Compare and contrast the goals and services provided to residents in nursing homes and rehabilitation environments.

KEY TERMS

almshouses
diagnosis-related
  groups (DRGs)
Frontier Nursing
  Service (FNS)
health maintenance
  organizations
  (HMOs)

Henry Street
  Settlement House
Hill-Burton Act
hospice
length of stay (LOS)
Lillian Wald
magnet hospital
  studies

Mary Breckinridge
Medicaid
Medicare
Occupational Safety
  and Health
  Administration
  (OSHA)
parish nursing
pesthouse

During the last half of the 20th century, the vast majority of U.S. nurses have practiced nursing in acute care inpatient hospitals. That is the kind of practice for which they were educated and the kind of practice they expected to engage in throughout their nursing careers. Moreover, it was not unusual for nurses to spend their entire careers in one or only a few hospitals. Also, nursing leaders within hospitals customarily rose through the ranks. Thus, it was not unusual for a good, committed nurse to start as a staff nurse and then to become an assistant nurse manager and then a nurse manager. Often the next step was that of supervisor, with the responsibility for several nursing units. At the top of the nursing hierarchy were the assistant directors of nursing and finally the director of nursing. All these positions often were filled through in-house promotions. However, as has been noted repeatedly throughout this book, U.S. society and U.S. health care are changing dramatically and rapidly, and nursing practice realities and expectations must change as well.

The National Advisory Council on Nurse Education and Practice has predicted a major shift as we enter the 21st century in both the focus of the health care system and the nature of nursing practice and responsibility:

> Earlier emphasis on acute care with substantial reliance on hospital-based care is shifting to a focus on disease prevention and modification of lifestyles. This shift promotes maintenance of individuals at home and treatment in ambulatory settings. (National Advisory Council on Nurse Education and Practice, 1996, p. 7)

The council noted that because of significant therapeutic and technological advances, there will be increased complexity of care and treatment in all care settings.

In 1997, the Division of Nursing reported that 60% of employed nurses were working in hospitals, 17% in community and public health settings, 8.5% in ambulatory care settings (eg, physicians' offices, nursing practices, and health maintenance organizations), and 8.1% in nursing homes or other extended care facilities (Division of Nursing, 1997). It will be interesting to note how those figures change over the next two decades. If current trends continue, the proportion of nurses employed in hospitals will decrease and the numbers employed in community and ambulatory care will increase.

In the immediate future, most nurses prepared for basic nursing practice still will be employed by acute care inpatient facilities, but health care cost containment will continue to define where and how health care personnel will practice. Thus, as patients' hospital stays shorten and the U.S. population ages, the need for highly skilled nursing care will extend rapidly beyond traditional inpatient hospitals. Given the increased importance and focus on a wide range of nursing care settings, recent graduate nurses should be prepared to explore a variety of practice settings. This will enable him or her to find the best fit between the scope and nature of nursing as it is practiced in each organization and his or her competencies, interests, and career goals.

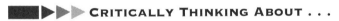 **CRITICALLY THINKING ABOUT . . .**

Most nurses are employed in hospitals. Is your goal to be a hospital nurse?

Nursing in Acute Care Hospitals

Despite repeated predictions that more and more nursing care will be moving beyond traditional inpatient hospital settings, hospitals as a category will remain the single largest employer of RNs in the immediate future. This is particularly true for recent graduates, because many of the practice opportunities and environments that will be described later require nursing experience or postbaccalaureate education or training. Hospitals also are a relatively familiar environment for recent nurse graduates because in most nursing education programs today the majority of the clinical education experiences are provided in traditional acute care hospital settings.

Development of Hospitals in the United States

As noted in Chapter 5, hospitals as they exist today are a relatively recent phenomenon. In the 1700s, most U.S. cities built public **almshouses,** or poorhouses, to provide food and shelter for the homeless poor. These almshouses were the only welfare system that was available to destitute people in that period. They became home to the aged, the disabled, the mentally ill, and the orphaned. Another type of institution also existed in that period—the **pesthouse**. Immigrants from Europe were flooding into America at that time, and it was common for people to contract highly contagious, potentially fatal diseases while aboard incoming ships. The concepts of hygiene and the nature of contagion were unknown. Therefore, contagious diseases such as smallpox, typhus, cholera, and yellow fever spread like wildfire, killing and disabling hundreds and thousands of people in weeks or months. Thus, when an outbreak occurred, a pesthouse would be opened to isolate the victims of that disease from the rest of the community until they either recovered or died. When the intensity of that particular epidemic ebbed, the pesthouse would be closed to await the next epidemic.

The conditions in almshouses and pesthouses were uniformly wretched. They were crowded, filthy, poorly heated, and poorly ventilated. Cross-infections were common and mortality was high.

The first hospitals *per se* were the Pennsylvania Hospital in Philadelphia (1751), the New York Hospital in New York City (1773), Massachusetts General Hospital in Boston (1816), and New Haven Hospital in Connecticut (1826). These hospitals cared for patients who were acutely ill or injured, but they did not care for the mentally ill; separate hospitals were established for this purpose. These included the Pennsylvania Hospital, founded in 1752, a second one established in Williamsburg, Virginia, in 1773, and the third, the Friends' Hospital near Philadelphia, in 1817.

Although the care provided in these early hospitals was superior to the conditions of the almshouses and pesthouses, it was still far from desirable. Linens were used for several different patients between launderings, open draining wounds were common, sanitation measures were poor, and, as one would expect, the stench often was overwhelming. People with sufficient funds arranged for medical and nursing care at home, and no self-respecting woman would ever have her baby in a hospital.

Factors Contributing to the Growth of American Hospitals

Time changed hospital conditions for the better. Ellis and Hartley (1995) have identified six major factors that served as forces in the development and improvement of hospitals and patient care in the United States within the last century and a half.

First, medical science has advanced rapidly. The discovery of anesthesia made possible the subsequent rapid developments in surgery. In addition, the development of germ theory quickly led to techniques and products that would sterilize or serve as antiseptics, diminishing the ever-present threat of hospital-acquired infections and cross-contamination. The development of medical technology closely followed earlier advances in medical science, including hospital laboratories (1889), x-ray equipment (1896), the electrocardiogram (1903), and the electroencephalogram (1929) (Haglund & Dowling, 1988).

Third, the quality of medical education in the United States underwent great improvement as a result of the 1910 Flexner report (see Chap. 1). Many medical schools of questionable quality were closed, and those that remained were strengthened. The role of hospitals was included in this upgrading of medical education, because the requirements to enter practice included extended clinical practice in hospitals in the form of internships and residencies. This improvement in the overall status of medical education and practice had a beneficial effect on the growth and increasing prestige of American hospitals.

A fourth factor contributing to the growth of hospitals was the availability of health insurance. Before 1929, most people did not have access to health insurance that would pay any part of the costs incurred during hospitalization care and treatment. Thus, only the wealthy could afford the increasingly prestigious medical care provided by American hospitals. However, in 1929, a hospital insurance plan was initiated at Baylor University Hospital to serve the needs of teachers in Dallas, Texas; this model was used as the basis for what would subsequently become the Blue Cross insurance plans all across the country (Raffel & Raffel, 1989). The availability of insurance plans meant that more and more people could afford hospital care, so the demand for hospitals rose.

The early 20th century was also a period of rapid growth in the size and power of labor unions in the United States. Although improvements in wages and working conditions were always basic targets of union demands and contracts, health insurance plans also became very important facets of the contracts that unions negotiated with the country's rapidly expanding industrial sector.

The federal government also contributed substantially to the growth of the American hospital industry. In 1935, as part of President Franklin Roosevelt's "New Deal," the government provided grants-in-aid to help establish public health and other programs to provide health assistance to the U.S. population. After World War II (1946), Congress enacted the **Hill-Burton Act**, which provided a massive infusion of funds for the construction of hospitals and related care facilities. In 1965, the Medicare and Medicaid plans were enacted. **Medicare** provides federal support for health care for men and women 65 years of age and over. **Medicaid** makes federal monies available to states for providing medical assistance to indigent persons, using various plans and strategies. Although in the early 20th century the federal government initiated many actions that contributed to the growth and expansion of hospitals, one of its subsequent actions has had a significant impact on the downsizing of that same industry: the establishment and implementation in 1982 and 1983 of diagnosis-related groups (DRGs). The concept of DRGs and their impact will be discussed later in this chapter and in Chapter 10.

Finally, the expansion of hospitals in the United States was made possible by the educational preparation of large numbers of well-trained, highly qualified nurses starting at the turn of the century (see Chap. 5). Typically, RNs are the single largest employee group in any hospital. Well-prepared nurses traditionally have enhanced the quality of patient care greatly and thus have played a significant role in the growth of the hospital industry in America.

As a result of the growth of hospitals, the upgrading of medical education and technology, the availability of health insurance, the enactment of Medicaid and Medicare, and the educational preparation of nurses, the public has been given access to more dependable, higher-quality medical care.

Entering Hospital Nursing: Evaluating the Environment

There is a great deal of variability within hospital nursing, and new nurses should carefully assess their preferences for work style and environment as well as their career goals and personal objectives. They should also become familiar with the employment opportunities that are available, starting by learning as much as possible about the hospitals they are considering.

Hospitals can be categorized in several ways. The most common descriptor of hospitals is in terms of number of beds. Knowing the number of beds gives an immediate rough image of the institution. A hospital with 1000 or more beds is quite large and bureaucratically complex; a 100-bed hospital is quite tiny. As the health care industry changes, the number of small hospitals is shrinking rapidly. Sometimes small hospitals that are acquired by larger corporate entities are converted to regional satellites or specialty service hospitals. More often, however, the smaller hospitals are simply closed if the larger corporate entity determines that the market for care in the community simply cannot make the small hospital profitable for the corporation.

Given all the changes in the structure and organization of hospitals today, a nurse looking for a position in a hospital should become familiar with the organizational structure in which patient care is carried out, the corporate environment, and the economic health of the community. This will allow the nurse to get the best idea of how secure employment is likely to be in any given institution.

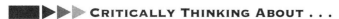 CRITICALLY THINKING ABOUT . . .

How many hospitals have you visited or worked in? What features distinguished them from each other?

Good Hospital Environments

Beyond the size of the hospital and its potential corporate viability, what should a nurse look for when seeking employment in a hospital? What is a "good" hospital, from a nursing perspective? What organizational characteristics enhance nurses' potential for engaging in the most professional practice? Some answers to these important questions were provided by the **magnet hospital studies** conducted in the 1980s. The motivation for conducting those studies was the nursing shortage that was troubling the health care industry at that time. Although there is no longer a nursing shortage in most parts of the country, the studies' findings as to what makes an environment enhancing to professional nursing remain valid more than a decade later.

The first study, sponsored by the American Academy of Nursing (McClure, Poulin, Sovie, & Wandelt, 1982), was designed to identify hospitals that had reputations for being good places to work and good places to practice nursing. The investigators conducted a detailed examination of 46 acute care hospitals, focusing on attraction and retention of nurses. Based on questionnaires and interviews, the investigators found that well-prepared nurse managers and chief nurse executives were vital components of the magnet hospitals. Nurse executives were seen as strong, supportive, and visible; they consistently enunciated high standards for practice and patient care. Magnet hospitals were characterized by participatory management, good personnel policies, competitive salaries, and good career development opportunities.

In the mid-1980s, Marlene Kramer and Claudia Schmalenberg (1988a and 1988b) conducted the second magnet hospital study, an in-depth follow-up study of 16 of those first magnet hospitals. These researchers used the framework developed by Peters and Waterman in their 1982 book *In Search of Excellence*. Peters and Waterman had identified eight characteristics that were common to the best-run companies in corporate America. Kramer and Schmalenberg wanted to determine the extent to which magnet hospitals possessed those same eight characteristics. They concluded that there were many areas of strong correspondence between the best-run companies and magnet hospitals.

Both successful companies and magnet hospitals were characterized by a "bias for action." That means that the organization is fluid and informal enough that communication is easy and exchange of information is achieved quickly and easily at all levels. Piles of paperwork were not the norm; instead, "management by walking about" was common, as were open-door policies among managers at all levels. These practices facilitated timely and creative communication. Bias for action also means that organizations are willing to try something new and will not punish experimenters if their innovations don't work out. "Management must promote a culture where the employee does not lose face to admit that something didn't work" (Kramer & Schmalenberg, 1988a, p. 17).

The second characteristic that was common to both well-managed companies and magnet hospitals was termed "close to the customer." This means a commitment to the consistent delivery of a product (patient care) of the highest quality. This commitment must be pervasive throughout the system. Three themes common to magnet hospitals were:

1. Intensive, active involvement of senior management
2. A very strong "people orientation"
3. Attention to measurement and feedback.

Several nurses in magnet hospitals commented that they routinely expected to receive answers to questions or concerns expressed to management within 48 hours, and this was very important to them. Moreover, caring for others extended not only to the clients and their families, but also to the nurses themselves. They felt the organization cared about them and acknowledged their successes openly and frequently.

The third principle that was operative in well-run companies and magnet hospitals was "autonomy and entrepreneurship." This principle is closely linked with a bias for action. Kramer and Schmalenberg cited the work of Dorothy Brooten and her associates at the University of Pennsylvania (1986) and that of Knaus, Draper, Wagner, and Zimmerman (1986), which clearly demonstrates the direct line between nurse autonomy and quality nursing care. Autonomy is the freedom to act based on what you know. It includes not only the freedom to act and succeed, but also the freedom to act and fail. Magnet hospitals were characterized by an environment that provided support for the staff to use their autonomy and initiative to devise new, unusual, and smart ways of providing care to patients. The magnet hospitals were known for their innovations (Kramer & Schmalenberg, 1988a).

The fourth characteristic shared by excellent companies and the magnet hospitals was "productivity through people." These organizations demonstrated true respect for the individual. People were treated with dignity, and rewards were associated with productivity and performance, not simply longevity in the system. Rewards for achievement often were accompanied by "a certain amount of 'splash' or 'hoopla'" (Kramer & Schmalenberg, 1988b, p. 11), so recognition was widely and publicly acknowledged. Some magnet hospitals had clinical ladders in place as a means of structuring the reward system; other had tried them and found that they did not work. The informal communication structure already mentioned also supported the "productivity through people" principle. Such a structure allows everyone in the organization to keep up to date and informed.

The fifth characteristic cited by Peters and Waterman was called "hands-on, value-driven." In excellent companies, the major role of leaders was seen as creating, instilling, and clarifying the company's value system. "The role of management was to generate enthusiasm down to the very last worker" (Kramer & Schmalenberg, 1988b, p. 13). When Kramer and Schmalenberg evaluated magnet hospitals against this criterion, they found that the nursing leaders in the magnet hospitals demonstrated the same kind of behavior. They were highly visible and accessible. They had national reputations, held national offices, and set value standards for nursing not only locally, but also regionally and nationally. Leaders in magnet hospitals were viewed as visionaries. The top-level nursing management teams were small (seldom more than three or four), very cohesive, enthusiastic about their roles, and very well educated.

▶▶▶ CRITICALLY THINKING ABOUT . . .

Is it economically feasible for smaller hospitals to attract the kind of nursing leaders that the magnet hospitals attracted? Why or why not?

Peters and Waterman found that excellent companies followed a sixth principle, "stick to the knitting," or stay with the business you know best. However, Kramer and Schmalenberg (1988b) found that this characteristic did not hold in nursing departments of the magnet hospitals because in the current health care arena, diversification is a survival tactic that keeps hospitals competitive.

The seventh characteristic applied to both excellent companies and magnet hospitals, "simple form, lean staff." Most organizations, as they grow, develop complex systems and structures for "top-down" management, with many levels of management between the top executives and the people who do the work. However, excellent companies and magnet hospitals shared several organizational characteristics that demonstrated that complex organizational hierarchies may not be the best organizational model. Excellent companies and magnet hospitals tended to be "radically decentralized." They had relatively few people at the top corporate levels, and there were minimal levels within the organization. The organizational structures of most of the magnet hospitals were characterized as flat, lean, and decentralized. This allowed for quick decisions and quality actions because of the flexibility and control of practice at the nursing unit level (Kramer & Schmalenberg, 1988b).

Finally, Peters and Waterman discovered that the best-run businesses operated according to an eighth characteristic, "simultaneous loose-tight properties." Magnet hospitals also demonstrated this principle. A firm central direction is established by a unifying set of values, values that are established and guarded by the nursing leadership. But at the same time the bedside nurse has autonomy, and decisions are made appropriately at the nursing unit level.

Kramer and Schmalenberg answered their original question, "Why do magnet hospitals excel?" by concluding that those hospitals were "infused with values of quality care, nurse autonomy, informal, nonrigid verbal communication, innovation, bringing out the best in each individual, value of education, respect and caring for the individual, and striving for excellence." They were "led by nurse leaders and managers who are zealots in holding and promulgating these values" (Kramer & Schmalenberg, 1988, p. 17).

The magnet hospitals studies provide us with a way of gauging a hospital's qualities. In addition to corporate viability, "good" hospitals are characterized by:

1. A bias for action
2. Closeness to customers
3. Autonomy and entrepreneurship
4. Productivity through people
5. Hands-on, value-driven
6. Simple form, lean staff
7. Simultaneous loose–tight priorities.

Hospital Nursing: Temporary Staffing Opportunities

Many nurses who wish to practice in hospitals but want some variety as well choose to work for a nursing staffing agency, also called a temporary nursing service. This is an attractive option for recent graduate nurses seeking a broad range of nursing experience, nurses who are pursuing advanced educational degrees, and nurses whose family responsibilities demand a flexible schedule. Nurses who have an even greater spirit of adventure may wish to become "flying nurses." Through an agency, these nurses make contract arrangements varying from a few weeks to several months with hospitals all over the United States and sometimes abroad.

Nursing in Ambulatory Care Settings

In general, ambulatory care refers to care provided to clients who come to the care facility for services. Ambulatory care is an area that is growing rapidly and promises to continue growing as long as it provides a cost-effective care delivery system that maintains high standards of quality and service to clients. Ambulatory care facilities are springing up all over the country, and their structure and services vary widely.

Office Practice

The most traditional form of ambulatory care is that administered by physicians and other independent health care providers in their offices. This includes general practice physicians, dentists, podiatrists, chiropractors, optometrists, and, more recently, advanced practice nurses. These providers may be engaged in a solo practice or in a joint practice with other health professionals with a similar practice specialty. RNs are often employed in these offices to provide assistance to the primary caregiver and to perform basic client assessments (eg, height, weight, blood pressure, pulse). Office nurses also administer prescribed medications and carry out other basic treatments. Nurses also may have responsibilities for conducting and recording basic laboratory work that is done in the office.

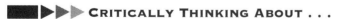 CRITICALLY THINKING ABOUT . . .

What do you see as the advantages and disadvantages for the nurse in office practice over hospital nursing practice?

A recent adjunct to the traditional individual and group practice of ambulatory care is the urgent care center. These centers typically are small outreach facilities located throughout the community that are owned and operated by hospitals in the community. The staff, including the physicians, are hospital employees. Clients typically are served on a walk-in, first-come-first-served basis, and diagnosis and care are given by a primary care provider such as a general practice physician, an advanced nurse practitioner, or perhaps a pediatrician. Urgent care centers are attractive options for clients whose injuries or illnesses are not serious enough to require emergency room treatment, but who require treatment in a more timely fashion than they might be able to obtain from their regular family physician, whose schedule is usually tightly packed with appointments. Moreover, the cost of treatment at an urgent care center may be 30% to 40% lower than the same treatment administered in a hospital emergency room (Kelly & Joel, 1996). The role of the office nurse in urgent care centers is much the same as in a regular professional practice office.

Outpatient Surgical Centers

Another rapidly growing segment of ambulatory care services provided by hospitals consists of outpatient clinics located within or near the hospital itself. These clinics commonly offer a wide range of surgical procedures that require less anesthesia and much less postoperative care than traditional inpatient surgical procedures. Outpatient surgical services have been established largely as a money-saving measure. The client goes to the clinic a day or two before the scheduled surgery for the necessary preoperative tests, then goes home with instructions about preparation for the surgical procedure (eg, when to return for the procedure, any preparations he or she should make). In inpatient surgery, those same preoperative tests typically are performed the day before surgery and the patient stays overnight in the hospital. Reducing the need for a preoperative overnight stay represents a significant savings in the cost of care.

After surgery, each patient is monitored to ensure safe recovery from anesthesia and to ensure that the surgical site is secure. An important role for RNs in outpatient surgical centers is teaching the patient and caregiver. Even in an outpatient setting, surgery still is an invasive procedure that can have serious consequences, and postoperative care still is required. However, postoperative care will be given not by nurses, but by a family member or friend, or perhaps even by the client. Thus, these people must understand:

1. Possible adverse side effects and how to monitor for them
2. How to care for the surgical site
3. How much rest and recovery time the postoperative client should have
4. How to administer postoperative medication, both prescribed and over-the-counter
5. Who to notify if any untoward events related to the surgery occur
6. When to return to the clinic for a follow-up assessment or treatment.

Community Health Centers

Community health centers commonly provide care to medically underserved populations. These people tend to cluster in ethnic urban enclaves, but more are appearing in small rural communities, which are also becoming medically underserved as general practitioners retire. These small rural communities often are economically depressed and have little appeal to younger practitioners, so the community is left without a full-time physician.

The models for urban community health centers emerged in the early 1970s and were supported largely by funding from the Office of Economic Opportunity, one facet of the "Great Society" mandate initiated by President Lyndon B. Johnson and the U.S. Congress in the late 1960s. The community health center was conceived of as a small, conveniently located facility (often a storefront) employing a salaried, full-time physician and staffed with a multidisciplinary health care team. Providing convenient, affordable (often free), culturally sensitive primary care was the goal. One of the hallmarks of these centers was significant community involvement in both their operations and policy making. To facilitate communication, efforts usually are made to staff community health centers with members of the ethnic groups served by the center. These centers can be freestanding or part of a community hospital system or public health department.

Most of the elements of President Johnson's Great Society gradually waned over time and disappeared, and so too did significant federal funding for community health centers. They now rely heavily on Medicare and Medicaid as sources of income, and their survival often depends on the ability of the director or staff to raise funds by writing proposals to a wide variety of private and government sources.

Care delivery in community health centers can be very demanding and often uncertain, but it can also be rewarding because the needs of the populations that are served are so great. Also, nurses have an opportunity to work in a truly interdisciplinary environment with a broad range of clients and whole families from a genuinely holistic perspective.

 CRITICALLY THINKING ABOUT . . .

> Have you received treatment in an outpatient surgical center or a community health center? From what you observed, what seemed to be the role of the nurse in that care setting?

One example of a nurse-managed community health center is the Community Free Clinic in Flagstaff, Arizona. This clinic began when two Flagstaff physicians decided to organize volunteer health care for people who fall through the cracks in our health care system—the so-called "notch" group. The people in a notch group work at minimum-wage jobs; their benefits are minimal, and most have no health insurance. Because they are employed, they do not qualify for welfare benefits. The large tourist industry in Flagstaff employs many minimum-wage workers, so the number of people in this notch group is substantial. These people simply do not earn enough to pay for health care for themselves and their families out of pocket, because minimum wage is barely enough to provide basic sustenance.

The Free Clinic emerged as a cooperative partnership between the county's public health department and the department of nursing at Northern Arizona University. One evening a week, a team consisting of a nurse practitioner, a community health nurse, nursing students, dental hygiene students, and volunteer nurses and office personnel operates a nursing center. This nursing center offers clients primary care, health promotion, disease prevention, and assistance in managing chronic health conditions. Thus, this nurse-managed clinic effectively meets its stated goals:

- ▶ It delivers health care services to an underserved population.
- ▶ It provides educational opportunities for students.
- ▶ It provides a site for nursing faculty to practice.
- ▶ It provides research opportunities for nursing practice. (Craig, 1996, p. 125)

Nursing in the Community

Nursing care in the United States is deeply rooted in the community. In the late 1800s and early 1900s, the early leaders of nursing in this country were profoundly committed to providing nursing and health care to clients in their own homes and in institutions situated within their communities. These women served thousands of new Americans—largely immigrants from Western and Southern Europe—and were, in effect, the foundation of health care for those people. These pioneers in community health also laid the foundation for advanced practice nursing as it is known today. Box 8-1 gives an historical overview of the achievements of these women.

Nurses can practice in a variety of areas within community nursing. These include home health nursing, hospice nursing, occupational nursing, school nursing, and parish nursing.

Home Health Care Nursing

A combination of changes in public policy regarding reimbursement for hospital care and changes in the demography of the United States have led to dramatic expansion of the home health care industry. In 1983, Medicare instituted the prospective pricing system and the use of **diagnosis-related groups (DRGs)** as a mechanism for reimbursing hospitals for patient care. Before time, the general practice was that hospitals billed Medicare for the care that was delivered after the patient's discharge and in general recovered most, if not all, of the costs that were incurred. Under this system, costs were rapidly escalating.

A study was undertaken by the federal government to determine what would be an expected **length of stay (LOS)** in the hospital for a patient admitted with a particular diagnosis and what the hospital costs would be for that LOS, assuming that medical and nursing care was carried out properly and the patient recovered success-

Box 8-1	
Pioneers in Community Health Nursing	

Lillian Wald and the Henry Street Settlement House

Lillian Wald, one of the founders of community health nursing, was born in 1867 and grew up in Rochester, New York. She obtained 3 years of nursing training at the New York Hospital School of Nursing and planned to continue her education at the Women's Medical College in New York. However, the desperate living conditions and health care needs of the urban immigrant populations came to her attention while she was still in her mid-20s. She was so moved by the misery she saw that she left her comfortable lifestyle and, with another nurse, Mary Brewster, began a career offering nursing care to needy people (Kalisch & Kalisch, 1995; Portnoy & Dumas, 1994).

Wald and Brewster's first endeavor was to set up a Nurses' Settlement House in a slum section of New York's Lower East Side. Wald and Brewster were not allied with a religious group. They provided care to those who could pay and to those who could not. They became known and trusted by their neighbors, and eventually by physicians, who increasingly referred patients to them.

> From the beginning, one of the basic principles underlying Lillian Wald's work held nursing care of the sick in their homes as the primary aim, with health instruction secondary . . . the visiting nurse was to respond to calls from the people themselves as well as from physicians and to act with as little delay as possible. (Kalisch & Kalisch, 1995, p. 175)

Within two years, the volume of work increased to the point that Wald and Beck urgently needed a larger facility and more nurses. So, in 1895, assisted financially by banker and philanthropist Jacob H. Schiff, they moved their Nurses' Settlement to 265 Henry Street, where it soon became known as the **Henry Street Settlement House.** By 1909, the staff at Henry Street had grown to 37 nurses, all of whom lived in the Henry Street headquarters. Nurses were very carefully selected for service at Henry Street, and only those who demonstrated a true understanding of the conditions and problems of the immigrants were retained.

Wald and her associates provided an extraordinary range of care. The *Annual Report of the Henry Street Settlement for 1905* showed that 5032 patients had been cared for in homes. Their report also showed that cases had been reported by families, physicians, and charitable agencies and that over half of them had been cured. The range of diagnoses was very broad, including 1735 that were "unclassified medical" and 602 more that were "unclassified surgical." Pneumonia and bronchitis, along with tuberculosis, accounted for more than 1200 of the patients treated by the Henry Street Settlement nurses in 1905. First-aid homes also were established in several densely populated sections of the city, where a daily nurse treated ailments such as minor surgical cases, ear problems, and eye problems, primarily among schoolchildren (Kalisch & Kalisch, 1995).

Mary Breckinridge and the Frontier Nursing Service

The **Frontier Nursing Service** (FNS) was another pioneering endeavor in American nursing that was committed to providing health care to needy people in their own homes and communities. **Mary Breckinridge,** the founder of FNS, was another of the great pioneers in public health. "The FNS is a model for nurse-managed care and provides a historical framework for the future of community health nursing" (Raines & Wilson, 1996, p. 123).

(continued)

BOX 8-1 (CONTINUED)

Mary Breckinridge was born into a Southern family in Memphis, Tennessee, in 1881. Her great-great-grandfather had served as attorney general under President Thomas Jefferson. She married at 23, but became a widow at 24. Searching for purpose in her life, she entered St. Luke's School of Nursing in New York City in 1907, completed nurse's training in 1910, and remarried. However, more tragedy awaited her: by 1918, an infant daughter and a 4-year-old son had both succumbed to illness and death, and her second marriage could not withstand the burden of the loss.

After volunteer service in France during the First World War, Breckinridge returned to the United States intent on following her dream of helping medically underserved mothers and children in the rural mountains of Kentucky. She went on to earn a Master of Public Health degree from Columbia University and completed the midwifery training program at the British Hospital for Mothers and Babies in London.

To complete her training, she traveled to Scotland to observe the Highlands and Islands Medical Service, which operated in a remote, isolated region much like Leslie County, Kentucky, where she planned to establish her practice. She founded the FNS using the principles of decentralized "district nursing" she had observed in Scotland (Raines & Wilson, 1996).

After her return to America, Breckinridge established a sound foundation of information about the region she planned to serve and gained support for her program to provide midwifery services to mothers and babies. She rode more than 600 miles on horseback, collecting statistics, observing, and giving and receiving advice. Breckinridge provided the initial funding for the first 3 years of the program using money she had inherited from a wealthy great-aunt.

Originally named the Kentucky Committee for Mothers and Babies, the FNS was officially established in 1925. The staff, consisting of Breckinridge and two British midwives trained in public health, traveled by horseback to hundreds of remote rural cabins providing prenatal care, deliveries, and preventive health care. They also instructed families in methods to improve sanitation in their homes (Raines & Wilson, 1996).

The challenges that faced Mary Breckinridge, such as demonstration of need, reimbursement, funding and public access to nursing care, are the same challenges that face today's nurse-managed care. . . . A successful nursing practice must be based on the needs of the community. . . . no place, no matter how remote, is inaccessible to community-based nursing care. (Raines & Wilson, 1996, pp. 126–127)

fully. Each DRG was assigned a fixed reimbursement amount. This allowed Medicare to anticipate what the cost should be for the care of a patient admitted with a particular diagnosis (along with other factors such as patient age, treatment, discharge status, and gender) (Oermann, 1997). Thus, a hospital receives a prepaid, fixed amount to cover the patient care delivered for each type of diagnosis, based on the expected LOS. If untoward events occur and the patient must stay in the hospital longer than the expected LOS, the hospital will not be reimbursed for the additional cost of care. If, on the other hand, everything goes extremely well and the patient is discharged sooner than the designated LOS, the hospital gets to keep the difference between the "real" cost of care and the "expected" cost of care.

Obviously, this reimbursement strategy provides a strong incentive for hospitals to discharge patients earlier. The impact of the prospective payment–DRG plan on home health care is clear: quite simply, patients are being discharged to home "quicker and sicker."

Several demographic and social factors also have an impact on home health care. The first is the rapidly increasing number of older Americans, with the largest growth still to come as the baby boom generation (Americans born between 1945 and 1965) approaches old age. Due to improved medical care and medical technology, these older adults will be living longer, and they will require care for an increasing number of chronic illnesses into very old age. Another significant social trend is the sharp rise in two-income families in the United States. This trend affects the demand for home care by significantly diminishing the number of available family caregivers in the home. Finally, there has been a steady movement toward the use of **health maintenance organizations (HMOs)** and managed care, both of which are associated with significantly lower utilization rates for hospitals (Joel, 1997). In short, there will be more people requiring care, and progressively less of that care will be delivered in hospitals. A sharply increased demand for home health care is bound to follow.

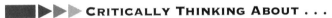 CRITICALLY THINKING ABOUT . . .

Can patients, who are being discharged from the hospital "quicker and sicker," be adequately cared for at home?

Home health care has traditionally been nurses' "turf." It is an excellent opportunity for nurses to provide quality care in a setting that is the most cost-effective and the most comfortable for patients—their homes (Campbell, 1997). Home health nurses must be extraordinarily competent and confident in their nursing skills, because, unlike nurses who work in a hospital, they do not have backup or consultation available from either physicians or other nurses. The demands on home care nurses also are escalating because many technical aspects of care that formerly were relegated to the hospital bedside have now come to the bedside at home. Intravenous pumps, chemotherapy, and ventilators are commonly used in the home today. Therefore, home health nurses must have up-to-date nursing knowledge.

Home health nurses must also have excellent assessment skills that apply not only to the patient but also to the family and the entire care environment. Good communication skills are a must, as is skill in identifying the patient's and family members' learning needs and fulfilling those needs (Campbell, 1997). Home health nurses must be knowledgeable about the networks that families can use to obtain support in the care of their sick or frail family member. Often home health nurses are called on to help families find their way through the maze of paperwork and "legalese" that surrounds the health care system. Families also may have financial burdens and problems about which only the home health nurse will know.

Home health nursing provides an extraordinary opportunity for nurses to establish ongoing therapeutic relationships with patients and families. Home health nurses practice with a great deal of autonomy and command great respect from their clients and the community they serve.

Hospice Care

Nursing as a part of hospice care could be considered a special type of home health care nursing. **Hospice** is generally defined as a coordinated, interdisciplinary program that provides palliative care for the dying. This means making the patient comfortable and free from pain in all dimensions, using a holistic, family-centered approach to care (Lazerowich, 1995). In other words, hospice provides pain and symptom control, as well as support services, for terminally ill people and their families. In the Middle Ages, hospices were places of refuge where weary travelers returning from the Crusades could find respite and comfort. Modern hospice care has its roots in 1967, when Dame Cicely Saunders founded St. Christopher's Hospice in London. Ten years later, the first U.S. hospice was established in New Haven, Connecticut. From there, the hospice movement grew slowly, relying primarily on volunteers and grassroots support. Because hospice services were largely outside the scope or consideration of mainstream medicine, there was little or no reimbursement available for hospice care.

In 1978, the National Hospice Organization was founded, and by 1982 federal legislation created a fully covered hospice Medicare benefit for hospices that met specified regulations. Hospices have grown rapidly since then. More than 75% of hospice programs are Medicare-certified, and 40 states have a Medicaid benefit to cover qualified hospice care. In 1996, there were nearly 2800 hospice providers in the United States, and there is continued rapid expansion among both for-profit and not-for-profit providers of hospice services. In 1995, approximately 390,000 people were cared for by hospices. This number represents 10% of deaths from all causes and 33% of deaths from cancer or acquired immunodeficiency syndrome (AIDS) (Hospice at Riverside and Grant, 1996).

Hospice services include the control of pain and spiritual, emotional, and psychological care of the patient. The hospice team also works closely with family members and significant others to meet their needs as well, both before and after the patient's death. A hospice program offers care to any person who has chosen not to continue curative treatment. Once the decision has been made to stop treatment and a prognosis of 6 months or less has been made, a patient is eligible for hospice care. There are many ways in which the decision to stop treatment may be made. Perhaps the physician decides that the current treatment is no longer effective and no other treatment options exist. In other cases, family members suggest the hospice option. The patient may also be the one to decide that although continuing treatment options may extend his or her life, they are simply too debilitating; the patient may feel that the hospice option offers a better quality of life for the time he or she has left to live. The decision to use hospice services is always a shared one, mutually agreed on by the patient, the family, and the physician.

The hospice team is usually medically directed and nurse-coordinated. The team typically includes the patient's own physician, nurses from the hospice agency, home health aides, social workers, chaplains, a psychologist, a nutritionist, a pharmacist, a physical therapist, and devoted volunteers. Pain management and symptom control are primary areas of expertise. Hospice nurses are not crisis-oriented; instead, they

> assist and empower patients and their families to anticipate pain and medicate effectively. Teaching patients and families to empower themselves and to feel in control of pain and suffering is the cornerstone of hospice work. . . . The concept of process is a critical one in the care of the dying person, for dying is a process with the phases

continually changing, integrating, and ultimately culminating in the final event. (Gurfolino & Dumas, 1994, p. 534)

With hospice, the plan of care is always relative and responsive to the patient's and family's wishes. The interdisciplinary team is responsible for the care of the patient and family 24 hours a day until death occurs. The team conducts a full assessment of the patient and family within 24 to 72 hours of the decision to select hospice. Hospice patients must (according to Medicare requirements) be seen by the coordinating nurse every 2 weeks at a minimum, and an interdisciplinary review of the plan of care is performed every 2 weeks. However, both patient visits and updates on the plan of care may take place more often.

An on-call nurse is available by beeper on a 24-hour basis. The nurse must be available to deal with any symptoms or clinical changes that develop during his or her time on call. The on-call nurse also is qualified to adjust dosages of pain medication (usually morphine) if necessary and is certified to pronounce death. Case loads are generally small (usually 10 to 12 patients at any one time), and the connections between the patient, family, and nurse are strong. This has a great deal to do with how well patient outcomes are achieved (Gurfolino & Dumas, 1994).

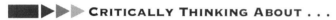 **CRITICALLY THINKING ABOUT . . .**

Would you consider working in a hospice?

Occupational Health Nursing

Occupational health nursing, considered a subspecialty of public health, has been serving the health needs of American workers for 100 years. In 1895, Fletcher D. Proctor introduced "district nursing" into several small villages in Vermont that were made up primarily of employees of the Vermont Marble Company, of which Proctor was the president. Proctor demonstrated a great deal of concern for the health and welfare of his company's employees and their families. He had been impressed with the care given by visiting nurses in other, larger cities, and hired two sisters, Ada Mayo and Harriet Stewart, to provide free nursing care to his employees and their families, as well as other townspeople who could not afford to pay for medical care (Kalisch & Kalisch, 1995).

Occupational health nurses are committed to working with employees and their families, employers, and other health and safety team members to attain and maintain a safe, healthy workplace. Employers have long known that a healthy workforce improves company profitability, because good health among employees reduces absenteeism, keeps insurance costs down, and diminishes the incidence of errors made by workers. Therefore, effective occupational health nurses are considered a financial asset to a company (Campbell, 1997).

Occupational health nurses often function in multiple roles within one job position, including clinician, educator, manager, and consultant (Burgel, 1994). The most common interaction between an employee and an employer is related to a health complaint. These complaints may be very wide-ranging (eg, wrist or back pain, problems related to a chronic health problem, a skin rash, recurrent headaches). In a large company, the occupational health nurse may develop a comprehensive program in support of employees' health, including health assessments, health histories, and other diagnostic measures. The occupational health nurse must be able to differentiate the normal from the abnormal and identify appropriate action and referrals.

Occupational health nurses often are responsible for programs of employee training, either in one-to-one or group settings. One purpose for such training sessions is to encourage workers to engage in safe work practices. Another is to heighten employees' level of understanding of workplace safety to the point where they can recognize potential on-the-job hazards. Occupational health nurses may also be responsible for interpreting material safety data sheets to employees and determining how to adjust work stations and work flow to diminish the number of trauma disorders related to repetitive forceful actions. Employees also can benefit from instruction on the long-term effects of noise and the need for hearing protection, as well as education regarding proper lifting techniques and back-strengthening exercises (Burgel, 1994). Occupational health nurses also can be active in establishing wellness programs to help employees reduce their health risks by emphasizing self-care and consumer responsibility.

The occupational health nurse must understand local, state, and federal regulations that govern employee health and workplace safety and must assist management in complying with those regulations. The major agency that protects the safety of workers is the **Occupational Safety and Health Administration (OSHA)**. Occupational health nurses must keep up to date on all OSHA regulations and ensure compliance with them within their organization. In sites (eg, hospitals) where there is a possibility of occupational exposure to blood or potentially infectious diseases, the occupational health nurse is responsible for ensuring the organization's compliance with the bloodborne pathogens standard that was adopted by OSHA in 1992. This OSHA standard mandates the use of universal precautions, provision of personal protective equipment by the employer, and safe needle-disposal containers. The employer is also required to provide, at no cost to employees, the hepatitis vaccine series. Should exposure occur, the occupational health nurse establishes postexposure policies and procedures in accordance with the OSHA standard (Burgel, 1994).

School Nursing

Lillian Wald, whose central role in the establishment of community health nursing is discussed in Box 8-1, also played a significant part in establishing school nursing in America. In New York City in the early 1900s, it was common for children to be sent home from school for health reasons. Most of the health problems were relatively minor and treatable (eg, head lice, ringworm, scabies), but the sick child had to be kept away from other children until the problem was cleared up. Wald suggested that having nurses in schools could supplement the work of local physicians and help solve the problem of absences from school due to health problems. Accordingly, she offered the services of one of her Henry Street Settlement House nurses, Lina L. Rogers, for a 1-month demonstration period. The experiment was a huge success, and the New York Board of Health soon appointed dozens of school nurses to assist Wald and her nurses with their work (Kalisch & Kalisch, 1995). The school nursing program in New York City was so successful in getting children healthy and back in school that by 1910, school nurses were employed in systems throughout the United States (Igoe, 1994).

Traditionally, school health encompasses three components: health services, health education, and a healthful school environment. In addition to these three components, the Centers for Disease Control and Prevention, Division of Adolescent and School Health, adds five more components: physical education, guidance and psychological services, food services, school and community health promotion activities, and site health promotion for faculty and staff (Igoe, 1994).

National health objectives that are targeted at the schools are presented in Box 8-2. These objectives provide additional structure to the framework within which school nursing is practiced and expand the role of the school nurse far beyond ensuring that every child's immunization record is complete and up to date. Examination of the national health objectives also reveals that achieving these objectives presents an interdisciplinary challenge that involves school nurses, faculty, and administrators as well as parents and community members.

School nurses require a strong working knowledge of human growth and development to detect developmental problems as early as possible. In addition, school nurses must be skilled in first aid and in the treatment of more severe injuries. A study by Sigsby and Campbell (1995) revealed that nearly 50% of the nursing activities performed by school nurses were directed toward alleviating pain; the second

---

Box 8-2

National Health Objectives Related to School Health

By the year 2000:

1. Increase to at least 50% the proportion of children in grades 1 to 12 who participate in daily physical education activities at school.
2. Increase to at least 90% the proportion of school lunch and breakfast programs with menus consistent with nutritional principles contained in Dietary Guidelines for Americans.
3. Increase to at least 75% the proportion of the nation's schools that provide nutrition education from preschool through 12th grade.
4. Include tobacco use prevention in the curricula of all elementary, middle, and secondary schools.
5. Provide children in all primary and secondary schools with educational programs on alcohol and other drugs.
6. Increase to at least 85% the proportion of people aged 10 to 18 who have discussed human sexuality with their parents or received information from parentally endorsed sources such as schools.
7. Increase to at least 50% the proportion of elementary and secondary schools that teach nonviolent conflict-resolution skills.
8. Provide academic instruction on injury prevention and control in at least 50% of public school systems.
9. Increase to at least 95% the proportion of schools that have age-appropriate HIV education curricula for children in grades 4 to 12.
10. Include in all middle and secondary schools instruction on preventing sexually transmitted diseases.

(*Healthy People 2000: National Health Promotion and Disease Prevention Objectives* [1991]. U.S. Department of Health and Human Services publication no. PHS91-50213.)

most common intervention was wound care and the promotion of wound healing. Many children turn to the school nurse with problems other than physical ones, so a school nurse must be sensitive and approachable and have solid counseling skills. Ensuring that all the children in the school are appropriately immunized, another responsibility of the school nurse, is an important way to protect public health. Should an outbreak of a communicable disease occur, the school nurse is responsible for educating students, parents, teachers, and staff about treatment of the disease and protection against further spread.

Federal law, under the Education for all Handicapped Children Act of 1975, requires public education systems to provide free, accessible education for handicapped children (Diers, 1997). This has resulted in the introduction of many physically challenged children into regular school classrooms. School nurses must be prepared to work closely with teachers and parents to provide the best and safest learning environment for these children and their classmates.

Lucille A. Joel sees an even broader role for school health programs and school nurses. She has advocated the establishment of full-service primary health care centers in inner-city schools. These centers would be staffed by advanced practice nurses whose specialty is school nursing. Several programs of this kind have already been established—largely with the support of foundations such as Robert Wood Johnson and the Kaiser Family Foundation—in Los Angeles, Chicago, and Detroit. Nurses in such centers serve as the primary care providers for the children and provide the necessary linkages with the rest of the health care system to ensure that each child receives comprehensive, appropriate health care. Joel has concluded:

> Linking primary health care services for children to the school is just common sense, like linking health care benefits to the workplace. Advanced practice nurses can deliver these services within networks that allow for ready referral and involvement in the full gamut of school activities. (Joel, 1994, p. 7)

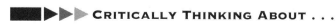 **CRITICALLY THINKING ABOUT . . .**

Does occupational or school nursing seem like an interesting career to you? Why or why not?

Parish Nursing

Parish nursing is a relatively new community-based area of nursing practice. The parish nursing role was developed in 1983 by Granger Westberg, a Lutheran chaplain. Leaders in many religious denominations support the parish nursing role because it is consistent with their vision of the church as a facilitator of healing and health. Churches play a significant role in the lives of their parishioners and the community at large and could have a far-reaching effect on health promotion and disease prevention. Many believe the time for church-based health promotion initiatives has come.

> Parish nurses have a unique opportunity to autonomously implement targeted, appropriate, population-based wellness interventions with measurable outcomes by applying community health nursing methods to their practice. As health care reform

---

BOX 8-3
Four Models of Parish Nursing

▶ *Institutional/Paid Model*—the parish nurse is employed by a hospital, community agency, or long-term care facility. The employing institution, in turn, contracts with one or more churches and provides the nurse's salary, benefits, and supervision.
▶ *Institutional/Volunteer Model*—the nurse volunteers his or her time to serve as a parish nurse. However, a relation exists between the church and an institution such as a religious order, so the church provides a stipend to the order in exchange for the nurse's service.
▶ *Congregational/Paid Model*—the parish nurse is employed directly by the congregation, and the church provides salary, benefits, and supervision.
▶ *Congregational/Volunteer Model*—the parish nurse is accountable directly to the congregation, but serves as a volunteer.

---

continues to heighten the focus on community health programs and health outcomes, perhaps nurses will seize this opportunity to develop effective leadership roles toward the advancement of community wellness. (Miskelly, 1995, p. 13)

Hands-on care is not a focus of parish nurses; rather, they provide education, advocacy, counseling, screening, volunteer training, and support group development and facilitation. Parish nurses also may serve as a liaison within the formal health care system and may refer clients to community resources. Providing health education, serving as a role model of holistic wellness, and offering health counseling also may be part of a parish nurse's responsibility (Miskelly, 1995). The nursing activities that a parish nurse could pursue are broad and varied.

There are several models for parish nursing (Box 8-3). Because parish nursing is relatively new, roles and organizational relationships are often ambiguous (Miskelly, 1995). A parish nurse must be flexible, diplomatic, and very knowledgeable about organizations and leadership theory and strategy.

 ▶▶▶ **CRITICALLY THINKING ABOUT . . .**

Should your church, synagogue, or other religious organization have a parish nurse?

Nursing in Long-Term Care Facilities

Increasing numbers of people require long-term care, including the rapidly growing number of older adults as well as persons with AIDS, traumatic head injuries, and progressive degenerative disorders. "Long-term care refers to the range of health and social services required to help people with functional deficits live as independently as possible" (Malone-Rising, 1994). Although illness or injury may have been a precipitating factor, the need for long-term services may or may not involve the treatment of a specific medical problem. Rather, it is the person's inability to perform activities of daily living (ADLs) and instrumental activities of daily living (IADLs) that sets up the need for long-term care (Box 8-4). Cognitive impairments also can create the need for long-term care.

The ability of a person to perform ADLs generally is considered the minimum level of functioning necessary to maintain independence. A person who cannot perform one or more ADLs would have a difficult time living alone. IADLs are also necessary, but they can be performed by persons outside of the home. Many older adults have demonstrated a great deal of ingenuity in establishing networks of assistance in IADLs, and even ADLs, to maximize the amount of time they can live independently in their own homes.

A great deal of long-term care actually takes place in the home, usually by unpaid caregivers such as family members, neighbors, and friends. As the caregiver's burden increases, he or she ideally obtains assistance from community and home health care services. However, the burden of care may simply become too much for the caregiver to manage, or he or she may die or become disabled, which leaves the ill person with no one to provide care. This is the most common path leading to admission to a nursing home.

Nursing Homes

Like hospitals in this country, nursing homes did not have very auspicious origins; they have their roots in the 19th-century almshouses and poorhouses. A person who was housed in a "county poorhouse" was there because he or she had no family to provide care and assistance, and no funds to live independently. The elderly poor faced the same fate. Eventually, however, various groups became concerned about the poor treatment of these needy segments of the population and took action. Churches and fraternal organizations began to sponsor homes to provide care for their elderly members, and the Social Security Act of 1935 provided legislation that permitted private, for-profit nursing homes to emerge during the late 1930s.

The federal government continued to support the expansion of the numbers of nursing homes. After World War II, the Hill-Burton Act, a piece of legislation that was highly instrumental in encouraging the construction of hospitals, was expanded in 1948 to include the construction of voluntary (not-for-profit) nursing homes as well. The federal government also has provided increasing support for nursing home care.

Box 8-4	
Factors Contributing to a Need for Long-Term Care Services	

Activities of Daily Living	**Instrumental Activities of Daily Living**
Eating and feeding oneself	Using the telephone
Bathing	Managing finances
Toileting	Shopping
Moving and transferring	Cooking
Dressing	Managing medications
	Doing laundry
	Light housework

"Since 1950, government funding for nursing home care has increased steadily and culminated in the 1965 Medicaid program, which now covers 40% of all nursing home costs" (Ellis & Hartley, 1995). About 75% of all nursing homes are now for-profit institutions that rely heavily on Medicare and Medicaid reimbursement for financial support. The nursing home industry has expanded significantly. In fact, Joseph Catalano (1996) noted that there were more beds in nursing homes than in hospitals.

A relatively recent trend in long-term care for older adults has been the rapid growth of "continuing care" environments or "life care" communities. Such environments provide a broad range of options regarding levels of care, depending on the needs of each resident. Older people may choose to enter a life care community while they are still healthy, active, and capable of being fully independent. In fact, there are financial incentives to do so; the fee to enter a life care community is much lower for a healthy person than it is for one who is already sick.

Healthy, active residents can live in independent apartments, obtaining the housekeeping services they want or need for a modest sum. Dining facilities are often the norm in such communities, although some units have kitchenettes. The dining facilities are often quite elegant; experienced chefs plan varied menus and prepare excellent cuisine, and guests are welcome.

Residents who suffer a decline in health or have a decreased ability to care for themselves can move to other units in the same community that better meet their care needs. Community residents are provided with a broad range of health and support services, up to and including skilled nursing care for those who require it. More and more of these communities are including care units specifically designed for the care of older adults suffering from Alzheimer's disease and other cognitive disorders.

Rehabilitation

Rehabilitation facilities are designed to provide care to patients who are being discharged from the hospital after recovering from an acute illness or injury but who still require more technical care and rehabilitation equipment and services than can be provided at home. This includes people (usually older adults) who have suffered cerebrovascular accidents and people (usually younger adults) who have suffered traumatic head injury or spinal cord injury. Nurses in facilities that have a strong rehabilitation component work as members of a highly integrated, interdisciplinary team that helps patients retain and maintain function, independence, and autonomy through a focused program of treatment and rehabilitation. The ultimate goal is that the patient will return to independent living in the community.

 CRITICALLY THINKING ABOUT . . .

> Have you had clinical experience in a nursing home or rehabilitation facility? Should nursing students have such experience as part of their undergraduate programs? Why or why not?

▶ CHAPTER SUMMARY

Nursing has played a significant role in the development of all American health care institutions. A large group of highly skilled nurses was one of the major contributing factors to the growth and improvement of hospitals in the United States. Nurses formed the very core of community health care and were instrumental in initiating programs of school health early in the 20th century. In addition, nurses' participation in ambulatory care settings is a critical factor contributing to the success of this rapidly growing segment of the U.S. health care delivery system.

One emerging issue that affects nursing is the downsizing of acute care hospitals. Although this opens the door to more nursing opportunities in the ambulatory care and community settings, many nurses and nursing leaders are very apprehensive about the effects of this trend. Many fear that when fewer nurses are available to provide expert clinical care to acutely ill hospitalized patients, the quality of patient care will be seriously compromised. In more and more cases, it has been shown that this fear is not unfounded—quite simply, too few qualified nurses in a hospital means a poorer quality of care. A sufficient number of well-prepared, professionally oriented nurses is necessary in acute care environments. Beverly Malone, president of the American Nurses Association, has articulated this concern:

> As the professional association representing the nation's registered nurses, ANA is concerned that too few people truly understand and recognize the value of RNs. The dangerous trend of replacing professional nurses with minimally trained aides is robbing patients of proper care and endangering their health and lives. A decade of research shows that when there are more RNs, patients experience fewer complications, lower readmission rates, and fewer deaths, and this means overall lower costs. (Canavan, 1997)

Thus, not only is cutting nursing care dangerous to patients, it also does not make good economic sense.

In short, a strong nursing presence is critical to the continuation of quality in all American health care institutions, and nurses must reiterate this fact at every opportunity. Nurses must give their enthusiastic support to nursing leaders who champion the cause of high-quality patient care. High-quality patient care is firmly grounded in the services of the most highly qualified of patient care experts—expert RNs.

KEY POINTS

▶ 1 The first hospitals were founded in the United States in the late 18th century, but they did not expand significantly until the late 19th and early 20th century due to six major factors: advances in medical science, advances in medical technology, improved medical education, widespread availability of insurance, financial support from the federal government, and availability of large numbers of highly trained RNs prepared in the hospital training schools.

▶ 2 Seven elements that make a hospital a good environment in which to practice nursing are an orientation to action, deep care for clients, encouragement of autonomy, demonstration of true respect for people, leadership that is closely involved in perpetuating the value system, a lean organizational structure, and a firm sense of direction combined with room for individual autonomy at the unit level.

▶ 3 Ambulatory care is one of the most rapidly expanding areas in the health care industry. Nurses play a central role in assessment, patient treatment and recovery, and patient teaching in ambulatory care centers.

▶ 4 Nurses can work in several areas in the community setting. Nurses who work in home health care must be confident and competent in their nursing skills because they make independent judgments all day. These nurses provide care to often very sick people and often work extensively with the client's family as well. Hospice nurses provide physical, spiritual, emotional, and psychological care to dying persons. These nurses also work closely with the patient's family members to meet their needs. Occupational nurses work with employees and families, employers, and other health and safety team members to attain and maintain a safe, health workplace. School nurses typically work with several components of school health: health services, health education, healthful school environment, physical education, guidance and psychological services, food services, school and community health promotion activities, and site health promotion for faculty and staff. Finally, parish nursing, a relatively new area of nursing, provides education, advocacy, counseling, screening, volunteer training, and support group development and facilitation.

▶ 5 Nursing homes typically are designed to provide lifetime, skilled nursing care for clients who cannot care for themselves or who are cognitively impaired. These people may or may not have an existing medical problem. Rehabilitation care is intended to provide skilled nursing care to clients who are out of the acute stage but still recovering from an illness or injury. The goal of rehabilitation care is to help the person retain and maintain function, independence, and autonomy.

REFERENCES

Brooten D, Kumer S, Brown LP, et al (1986). A randomized clinical trial of early hospital discharge and home follow-up of very-low-birth-weight infants. *N Engl J Medicine, 315*, 934–939.

Burgel BJ (1994). Occupational health: Nursing in the workplace. *Nursing Clinics of North America, 29*, 431–441.

Campbell C (1997). Nursing today. In Chitty KK (Ed.), *Professional Nursing: Concepts and Challenges* (2nd ed.). Philadelphia: WB Saunders.

Canavan K (1997, May–June). Media embraces ANA's concerns about unsafe patient care. *The American Nurse*, pp. 1, 12.

Catalano JT (1996). *Contemporary Professional Nursing*. Philadelphia: FA Davis.

Craig CE (1996). Making the most of a nurse-managed clinic. *Nursing and Health Care, 17*, 124–126.

Diers D (1997). What is nursing? In McCloskey JC, Grace HK (Eds.), *Current Issues in Nursing* (5th ed.). St. Louis: Mosby.

Division of Nursing (1997). *Advance Notes from the National Sample Survey of Registered Nurses, March 1996*. Rockville, MD: Author.

Ellis JR, Hartley CL (1995). *Nursing in Today's World: Challenges, Issues, and Trends* (5th ed.). Philadelphia: JB Lippincott.

Gurfolino V, Dumas L (1994). Hospice nursing: The concept of palliative care. *Nursing Clinics of North America, 29*, 533–546.

Haglund CL, Dowling WL (1988). The hospital. In Williams SJ, Torrens PR (Eds.), *Introduction to Health Services* (3rd ed.). New York: John Wiley & Sons.

Hospice at Riverside and Grant (1996). *Hospice at Riverside and Grant: History and overview.* Columbus, OH: Author.

Igoe JB (1994). School nursing. *Nursing Clinics of North America, 29*, 443–458.

Joel LA (1994). Closing the school health safety net. *AJN*, February, p. 7.

Joel LA (1997). Moving the care site from hospital to home: Whose turf? In McCloskey JC, Grace HK (Eds.), *Current Issues in Nursing* (5th ed.). St. Louis: Mosby.

Kalisch PA, Kalisch BJ (1995). *The Advance of American Nursing* (3rd ed.). Philadelphia: JB Lippincott.

Kelly LY, Joel LA (1996). *The Nursing Experience: Trends, Challenges, and Transitions* (3rd ed.). New York: McGraw-Hill.

Knaus W, Draper E, Wagner D, Zimmerman J (1986). An evaluation of outcomes from intensive care in major medical centers. *Annals of Internal Medicine, 104*, 410–418.

Kramer M, Schmalenberg C (1988a). Magnet hospitals: Part I. Institutions of excellence. *J Nursing Administration, 18* (January), 13–24.

Kramer M, Schmalenberg C (1988b). Magnet hospitals: Part II. Institutions of excellence. *J Nursing Administration, 18*(February), 11–19.

Lazerowich V (1995). Development of a patient classification system for a home-based hospice program. *J Community Health Nursing, 12*, 121–126.

Malone-Rising D (1994). The changing face of long-term care. *Nursing Clinics of North America, 29*, 417–429.

McClure M, Poulin M, Sovie M, Wandelt M (1982). *Magnet hospitals: Attraction and retention of professional nurses.* Kansas City, MO; American Nurses Association.

Miskelly S (1995). A parish nursing model: Applying the community health nursing process in a church community. *J Community Health Nursing, 12*, 1–14.

National Advisory Council on Nurse Education and Practice (1996). *Report to the Secretary of the Department of Health and Human Services on the Basic Registered Nurse Workforce* (U.S. Department of Health and Human Services, Health Resources and Services Administration, Bureau of Health Professions, Division of Nursing). Washington DC: U.S. Government Printing Office.

Peters TJ, Waterman RH (1982). *In Search of Excellence.* New York: Harper & Row.

Portnoy FL, Dumas L (1994). Nursing for the public good. *Nursing Clinics of North America, 29*, 371–376.

Raffel MW, Raffel NK (1989). *The U.S. health system: Origins and functions* (3rd ed.). Delmar Publ.

Raines KH, Wilson A (1996). Frontier Nursing Service: A historical perspective on nurse-managed care. *J Community Health Nursing, 13*, 123–127.

Sigsby LM, Campbell DW (1995). Nursing interventions classification: A content analysis of nursing activities in public schools. *J Community Health Nursing, 12*, 229–237.

RECOMMENDED READINGS

Bocchino C (1993). Federal initiatives focus on fetal and childhood development and school nursing. *Pediatric Nursing, 19*, 398–399.

Granneman S, Russell CL (1997). Improving patient follow-up through implementation of an ambulatory care program. *J Nursing Care Quality, 11*(3), 62–67.

Haas S, Gold C (1997). Supervision of unlicensed assistive workers in ambulatory settings. *Nursing Economics, 15*, 57–59.

Hill-White D, Christansen HT (1987). The declining status of school nurses in New York. *J School Health, 57*, 137–143.

Magilvy JK, Brown NJ (1997). Parish nursing: Advanced practice nursing model of healthier communities. *Advanced Practice Nursing Quarterly, 2*(4), 67–72.

Martin LB (1996). Parish nursing: Keeping body and soul together. *Canadian Nurse, 92*, 25–28.

Miskelly S (1995). A parish nursing model: Applying the community health process in a church community. *J Community Health Nursing, 12*, 1–14.

Ramsey PW, McConnell P, Palmer BH, Glenn LL (1996). Nurses' compliance with universal precautions before and after implementation of OSHA regulations. *Clinical Nurse Specialist, 10*, 234–239.

Reed S, Peterson C (1996). Washington watch. Workplace hazards: ANA members help save OSHA unit. *AJN, 96*(12), 20.

Schank MJ, Weis RM (1996). Parish nursing: Ministry of healing. *Geriatric Nursing, 17*, 11–13.

Sheppard A (1992). Career development in intensive care, part 1. *Br J Nursing, 1*, 467–469.

9

Advanced Nursing Practice: Expanding Opportunities for Professionalization

CHAPTER OUTLINE

Evolution of Advanced Nursing
    Practice
Models of Advanced Nursing
    Practice
Role Responsibilities of APNs

Chapter Summary
Key Points
References
Classic References
Recommended Readings

LEARNING OBJECTIVES

▶ **1** Describe the evolution of the role of nurse anesthetists in the United States.

▶ **2** Describe the development of the role of nurse-midwives in the United States.

▶ **3** Discuss the development of the role of clinical nurse specialists.

▶ **4** Describe the development of the role of nurse practitioner.

▶ **5** Explain the reasons for the possible unification of the clinical nurse specialist and nurse practitioner roles.

▶ **6** Describe two examples of practice models in which advanced practice nurses are delivering care to clients within the community.

▶ **7** List the general role responsibilities expected of advanced practice nurses and the elements of a knowledge base necessary for advanced nursing practice.

KEY TERMS

advanced nursing
  practice

anesthetizers

certified nurse-
  midwife (CNM)

clinical nurse
  specialist (CNS)

certified registered
  nurse anesthetist
  (CRNA)

general systems
  theory

Hildegard Peplau

Loretta Ford

migration history

nurse practitioner
  (NP)

1965 Nurse
  Training Act

1971 Nurse
  Training Act

organizational
  theory

patient–clinician
  partnership

primary care

role theory

SAS Health Care Center

state nurse practice
  acts

teaching–learning
  theory

Chapter 1 pointed out that nursing has yet to achieve the status accorded a true profession, but that progress is being made in that direction. One area in which great strides have been made since the 1960s—notably in the 1980s and 1990s—is **advanced nursing practice**. The American Nurses Association (ANA)'s social policy statement characterizes advanced nursing practice as:

> The scope of advanced nursing practice is distinguished by autonomy to practice at the edges of the expanding boundaries of nursing's scope of practice. One hallmark of advanced practice nursing—whether in the primary care setting, the community, or the hospital—is the preponderance of self-initiated treatment regimens, as opposed to dependent functions . . . Because of the expanded practice and knowledge base, advanced practice nursing is also characterized by a complexity of clinical decision making and a skill in managing organizations and environments greater than that required for the practice of nursing at the basic level. (ANA, 1995, p. 16)

Significant growth in the numbers of advanced practice nurses (APNs) and their proper use within the changing American health care system bode well for the continuing professionalization of nursing. In 1996, 6.3% of the RN population was prepared for advanced practice. Of these 161,711 APNs, the largest group were nurse practitioners, the second largest clinical nurse specialists. About 20% were nurse anesthetists, and the smallest group of APNs were nurse-midwives (Division of Nursing, 1996) (Fig. 9-1). The largest number of APNs were employed in health maintenance organizations and community health care settings—18% and 14%, respectively (Division of Nursing, 1996).

Chapter 6 discussed the general nature of and educational preparation requirements for advanced nursing practice positions and provided an introduction to this exciting and rewarding facet of nursing practice. This chapter expands on that discussion by presenting the historical development of four established advanced nursing practice groups: nurse anesthetists, nurse-midwives, clinical nurse specialists, and nurse practitioners. There are other groups of APNs, such as case managers, but the four groups discussed here comprise the vast majority of APNs. The development history is followed by a discussion of alternative models of practice by which APNs

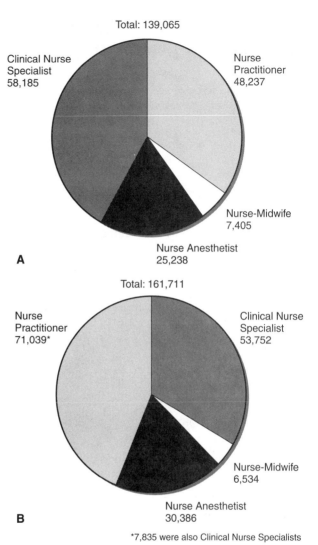

Figure 9-1. Number of advanced practice nurses in the United States in **(A)** 1992 and **(B)** 1996. (U.S. Department of Health & Human Services, Division of Nursing [1992]. *National Sample Survey of RNs;* American Nurses Association [1993]. Advanced practice nursing: A new age in health care. *Nursing Facts.* Washington DC: American Nurses Publishing.)

may pursue their career goals and the roles and activities generally expected of nurses in advanced practice positions. The chapter concludes with a discussion of the general theoretical foundations (beyond nursing theory) that an APN must command to practice successfully.

◼ ▶▶▶ **CRITICALLY THINKING ABOUT . . .**

Do you know any APNs? Have they told you about their work? What is your reaction? Would you like to follow in their steps?

Evolution of Advanced Nursing Practice

Nurse Anesthetists

Major advances in anesthesia science in the mid-1800s paved the way for the development of **certified registered nurse anesthetists** (CRNAs), the oldest of the advanced nursing specialities. Surgical procedures were growing in numbers and complexity, capturing the interest of physicians to a much greater extent than did the administration of the anesthesia that made surgery possible. **Anesthetizers** were originally unpaid or minimally paid surgeons in training. There was little motivation for physicians to specialize in anesthesia science, but experts in the area were essential to the continuing expansion and improvement of surgical procedures (Diers, 1991). Accordingly, nurses were recruited and trained for that purpose. Surgeons readily accepted the nurse anesthetists because they offered more stability over time and directed their full attention to the anesthesia process and the patient's response to anesthesia. The early nurse anesthetists also were welcome because they were, for the most part, religious sisters who did not expect payment for their services (Bigbee, 1996).

Nurse anesthesia became separated from mainstream nursing very early in its history, and that alienation still exists. Late in the 19th century, the Sisters of the Third Order of St. Francis developed a network of hospitals throughout the Midwest as part of a contract negotiated with the Missouri Pacific Railroad. One of those hospitals was the Mayo Clinic, where nurses administered all the anesthesia. Alice Magaw, an early nurse anesthetist at the Mayo Clinic, became known as the "mother of anesthesia." She believed that nurse anesthesia should not be under the jurisdiction of nursing service administration because it was a specialized field, which nursing was not at that time. Moreover, Magaw argued that anesthesia required education and recognition that would not be possible if it were under a department of hospital nursing (Bigbee, 1996).

Because of the trauma-related nature of much of the practice of anesthesia, nurse anesthesia has always been strongly influenced by wars. The visibility of and public enthusiasm for nurse anesthetists were greatly enhanced when it was demonstrated that battlefield mortality rates were substantially reduced due to the anesthesia care provided by hospital-sponsored medical units.

Physicians started specializing in anesthesia around the turn of the century. Because medical anesthesia was then a low-status, low-paying specialty area, it attracted primarily women physicians. These women physicians typically were opposed to nurse anesthetists, even though both groups experienced much of the same gender discrimination and stereotyping (Bigbee, 1996).

Nurse anesthetists were leaders in achieving a strong national presence. Agatha Hodgins formed the American Association of Nurse Anesthetists (AANA) in 1931. At their first meeting, the group voted to affiliate with the ANA. Their application was refused, purportedly because the ANA feared assuming legal responsibility for a group that could be charged with practicing medicine (Thatcher, 1953). Immediately after World War II, the AANA initiated a certification program, the first nursing specialty to do so.

Many things have changed within the past century for nurse anesthetists. First, they have not remained as welcome in operating rooms as were their religious-order predecessors. As medical anesthesiologists have increased their control over anesthesia practice, CRNAs have faced considerable interprofessional conflict, engaging in courtroom and legislative skirmishes at the state level from New York to California since the early 1900s. Legislatively, the AANA waged a complex battle from 1977 to 1989 to secure third-party reimbursement under Medicare. Nurse anesthesia has become increasingly attractive to men in nursing, more than any other nursing specialty: about 40% of all practicing CRNAs are men. Finally, nurse anesthetists now have the highest average salaries of any of the advanced nursing specialties (Bigbee, 1996).

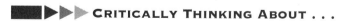 **CRITICALLY THINKING ABOUT . . .**

Was it proper for physician anesthesiologists to replace nurse anesthetists? Why or why not?

Nurse-Midwives

Nurse-midwifery was the second of the four major advanced practice nursing specialties to develop in the United States, even though midwifery has been an integral aspect of the health and wellbeing of communities for many centuries in many cultures. However, in America in the early 20th century, midwives were largely discredited for a number of reasons. The status of women in general was very poor; they were generally seem as economically exploitable and socially and politically incompetent. Moreover, midwives were discredited because of overly conservative religious attitudes and were replaced by physicians. Midwives often were falsely blamed for poor maternal-child health outcomes when the fault actually lay with inadequate hospital resources for complicated deliveries, inadequate preparation of physicians in obstetric care, and lack of prenatal care.

In response to the tremendous maternal-child health needs of the rapidly growing immigrant population in New York City, the Children's Bureau and the Maternity Center Association were established in 1912. Under the direction of Lillian Wald, the Children's Bureau conducted studies of infant and maternal mortality and demonstrated the importance of early and continuous prenatal care. However, negative attitudes toward midwives persisted, peaking around 1912. There were heated debates surrounding the licensing and control of midwives, medicine was assuming more and more control over obstetric care, and there was a mass movement away from home births (Bigbee, 1996).

Nurse-midwifery in general languished until the late 1960s and early 1970s. At that time, the demand for the services of well-prepared nurse-midwives increased dramatically, due partly to the influence of the women's movement in all issues pertaining to women's health, including birthing issues. Birth rates were rising rapidly as the baby boomers started having their own children, and the number of obstetricians was inadequate to meet the demand. In the early 1970s, middle- and upper-income families "discovered" midwives, and private midwifery practice flourished. Additionally, **certified nurse-midwives (CNMs)** were being increasingly used in federally funded health projects, and the American College of Obstetricians and Gynecologists gave official recognition to CNMs in 1971.

More recently, nurse-midwifery practice and education have continued to expand for many of the same reasons that other advanced nursing practice specialties are expanding, including shortage of physicians, the availability of federal funding, and changes in nurse practice acts. In addition, the women's movement, including the demands of sensitive and caring approaches to women's health care, has fueled the success of nurse-midwifery in the United States. (Bigbee, 1996, p. 11)

Nurse-midwives have been very active and well organized since the 1920s. The first organization was an outgrowth of Mary Breckinridge's Frontier Nursing Service (see Chap. 8). This was the Kentucky State Association of Midwives, which subsequently became the American Association of Nurse-Midwives, founded in 1928. The American College of Nurse-Midwifery was incorporated in 1955 to serve as an independent specialty nursing organization. In 1956 it merged with the American Association of Nurse-Midwives to form the American College of Nurse-Midwives (ACNM). This organization grew quickly, establishing an accreditation process by 1962 and implementing a certification examination and process by 1971. The ACNM also began publishing the *Journal of Nurse-Midwifery*. The ACNM has also been politically active. In 1971, it approved a statement prohibiting CNMs from performing abortions, and in 1980 it issued a statement allowing CNMs to practice in a variety of settings, including hospitals, homes, and birthing centers (Bigbee, 1996).

The education of American nurse-midwives has evolved and expanded over time as well. The first nurse-midwifery training program was established in connection with the Maternity Center of New York in 1932 and was known as the Lobestine Midwifery School. Its primary objective was to prepare public health nurses to instruct and supervise traditional midwives as well as public health nurses with limited obstetric training. The school graduated 320 students between 1933 and 1959. The second formal program for training nurse-midwives was established by the Frontier Nursing Service in 1939. The Frontier Graduate School of Midwifery graduated 460 nurse-midwives by 1976 and continues to operate today. As of 1995, there were 44 CNM programs, including 31 that offer a master's degree (Bigbee, 1996).

 CRITICALLY THINKING ABOUT . . .

What would be the advantages and disadvantages of a career as a CNM?

Clinical Nurse Specialists

The evolution of the **clinical nurse specialist (CNS)** as an APN differs from that of both nurse anesthetists and nurse-midwives. The origins of both the title and the concept of the CNS are controversial. Hildegard Peplau (1965) contended that the title actually originated as early as 1938. Norris (1977) stated that the CNS concept was introduced in 1944 in connection with the National League for Nursing's Committee to Study Postgraduate Clinical Nursing Courses. Shirley Smoyak (1976) offered yet another explanation. She traced the concept's origin to a national conference of directors of graduate nursing programs held at the University of Minnesota in 1949.

Regardless of the exact origin of the CNS title and concept, the important fact is that educating nurses in university graduate programs for advanced clinical practice originated in the mid-20th century and differed from graduate education for nurses before that time. In the earlier era, the diploma was considered the preferred (and sufficient) preparation for clinical nursing practice. Thus, students in graduate programs focused on functional areas of specialization that would provide leadership within the nursing education and nursing practice environment. These functional areas included administration, education, and supervision.

The development of the CNS role allowed nurses to focus on specific clinical areas of practice. Today, CNSs function in a broad range of clinical areas, but initially the CNS role developed in the area of psychiatric/mental health nursing. The first training program in America for psychiatric nurses was opened at McLean Hospital in Massachusetts in 1880. At that time, the nurse's role in mental health was largely custodial and under the direct supervision of physicians. In the early 1900s, psychiatric nursing emerged as an identifiable specialty area, and great strides in the practice of psychiatry were made between 1900 and 1930, primarily due to the influence of the writings of Sigmund Freud. Starting in 1930, the writings of Harry Stack Sullivan began to have a significant impact on psychiatric nursing. He emphasized interpersonal interactions with patients, and his work led to psychiatric nurses' playing a more direct role in the psychiatric care of hospitalized patients. Another reason for the growth in psychiatry was the public's increasing recognition of mental health concerns, spurred perhaps by soldiers returning from World Wars I and II with stress-related disorders (Bigbee, 1996).

Hildegard Peplau established the first psychiatric master's degree program for nurses at Rutgers University in 1954. She also proposed the first conceptual framework for psychiatric nursing. The writings of Sullivan, Peplau, and other scholars generated a body of knowledge that

> provided the support for psychiatric nurses to begin exploring new leadership roles in the care of mental health clients in both in-patient and out-patient settings . . . By 1970, a cadre of graduate-prepared psychiatric CNSs assumed roles as individual, group, family, and milieu therapists and obtained direct third-party reimbursement for their services. (Bigbee, 1996, p. 15)

Shortly thereafter, psychiatric nurses identified minimal educational and clinical criteria for CNSs and established national specialty certification through the ANA.

The success of the psychiatric nurses in developing the CNS role in their specialty encouraged nurses in other specialty areas to follow suit. This movement was encouraged by the passage of the **1965 Nurse Training Act**, which made funding available for graduate study by nurses. As more nurses entered graduate study, more attention was given to developing programs of study in clinical specialties; in contrast, earlier programs had emphasized education and administration alone. The goal of these programs was to prepare specialists who would provide a high level of nursing care in the specialty and assist nurses and others in hospitals to improve their practice through role modeling and consultation with other health care providers (Christman, 1991). Studies conducted through the 1970s and into the 1980s demonstrated the positive effects of introducing CNSs into the clinical environment in terms of improved patient outcomes (Georgopoulos & Sana, 1971; Ayers, 1971; Linde & Janz, 1979; Brooten et al, 1991).

When the CNS role was still new, employment opportunities were limited, so many early CNSs (like CNMs before them) assumed roles in administration and education. As time passed, however, the CNS role became more institutionalized, especially in larger hospitals. In 1992, the ANA reported that CNSs made up the largest single group of APNs (Bigbee, 1996). However, recent changes in the American health care system have had a profound impact on many CNSs. One can see from Figure 9-1 that by 1996 the number of nurse practitioners had surpassed the number of CNSs. The impact of these changes will be described later in this chapter.

Unlike the two advanced practice areas previously discussed (nurse anesthetist and nurse-midwife), CNSs did not experience serious opposition from physicians in the development of their roles and responsibilities. Bigbee (1996) suggested that one reason for this general lack of opposition was that the CNSs' preparation was, from the outset, placed within graduate education. The roots of both nurse anesthetists and nurse-midwives were in earlier practices that did not require graduate education—in fact, not even baccalaureate education. One also could surmise that physicians were more cooperative regarding the advanced practice role of the CNSs because in the hospital environment, the role of the CNS complemented the role of the physician; nurse anesthetists and nurse-midwives, on the other hand, were perceived as competitors to physicians, attempting to control the practice and the patients receiving anesthesia and obstetric care.

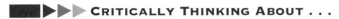 CRITICALLY THINKING ABOUT . . .

Would you consider a career as a CNS? Why or why not?

Nurse Practitioners

Nurse practitioners (NPs) are the newest group of APNs to emerge in America. They are also the fastest-growing group of APNs. The success of the NP movement since its inception in the mid-1960s has been nothing short of phenomenal. Many sociopolitical factors have contributed to the growth in numbers and the dramatic expansion of the role of NPs in a wide variety of clinical specialties. **Loretta Ford**, who was instrumental in establishing the first NP program in pediatrics at the University of Colorado, noted:

> The nurse practitioner movement is one of the finest demonstrations of how nurses exploited trends in the larger health care system to advance their own professional agenda and to realize their great potential to serve society. (Ford, 1991, p. 287)

Some of the sociopolitical factors that contributed to the growth of the NP movement included an acute shortage of primary care physicians in the 1960s and 1970s; physicians were choosing the more lucrative medical specialties over primary care practice. At the same time, the United States was undergoing a period of rapid social change due to the Vietnam War and movements that promoted racial and gender equity and rights. The consumer movement had become strident in its demand for more accessible, more affordable, more sensitive care for more people. Health care delivery costs were escalating 10% to 14% annually. One response to the shortage of physicians was the introduction of the physician's assistant role in the 1960s. This move was not viewed favorably by nursing leaders, who believed that well-prepared nurses were more logically suited to provide patient care than physician's assistants, whose preparation could be highly variable. The emphasis on primary care in the 1970s and 1980s also favored the growth of the NP movement, as did the movement toward ambulatory, interdisciplinary, family-centered care.

The first NP program was established in 1965 as a postbaccalaureate certificate program at the University of Colorado by Loretta Ford and Henry Silver. This was a demonstration project supported by the Commonwealth Foundation. Its purpose was to prepare professional nurses to "provide comprehensive well-child care as well as to manage common childhood health problems. Family dynamics and community cultural values were strongly emphasized" (Bigbee, 1996, p. 18). An evaluation study conducted by the Bureau of Sociological Research at the University of Colorado found that the pediatric NPs who completed the program were competent in assessing and managing the care of 75% of well and ill children who came to community health stations. Moreover, pediatricians who used pediatric NPs as part of their staff found that 33% more patients could be seen (Ford & Silver, 1967). Clearly, the demonstration program proved to be a success.

In the early 1970s, the movement to expand the traditional nursing role picked up considerable momentum from a report prepared by a group of health care leaders at the request of Elliott Richardson, then the Secretary of Health, Education, and Welfare. This report, *Extending the Scope of Nursing Practice*, concluded that "enlarging the nurse's role was essential for providing equal access to health services to all citizens" (Kalisch & Kalisch, 1996, p. 454). The committee recommended several primary care functions for which nurses should be prepared, including:

- Routine health assessment for persons and families
- Provision of care during normal pregnancies and deliveries
- Management of care for selected patients
- Consultation and collaboration with other health care professionals (U.S. Department of Health, Education, and Welfare, 1972).

Additional impetus for the expansion of advanced nursing practice and the preparation of nurses qualified to practice advanced nursing was the **1971 Nurse Training Act**. In providing authority for special grants and contracts, the act stated that funds should be used to establish training programs to prepare pediatric NPs or other types of NPs. Thus, the NP program in the United States was no longer an experimental alternative method of health care provision; it had become a model of health care delivery that was widely accepted by physicians and patients alike (Kalisch & Kalisch, 1996). By the mid-1980s, NPs were practicing widely in the very settings the movement's founders had envisioned: outpatient clinics, health maintenance organizations, health departments, neighborhood and rural health centers, schools, homes, and private medical practices.

Regulation of advanced nursing practice varies widely among the states. Three major elements affect what legally constitutes advanced nursing practice in each state:

1. Legal authority—authority under which the NP engages in practice
2. Reimbursement—the extent to which, or the conditions under which, NPs are eligible for direct reimbursement for services from third-party payers
3. Prescriptive authority—extent of NP's authority in prescribing medications for clients.

Despite strong opposition from many state medical associations to the revision of **state nurse practice acts**, which give NPs a greater scope of practice and autonomy, as of January 1997 all 50 states had revised their nurse practice acts or issued regulations to extend the functions that qualified nurses could perform (Fig. 9-2). In 26 states, NPs practice under the sole authority of the state board of nursing, with

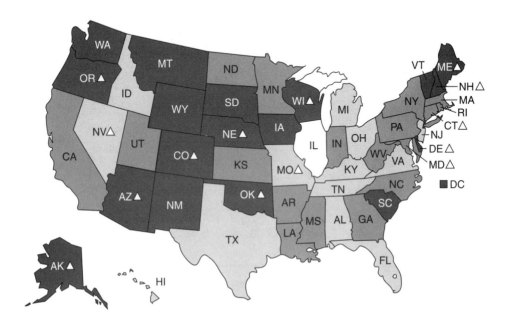

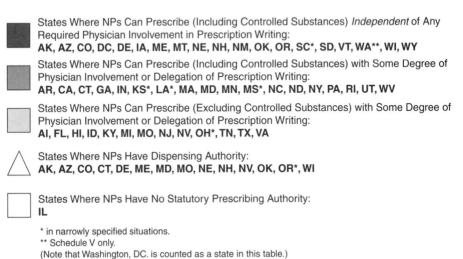

■ States Where NPs Can Prescribe (Including Controlled Substances) *Independent* of Any Required Physician Involvement in Prescription Writing:
AK, AZ, CO, DC, DE, IA, ME, MT, NE, NH, NM, OK, OR, SC*, SD, VT, WA**, WI, WY

▨ States Where NPs Can Prescribe (Including Controlled Substances) with Some Degree of Physician Involvement or Delegation of Prescription Writing:
AR, CA, CT, GA, IN, KS*, LA*, MA, MD, MN, MS*, NC, ND, NY, PA, RI, UT, WV

▢ States Where NPs Can Prescribe (Excluding Controlled Substances) with Some Degree of Physician Involvement or Delegation of Prescription Writing:
Al, FL, HI, ID, KY, MI, MO, NJ, NV, OH*, TN, TX, VA

△ States Where NPs Have Dispensing Authority:
AK, AZ, CO, CT, DE, ME, MD, MO, NE, NH, NV, OK, OR*, WI

☐ States Where NPs Have No Statutory Prescribing Authority:
IL

* in narrowly specified situations.
** Schedule V only.
(Note that Washington, DC. is counted as a state in this table.)

Figure 9-2. Summary of nurse practitioner statutory prescribing authority. (Pearson L [1997]. Annual update of how each state stands on legislative issues affecting advanced nursing practice. *The Nurse Practitioner 22*[1]:25.)

no requirements for physician collaboration or supervision. In 16 states, NPs practice under the sole authority of the board of nursing, but there is a requirement for physician collaboration or supervision. The laws regarding reimbursement to NPs are important because they bear directly on the professional issue of autonomy. Without laws that permit direct reimbursement, NPs must retain the status of employees of (or, at best, consultant to) physician practices. The physicians receive the reimbursement for NP services, which they then pass on to the NP who provided the services. Prescriptive privileges are always an issue when establishing state nursing practice and medical practice laws. The laws of 16 states allow NPs to prescribe (including controlled substances) with some degree of physician involvement; in 12 states, NPs can legally prescribe (excluding controlled substances) with some degree of physician involvement.

Although there is variation, the general pattern is that western states tend to provide legal authority for the broadest scope of advanced nursing practice (Pearson, 1997). States with a strong medical presence allow the narrowest scope of practice for NPs. For example, Ohio has the highest number of medical schools per capita in the United States, and it was the last state to revise its nurse practice act to recognize NPs.

 CRITICALLY THINKING ABOUT . . .

Should NPs be allowed to prescribe medications for their clients? Why or why not?

The CNS Dilemma: A Contemporary Challenge in Advanced Practice

For the most part, the role of the CNS has evolved within the acute care hospital environment. CNSs were expected to practice as specialists who would provide a high level of nursing care in their specialties and assist nurses and others in hospitals to improve their practice by serving as role models and consulting with other health care providers. Although such a broad definition is troublesome for some, it often has served CNSs and the hospitals that employ them very well because it has allowed flexibility in the CNS role. However, that same flexibility is proving to be a danger to many CNSs in the contemporary acute care environment, which is characterized by cost-cutting, downsizing, and managed care systems that require extensive, detailed documentation of reimbursable services. For many CNSs, their colleagues, and their patients, the broad definition of the CNS role has been a source of role confusion and ambiguity, and this may prevent CNSs from optimizing their knowledge and skills (Holt, 1997; Redekopp, 1997). As Frieda Holt, a contemporary nursing educator involved in the graduate preparation of CNSs, has said:

> The CNS is patient care expert, consultant, teacher, administrator, staff developer, and researcher—a combination that varies with the institution, the individual CNS, and the particular day one is examining. The flexibility of the Master's degree nurse has been considered an asset since the CNS evolved, yet today it may put the CNS's job in jeopardy. With the focus in the health care arena on cost, outcome, and accountability, the CNS role may be easier to eliminate than document. (Holt, 1997, p. 40)

Up to now, CNSs have been in the enviable position of fashioning their practice in direct response to the needs of patient care units, their own expertise, and expectations of nursing administrators. Thus, almost every CNS's career has been unique. Although this career pattern has proved to be challenging and rewarding to many CNSs, it also has been largely undocumented. In today's health care setting, there is pressure to decease length of stay and increase the use of unlicensed personnel, all to decrease costs. This is a time when CNSs are needed to ensure quality care, but because CNSs play such a variety of roles to a variety of people, their worth is being questioned (Holt, 1996).

Creative approaches are being initiated to deal with this serious challenge to the existence of the CNS role in the American health care system. David Picella (1996) has proposed the use of a computer program to document the various activities of CNSs. The use of such a database would allow administrators and CNSs to quantify CNSs' contribution to high-quality patient services. At the University of Iowa Hospitals and Clinics, a CNS task force conducted a study of CNS activities and proposed a change in titles of the APNs in that system. Five titles and the primary role components of each title were identified: advanced registered NP, CNS, education nurse specialist, research nurse specialist, and informatics nurse specialist. These APNs believed that retitling their job function helped to identify the major responsibilities of their position, clarify their role expectations, and create tools to evaluate their job role worth (Chase, Johnson, Laffoon, Jacobs, & Johnson, 1996).

Several leaders in nursing, including the ANA and a conference group of the American Association of Colleges of Nursing, have recommended that the functions of the CNS and the NP should be combined (Fenton & Bryckzynski, 1993; Giovinco, 1993; American Association of Colleges of Nursing, 1995; Payne & Baumgartner, 1996). Many CNSs are responding to that recommendation by doing additional graduate work toward NP qualification. Many universities offer a post-master's course of study to meet that specific need. A nurse qualified as a CNS/NP has experience in acute-level environments as well as the knowledge and skills necessary to engage in the preventive models of care emphasized for NPs. Such nurses can practice holistically, improve quality of care, and decrease costs. Nurses with skills in both health promotion and acute illness care will be needed in ever-increasing numbers (Busen & Engleman, 1996; Hester & White, 1996; Zwanziger et al, 1996).

 Critically Thinking About . . .

What advantages and disadvantages do you see in combining the CNS and NP roles?

Models of Advanced Nursing Practice

APNs, depending on their graduate study, are qualified to practice with a substantial degree of autonomy in many health care settings. In this section, two models in which APNs may provide care are discussed, and an example of each model is described.

The first model is primary care. This concept has grown in popularity in the last quarter of the 20th century as cost containment has become a focus of the health care system. The overall goal of primary care is to improve health promotion and disease prevention for persons, families, and communities.

The second model, actually a special case of primary care, focuses on the management of high-risk and vulnerable populations in the community. These populations include many different groups, such as ethnically diverse or immigrant populations, elderly adults with multiple chronic health problems, or people who require care in their homes for any number of reasons. APNs have much to contribute to meeting the care needs of persons and families in such circumstances.

Primary Care

The National Academy of Sciences Institute of Medicine has defined **primary care** as:

> the provision of integrated, accessible healthcare services by clinicians who are accountable to addressing a large majority of personal healthcare needs, developing a sustained partnership with patients, and practicing within the context of family and community. (Donaldson, Yordy, & Vanselow, 1994, p. 15)

A significant aspect of this definition of primary care is the concept of the **patient–clinician partnership**. Like any partnership, each party has clearly understood responsibilities to fulfill, and decision making is a shared process. Moreover, this partnership is forged against the backdrop of the client's personal context, including family, community, living conditions, work situation, and cultural background. Obviously, the primary care model of practice requires that a clinician approach client care from a holistic perspective. This perspective is a major focus in the preparation of all nurses, and especially nurses prepared for advanced practice.

There are two conditions under which a primary care clinician enters into a health partnership with a client. First, the relationship is expected to continue over time. Second, the clinician is expected to use a recognized, scientifically sound knowledge base as the foundation for the care that is delivered.

Although the patient–clinician partnership is at the heart of primary care, care is customarily delivered by primary care teams as part of an integrated delivery system that serves a defined population, such as a neighborhood, a school, or a business (Venegoni, 1996).

 CRITICALLY THINKING ABOUT . . .

As long as physicians control the diagnosis and treatment of health problems, can patients and nurse clinicians truly engage in a productive partnership?

Industry-Sponsored Comprehensive Health Care in the Workplace

Jimmie Butts (1996) has described his participation in establishing a nurse-managed health care facility in a corporate setting that became a model for other companies. In 1984, the director of human resources at SAS Institute Incorporated, a 300-employee software development company in North Carolina, determined that the rapidly rising cost of health insurance was cutting into company profits at an alarming rate. The employees of SAS were largely young and healthy, and the insurance costs in no way matched the payouts for hospital care that would be expected in a company with older employees experiencing more health problems. SAS needed to find a more cost-effective alternative. One of these alternatives was to hire an NP to develop an onsite primary care and wellness program to encourage healthy lifestyles among employees.

Butts had completed a family NP program at the University of North Carolina at Chapel Hill School of Nursing in 1976. After discussions with the director of human resources, Butts was hired in April 1984 and given

> the opportunity to design a program that included health education, preventive medicine, quality nursing, early identification of risk factors, and the opportunity to document the value of those services using an SAS Institute-developed software system—a nurse-managed program that most nurses only dream about. (Butts, 1996, p. 271)

The **SAS Health Care Center** had four aims:

1. To provide comprehensive assistance to employees and their families to meet health care needs
2. To contribute to developing a healthy working environment
3. To provide reliable, current health information for all age groups
4. To empower employees and their families to become wise consumers of health care.

After more than 10 years of experience, the system was still working well. Health care providers in the SAS Health Care Center included full-time NPs, contract NPs, a licensed practical nurse, nursing assistants, medical technologists, a nutritionist, and a work–family administrator. They also had a support staff to provide clerical and managerial services. They contracted for special services with a geriatric counselor, geriatric NPs, and a certified psychological counselor. A physician also served as a consultant, coming in about 4 hours a week to provide teaching and counseling, to review medical notes, and occasionally to see a patient at the NP's request. The physician could also arrange hospital admission if required.

The center provides various types of care, including acute care (eg, visits for colds, flu, and various other complaints), blood pressure checks, and regular routine visits. The center also provides comprehensive physical examinations, including laboratory tests, health risk appraisals, health histories, and electrocardiograms. Employees and families also may obtain allergy injections and immunizations at the center. Emergency care may be obtained from the nurses in the center or from a physician in the community. In addition, a wide range of counseling is available, as are referrals to appropriate care providers in the community. Employees must subscribe to an insurance provider for care received outside the center (eg, hospital care); the center provides employees with information to help them chose an insurance provider.

This nurse-managed center provides many benefits to the company and employees alike. First, it is convenient: an employee can be seen at the center and be back to work within 30 to 60 minutes, a fraction of the time it would take to see a practitioner off the premises. Second, regular and early examinations often reveal risk factors that can be reduced through early treatment. Long before health care received so much press, SAS and its self-funded insurance plan paid for physical examinations, mammograms, and well-baby care. Wellness programs for employees and their families have always been a benefit offered by the center. In 1996, it provided about 50 programs a year, and as many as 10,000 people have participated in programs in a year.

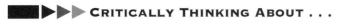 CRITICALLY THINKING ABOUT . . .

Think of employed adults you know. Does their employer offer wellness programs? If so, describe how your friend or relative uses it.

Management of High-Risk and Vulnerable Populations in the Community

Delivering high-quality, timely, and effective primary care to vulnerable populations is one of the most important challenges for health care providers. Since the 1960s, NPs have been an integral part of providing community-based care to underserved and at-risk populations. One model of delivering care to medically underserved populations was described briefly in Chapter 8: the Community Free Clinic in Flagstaff, Arizona. This chapter describes a model of primary care for another at-risk population: a system to provide transcultural care for immigrant families in the San Francisco area.

NPs must constantly be attuned to the importance of providing culturally sensitive care to their clients. This is especially important for the NP who one serves a community that is home to many recent immigrants and refugees. Shotsy Faust (1996) has provided guidelines for working with immigrants and refugees as they make the transition to a new world, a new culture, and a new life. Faust explains that because the traditional Western medical model teaches practitioners to focus on the patient's complaints and the underlying pathophysiology, the broader context of the patient's health beliefs or practices may be ignored. When working with another culture, a nurse has few guidelines or experiences to assess the context or culture of the complaint, so it is simply easier to focus on the measurable processes of the body.

> Unfortunately, a focus on the disease alone can lead to frustration for both patient and practitioner. Symptoms and conditions that cannot be explained by our medical tradition and are not readily quantifiable by examination or laboratory testing are easily overlooked or dismissed. (Faust, 1996, p. 287)

Two aspects of eliciting a patient's history and subjective information are unique to working with immigrants or refugees. One is the newcomer's migration status (an immigrant or a refugee), and the other is his or her migration history and psychological stage within the migration process.

First, it is useful to understand the differences between immigrants and refugees and the implications this has for their health and plans for their care. Immigrants have come to a new land seeking opportunities and a better life for themselves and their families. They had time to plan their emigration, and they chose their new homeland. They brought their possessions, their money, and their families with them. In contrast, refugees fled for their lives; they had no opportunity to plan for the emigration and usually little or no choice about where they would go. Many refugees, and the families they were forced to leave behind, experienced persecution and torture before fleeing their homeland. Additionally, many spent time—sometimes years—in detainment camps awaiting asylum. Because of these hardships, refugees are at higher risk for physical and emotional crises soon after arrival than are immigrants.

The practitioner's focus during the first visit should be on the client's migration status (immigrant or refugee), motivation for emigrating, and emotional status. The client's political or legal status is not at issue.

> Many undocumented newcomers or illegal aliens fear that questions about immigration status could result in deportation or reprisal. Consequently, it is important that the nurse practitioner explain that legal status is not germane to the clinic visit, and will not be reported or documented. (Faust, 1996, p. 288)

After determining the client's migration status, it is important to determine the client's migration history and psychological stage. Carlos Sluzki, a physician who worked with migrant families for many years, developed the **migration history** model (Sluzki, 1979, 1992), a helpful tool in collecting historical information from patients and families and a useful predictor of potential patient stress. Sluzki divided migration into five stages:

1. Planning stage
2. Act of migration
3. Period of overcompensation
4. Period of decompensation
5. Resolution stage or stage of intergenerational support.

In the planning stage, people make their plans to emigrate. For immigrants, this can be a long time; for refugees, it may encompass only days or even a few hours. The act of migration refers to the length of time of transit from one country to another, including any time spent in a refugee or detention camp. The period of overcompensation occurs soon after the newcomer arrives, when he or she focuses on obtaining housing, using public transportation, receiving welfare assistance, enrolling children in school, and finding health care. The period of decompensation occurs about 6 months to a year after arrival, when the reality of making a life in the new country becomes more apparent. Newcomers speak little if any English, and they may have no transferable job skills. Their housing may be limited to overcrowded, low-income areas. Fond memories of the homeland and relatives left behind emerge. Newcomers often experience hopelessness and despair at this point and may come to the clinic with complaints of weakness, headache, dizziness, or fatigue. In addition, symptoms of preexisting conditions often flare up at this point. Finally, resolution comes about in the stage of intergenerational support. In this final stage, families can come together, providing strength and support to the members. Many of the earlier crisis-related symptoms subside, and the client no longer needs the interventions of the clinician.

Faust describes how the migration history model can be used to obtain and interpret client data and develop appropriate clinical care plans for each client. Practitioners must also be aware that most of their clients will be dual users of health systems—that is, they will seek help from Western practitioners but also will continue to consult folk or traditional healers and use traditional healing methods. Including the family in the plan of care is of great importance, because the family is the most important unit of care in most cultures. "Including the family according to the patient's beliefs and wishes demonstrates the practitioner's respect for cultural values and enhances the prospects of compliance with the therapeutic regimen or plan" (Faust, 1996, p. 293).

Clearly, unique opportunities and challenges await the skilled NP who can practice in a multicultural milieu such as the one Faust describes.

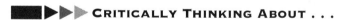 **CRITICALLY THINKING ABOUT . . .**

The Los Angeles school system offers instruction to students in more than 100 languages, reflecting the cultural heterogeneity of the community. How can nurses best provide culturally sensitive care in such a complex environment?

Role Responsibilities of APNs

So far, advanced nursing practice has been described in terms of the educational programs available to prepare advanced practitioners, the populations APNs serve, and the settings in which they deliver patient care. This section focuses on the nature of the expectations for performance among APNs. In other words, what roles are APNs expected to perform, and what are their responsibilities?

Traditionally, CNS positions have had five components:

1. Direct patient care at an expert level
2. Consultation and collaboration with nurses and other members of the health care team
3. Education of patients, families, and members of the health care team
4. Research
5. Leadership within the institution.

CNSs have typically carried out these responsibilities in inpatient acute care hospitals.

The expectations for NPs have been somewhat different. There is more focus on assessment and direct care, usually at the individual patient level, and less on the leadership component. Also, NPs generally work with physicians as practice partners; CNSs generally supervise and collaborate with other nurses. Thus, NPs and CNSs tend to have different views of their relationships with physicians.

General Role Responsibilities of APNs

The roles of CNS and NP have evolved separately, but it is increasingly likely that they will become blended as the American health care industry continues to evolve. Accordingly, the ANA has issued guidelines for expectations for APNs regardless of the focus of their clinical work (Box 9-1).

To accomplish these expectations, APNs must assume multiple roles. In their role as caregivers, APNs assist clients in changing situations that support illness and are harmful to health. The APN's teaching role "focuses on assisting individuals in attaining and maintaining healthy lifestyles" (Creasia, 1996, p. 89). When APNs serve as client advocates, they protect their clients and mediate between the clients and their environment, all the while acting on behalf of their clients. As a quality improvement coordinator, the APN coordinates activities that will improve the system of care delivery. APNs also may assume managerial roles at different levels in their organization.

BOX 9-1

Guidelines for Expectations for Advanced Practice Nurses (APNs)

APNs work with individuals, families, groups, and communities to:

Assess health needs
Develop diagnoses
Plan, implement, and manage care
Evaluate outcomes of care.

Within their specialty area, APNs may:

Plan and advocate care that promotes health and prevents disease and disability
Direct care or manage systems of care for complex patient, family, and community populations
Manage acute and chronic illness, childbirth, and the care of patients before, during, and after anesthesia
Prescribe, administer, and evaluate pharmacologic treatment regimens.

APNs also:

Serve as mentors, consultants, and educators of nurses in basic practice
Conduct research to expand the knowledge base of nursing practice
Provide leadership for practice changes
Contribute to the advancement of the profession, the health care sector, and society as a whole.

Knowledge Base for APNs

APNs must be expert clinicians, so they must be firmly grounded in the basic biologic and physical sciences as well as in advanced areas such as physiology, pathophysiology, and pharmacology. APNs also must have a thorough theoretical and clinical understanding of their speciality area: the disease processes they are likely to encounter, the interventions that are most appropriate, and the developmental and socioemotional aspects of the clients with whom they work. Strong assessment skills are a must, as are skills in differentiating the normal from the abnormal. Beyond these basics of clinical excellence, however, APNs also need a theoretical knowledge base; this is vital to the effective performance of APNs in the demanding circumstances in which they practice.

The first two theoretical foundations for successful advanced nursing practice were identified in Chapter 2 as the basics for the general knowledge base for nursing science. These are **general systems theory** and **role theory**. Using general systems theory helps the APN analyze the part of the health care system where he or she practices and determine how it fits into the rest of the health care system and the community in general. It also permits the APN to analyze the work environment in terms of its subsystems and the links that make them work together to provide maximum benefit for its clients.

A clear understanding of role theory is a key component for an APN in establishing and continuing an advanced role. APNs are the most professional of nurses. They are accorded more autonomy in practice than nurses who have less education and clinical preparation. However, the role of an APN is a reciprocal one: it is highly dependent on others, such as families, physicians, and ancillary health care personnel (Cresia, 1996). Therefore, the way the APN performs the advanced role depends not only on his or her conception of the role, but also on the expectations of others and the context in which the role is enacted. In short, for an APN to perform successfully in the role, there must be agreement among all parties that his or her behaviors are appropriate to the role as they understand it.

Understanding role theory is especially important to nurses who are entering APN roles that may be new to them, new to their clients and colleagues, new to the community in which they establish their practice, and even new to the health care system. These APNs would be at most risk for experiencing role ambiguity (the stressor that results when role expectations are unclear) and role overload (which results when too much work is expected in the allotted time or the role becomes too complex). An understanding of role theory allows the APN to recognize the signs of role stress and strain, identify its sources, and take action to resolve it. Otherwise, the probability of classic burnout is very high.

Organizational theory also provides information that can contribute to an APN's success. Put simply, anyone who is employed functions within an organization. The better one understands the nature and functions of organizations, the more likely it is that one will experience personal success and contribute to the success and development of the organization as well. Most current health care organizations are highly bureaucratic. The limiting effect of bureaucracies on truly professional practice was addressed in Chapter 1. Ideally, as the health care system decentralizes from the highly bureaucratized hospital environment, the new, smaller health care delivery systems will be less stultifying and will encourage autonomy and self-responsibility. An understanding of organizational theory and behavior can enable an APN to be proactive and to ensure that these new environments enhance professionalization rather than retarding it.

One of the primary functions of an APN is effective teaching. The APN's clients must have a clear understanding of their health status and the options that are available to them to maximize their health and that of their family and community. This can be achieved through effective teaching by health care practitioners. Traditionally, APNs have been consistently cited as providing the best education of all the primary care providers. To achieve excellence in teaching with both clients and colleagues, the APN must have a thorough understanding of **teaching–learning theory** and practice. Most APNs teach adults; therefore, they must clearly understand and be able to apply the concepts that underlie adult learning processes and motivation. APNs also must be prepared to evaluate the outcomes of their teaching—that is, the extent to which client behavior changed in the desired manner.

Finally, the successful APN must be able to apply to the advanced practice role the theories, concepts, and principles inherent in some key processes. These processes include leadership, communication, and consultation. A nurse does not become an effective leader, communicator, or consultant overnight. He or she brings these processes to the advanced practice role by developing a clear understanding through study and diligent application of underlying principles. The same is true for the processes of collaboration, decision making, and conflict resolution. These and many other interpersonal processes are involved in the effective implementation of any advanced practice role. APNs must strive to enhance their understanding of the processes and refine their application of the processes throughout their professional nursing career.

 CRITICALLY THINKING ABOUT . . .

> Incorporating role theory, systems theory, and organizational theory into the curriculum designed to prepare APNs reflects which kind of nursing knowledge discussed in Chapter 2?

▶ CHAPTER SUMMARY

Currently, and for the foreseeable future, advanced nursing practice affords an opportunity to move American nursing toward fully professional status faster than at any other time in our history. Limited autonomy, one of the primary elements of a profession, has until now eluded most nurses in their practice. However, all 50 states gradually have revised their nurse practice acts to acknowledge APNs and provide for direct reimbursement for their services by third-party payers. Also, several states' nurse practice acts permit nurses to prescribe medications for clients. This is a significant element in the control an APN has over the care of his or her client, and it is the component in nurse practice acts that is usually resisted the most vigorously by state medical associations.

As the American health care system decentralizes and moves away from the dominance of bureaucratic, hierarchical hospitals and into the community, APNs will be very well positioned to assume roles and responsibilities that have not been afforded nursing before. Advanced nursing practice in America has its roots firmly planted in the community, building on the proud heritage of nurses such as Lillian Wald and Mary Breckinridge. The opportunity to return to these roots should be welcomed. But this time, nurses have a lot more tools in their "little black bag"—the symbol of early nurses who ventured out to care for their patients. Today, there is better science, a broader understanding of the theoretical constructs that underlie nursing practice, and health care technology of which nursing's founders could never have dreamed. Today's APNs are prepared to practice with autonomy, authority, and responsibility. As more and more nurses join the ranks of those already practicing in advanced roles, the discipline and practice of nursing will benefit, the American health care system will benefit, and the clients served by the system will benefit most of all.

KEY POINTS

▶ 1 **The CRNA is the oldest of the advanced nursing specialities. Nurses were predominately the early anesthetists: surgical procedures became more complex and required experts in administering anesthesia, but physicians were not interested in this aspect of care. Nurse anesthesia became separated from mainstream nursing very early on and remains so today. Nurse anesthetists have faced challenges from medical anesthesiologists but remain a strong, viable advanced nursing practice role.**

▶ 2 Nurse-midwifery was the second of the four major advanced practice nursing specialities to develop in the United States. Early in the 20th century, American midwives were largely untrained and generally discredited. However, the educational requirements of nurse-midwives have been raised over the years, and many nurse-midwife programs today are at the graduate level. Nurse-midwifery languished until it was rediscovered in the late 1960s as part of the women's health movement. Since that time, it has been a growing enterprise.

▶ 3 The CNS role developed largely within hospital systems in response to the need for additional expertise and leadership in clinical nursing. Psychiatric/mental health nurses led the way in developing the CNS role in the mid-1950s. The purpose of CNSs was to provide a high level of nursing care in the specialty and to serve as a change agent in hospitals by serving as role models and consulting with other health care providers. CNSs generally were not opposed by physicians (the way nurse anesthetists and nurse-midwives were) because they were viewed as complementary to physicians rather than competitive.

▶ 4 NPs are the newest advanced practice nurses to emerge in America and the fastest-growing group of APNs. Factors that impelled the growth of the NP movement included a physician shortage in the 1960s and 1970s and rapid social changes in the same period. The federal government provided financial support for graduate education for APNs, and states have revised their nurse practice acts to permit APNs to function more broadly and more independently than they had ever done.

▶ 5 The role of CNSs has evolved in hospitals, but as hospitals are downsizing, that role is being seriously challenged. Because of the diverse expectations for CNSs, many have experienced role ambiguity, and their contributions to patient care have often gone undocumented. CNSs have responded to the challenge in many ways, one of which is obtaining additional graduate education to qualify for nurse practitioner certification. This preparation would produce an APN with highly developed acute care skills as well as health promotion skills.

▶ 6 APNs are qualified to practice in many settings, including industry-sponsored, nurse-managed health care centers and community clinics that serve the special needs of immigrants and refugees.

▶ 7 Some of the general role responsibilities expected of APNs (depending on their specialty) include assessing health needs; planning, implementing, and managing care; managing acute and chronic illness and childbirth; caring for patients before, during, and after anesthesia; prescribing, administering, and evaluating pharmacologic treatment regimens; serving as mentors, consultants, and educators of nurses in basic practice; and providing leadership for practice changes. In addition to these role responsibilities, the elements of a knowledge base necessary for APNs include general systems theory, role theory, organizational theory, teaching–learning theory, and the key processes of leadership, communication, and consultation.

REFERENCES

American Association of Colleges of Nursing (1995). Summary of work group activities. *Role Differentiation of the Nurse Practitioner and Clinical Nurse Specialist: Reaching Toward Consensus.* Proceedings of the Masters Education Conference, December 8–10, 1994, San Antonio, Texas. Washington DC: Author.

American Nurses Association (1995). *Nursing's Social Policy Statement.* Washington DC: Author.

Bigbee J (1996). History and evolution of advanced nursing practice. In Hamric AB, Spross JA, Hanson CM (Eds.), *Advanced Nursing Practice: An Integrative Approach.* Philadelphia: WB Saunders, pp. 3–24.

Brooten D, Gennaro S, Knapp H, Jovene N, Brown L, York R (1991). Functions of the CNS in early discharge and home follow-up of very low birth weight infants. *Clinical Nurse Specialist, 5,* 196–201.

Busen NH, Engleman SG (1996). The CNS with practitioner preparation: An emerging role in advanced practice nursing. *Clinical Nurse Specialist, 10,* 145–150.

Butts JK (1996). Industry-sponsored comprehensive healthcare in the workplace. In Hickey JV, Ouimette RM, Venegoni SL (Eds.), *Advanced Practice Nursing: Changing Roles and Clinical Applications.* Philadelphia: Lippincott-Raven, pp. 270–275.

Chase LK, Johnson SK, Laffoon TA, Jacobs RS, Johnson ME (1996). CNS role: An experience in retitling and role clarification. *Clinical Nurse Specialist, 10,* 41–45.

Christman L (1991). Advanced nursing practice: Future of clinical nurse specialists. In Aiken LH, Fagin CM (Eds.), *Charting Nursing's Future: Agenda for the 1990s.* New York: JB Lippincott, pp. 108–120.

Creasia JL (1996). Professional nursing roles. In Cresia JL, Parker B (Eds.), *Conceptual Foundations of Professional Nursing Practice* (2nd ed.). St. Louis: Mosby, pp. 67–91.

Diers D (1991). Nurse-midwives and nurse anesthetists: The cutting edge in specialist practice. In Aiken LH, Fagin CM (Eds.), *Charting Nursing's Future: Agenda for the 1990s.* New York: JB Lippincott, pp. 159–180.

Division of Nursing (1996). *Report to American Association of Colleges of Nursing.* Washington DC: Division of Nursing, Bureau of Health Profession, Health Resources and Services Administration, Public Health Service, U.S. Department of Health & Human Services.

Donaldson M, Yordy K, Vanselow N (Eds.) (1994). *Defining Primary Care: An Interim Report.* Washington DC: National Academy Press.

Faust SC (1996). Providing including healthcare across cultures. In Hickey JV, Ouimette RM, Venegoni SL. *Advanced Practice Nursing: Changing Roles and Clinical Applications.* Philadelphia: Lippincott-Raven, pp. 287–297.

Fenton MV, Brykczynski KA (1993). Qualitative distinctions and similarities in the practice of clinical nurse specialists and nurse practitioners. *J Professional Nursing, 9,* 313–326.

Ford LC (1991). Advanced nursing practice: Future of the nurse practitioner. In Aiken LH, Fagin CM (Eds.), *Charting Nursing's Future: Agenda for the 1990's.* New York: JB Lippincott, pp. 287–289.

Giovinco G (1993). Critique of qualitative distinctions and similarities in the practice of clinical nursing specialists and nurse practitioners. *Nursing Scan in Research, 7*(2), 4–5.

Hester LE, White MJ (1996). Perceptions of practicing CNSs about their future roles. *Clinical Nurse Specialist, 10,* 190–193.

Holt FM (1996). Is CNS flexibility in a cost-conscious world a liability? *Clinical Nurse Specialist, 10,* 40.

Holt FM (1997). Our continuing fight for clarity and simplicity. *Clinical Nurse Specialist, 11,* 86.

Kalisch PA, Kalisch BJ (1996). *The Advance of American Nursing* (3rd ed.). Philadelphia: Lippincott-Raven.

Payne JL, Baumgartner RG (1996). CNS role evolution. *Clinical Nurse Specialist, 10,* 46–48.

Pearson LJ (1997). Annual update of how each state stands on legislative issues affecting advanced nursing practice. *The Nurse Practitioner: The American Journal of Primary Health Care, 22,* 19.

Picella DV (1996). Use of a relational database program for quantification of the CNS role. *Clinical Nurse Specialist, 10,* 301–308.

Redekopp MA (1997). Clinical nurse specialist role confusion: The Need for identity. *Clinical Nurse Specialist, 11,* 87–91.

Sills GM (1983). The role and function of the clinical nurse specialist. In Chaska NL (Ed.), *The Nursing Profession: A Time to Speak.* New York: McGraw-Hill, pp. 563–579.

Sluzki C (1979). Migration and family conflict. *Family Process, 18*(4), 379–390.

Sluzki C (1992). Disruption and reconstruction of networks following migration/relocation. *Family Systems Medicine, 10*(4), 359–363.

Smoyak SA (1976). Specialization in nursing: From then to now. *Nursing Outlook, 24,* 676–681.

Thatcher VS (1953). *A history of anesthesia: With emphasis on the nurse specialist.* Philadelphia: J.B. Lippincott.

Venegoni SL (1996). Primary care: Improving health promotion and disease prevention. In Hickey JV, Ouimette RM, Venegoni SL (Eds.), *Advanced Practice Nursing: Changing Roles and Clinical Applications.* Philadelphia: Lippincott-Raven, pp. 255–256.

Zwanziger PJ, Peterson RM, Lethlean HM, et al (1996). Expanding the CNS role to the community. *Clinical Nurse Specialist, 10,* 199–202.

Classic References

Ayers R (1971). Effects and development of the role of the clinical nurse specialist. In Ayers R (Ed.), *The Clinical Nurse Specialist: An Experiment in Role Effectiveness and Role Development.* Duarte, CA: City of Hope National Medical Center.

Ford LC, Silver HK (1967). The expanded role of the nurse in child care. *Nursing Outlook, 15*(8), 43–45.

Georgopaulus BS, Sana M (1971). Clinical nursing specialization and intershift report behavior. *AJN, 71,* 538–545.

Linde BJ, Janz NM (1979). Effect of a teaching program on knowledge and compliance of cardiac patients. *Nursing Research, 28,* 282–286.

Norris DM (1977). One perspective on the nurse practitioner movement. In Jacox A, Norris C (Eds.), *Organizing for Independent Nursing Practice.* New York: Appleton-Century-Crofts, pp. 21–33.

Peplau HE (1965). Specialization in professional nursing. *Nursing Science, 3,* 268–287.

U.S. Department of Health, Education, and Welfare, Secretary's Committee to Study Extended Roles for Nurses (1972). *Extending the Scope of Nursing Practice.* Washington DC: U.S. Government Printing Office.

RECOMMENDED READINGS

Dunn L (1997). A literature review of advanced clinical nursing practice in the United States of America. *J Advanced Nursing, 25,* 814–819.

Garde JF (1996). The nurse anesthesia profession. *Nursing Clinics of North America, 31,* 567–580.

JCAHO medical staff standards: Impact on clinical privileges for nurse-midwives. *J Nurse-Midwifery, 41,* 43–46.

Lichtman R (1996). Entry-level degrees for midwifery practice. *Journal of Nurse-Midwifery, 41,* 47–49.

Nugent KE, Lambert VA (1997). Evaluating the performance of the APN. *Nursing Management, 28*(2), 29–32.

Page NE, Arena DM (1994). Rethinking the merger of the clinical nurse specialist and the nurse practitioner roles. *Image: J Nursing Scholarship, 26,* 315–318.

O'Flynn AI (1996). The preparation of advanced practice nurses: Current issues. *Nursing Clinics of North America, 31,* 429–438.

Pinelli JM (1997). The clinical nurse specialist/nurse practitioner: Oxymoron or match made in heaven? *Canadian J Nursing Administration,* Jan–Feb, 85–105.

Urban N (1997). Managed care challenges and opportunities for cardiovascular advanced practice nurses. *AACN Clinical Issues, 8,* 78–89.

Ventre F, Spindel PG, Bowland K (1995). The transition from lay midwife to certified nurse-midwife in the United States. *J Nurse-Midwifery, 40,* 428–437.

10

Issues in Nursing Practice: Changing Opportunities in a Changing Health Care Environment

CHAPTER OUTLINE

The Managed Care Environment
The Managed Care Environment
  and Nursing
Thriving in the Managed Care
  Environment

Chapter Summary
Key Points
References
Recommended Readings

LEARNING OBJECTIVES

▶ **1** Identify factors that have contributed to the financial crisis that faces the health care system in the United States.

▶ **2** Describe the major elements of a managed care system.

▶ **3** List at least five effects of managed care that nurses have identified in the *American Journal of Nursing*'s patient care survey.

▶ **4** Discuss why RNs are concerned about the use of unlicensed assistive personnel in hospital nursing care.

▶ **5** Explain the implications of the managed care environment for advanced nursing practice.

▶ **6** Describe examples of creative strategies that nurses can use to adapt their practice to the managed care environment and still maintain quality of care.

▶ **7** Summarize the actions that nurses should be taking to become a more proactive voice in the health care debate and ensure the future of nursing in the health care system.

KEY TERMS

American Nurses
    Association's
    (ANA's) report
    card study
fee-for-service
health maintenance
    organizations
    (HMOs)
home health care

managed care
managed care
    organizations
    (MCOs)
Medicaid
Medicare
patient care
    survey

perioperative
preferred provider
    organizations (PPOs)
prospective payment
unlicensed assistive
    personnel (UAP)
utilization review

The radically changing American health care system presents unparalleled challenges and opportunities for nurses and the nursing practice enterprise. Some nurses who are disturbed by the changes they see take solace in the fact that there have been ups and downs before in the history of American nursing. They feel that things will eventually return to normal and that the serious challenges to nursing will fade away. This is not likely to happen, for reasons tied to technology, the economy, and demography.

Advances in technology have led to the treatment and cure of diseases and conditions that were never treatable or curable before now. In addition, the American taste for the very best in health care has led society to believe that it deserves to have access to these advances. This expectation has carried an extremely high price tag and has generated a steep escalation in national health care costs. The proportion of the nation's gross domestic product devoted to health care rose from 5.9% in 1965 to 14.1% in 1995. The Congressional Budget Office has estimated that health care spending will climb to 18% of the gross domestic product by 2005 (Buerhaus, 1997; Congressional Budge Office, 1995).

The demographic reality that will have the most dramatic impact starting early in the 21st century will be the sharp rise in the number of older Americans, as the baby boom generation ages. Moreover, due to technology, a larger number of old people will live even longer than preceding generations of Americans. We will have more "old-old" people than ever before.

These pressures on health care costs will continue: technology will still be available and will probably continue to improve, and Americans will continue to become old in larger numbers than ever before. Thus, the health care system in America must undergo a major overhaul in terms of strategies for health care delivery and health care financing.

In 1994, President Bill Clinton proposed a program of comprehensive health care reform that was to bring costs under control while maintaining quality of care and improving access to health care for all Americans. The American Nurses Association (ANA) strongly supported President Clinton's proposals, but the program failed dismally due largely to political factors.

▶▶▶ CRITICALLY THINKING ABOUT . . .

What role, if any, should the government take in reducing the cost of health care?

Nonetheless, health care reform in the United States has proceeded rapidly in the 1990s, largely without major federal intervention as the primary driving force. Peter Buerhaus, a prominent health policy expert, has identified five interrelated economic pressures that have driven the evolution of the health care system in the 1990s and will continue to do so in the foreseeable future:

1. Efforts to reduce the rate of increase in national spending on health care
2. Actions to reduce the federal budget
3. The growth of managed care organizations (MCOs)
4. Growing economic competition among MCOs
5. The evolution of integrated health delivery systems.

As a result of these factors, the American system of health care has embarked on a journey of sorely needed change from which it will never return. The factors listed above are changing how organizations are paid for delivering health care. This, in turn, affects health care employers' demand for nursing services and dramatically changes the environments in which nurses work (Buerhaus, 1997).

Nursing is a vital part of the health care system and has a great deal to offer, much of which has until now gone unnoticed. Thus, nursing must strive to become a key player in the political and corporate decision-making processes that will propel the health care system into and through the 21st century.

This chapter describes the factors driving the changes in the American health care system, the changes themselves, and their impact on nursing. Many nurses and nursing organizations already have taken actions to deal with the challenges presented by the changing health care delivery system, and some of these actions will be considered. Finally, we will examine some strategies nurses should use to emphasize their contributions to the American health care system and to become more proactive in shaping that system to benefit themselves, their clients, and society.

The Managed Care Environment

The closing decade of the 20th century has been turbulent for all people touched by the American health care system. Changes have affected employers, employees, unemployed persons, and health care providers. People have been forced to find new ways to obtain health care and pay for it, and health care providers have been forced to deliver care in new ways, not always to their liking. Employers and third-party payers, including private and public insurers, demand more accountability and cost-effectiveness from all aspects of the health care delivery system. This has happened because health care costs were, quite simply, spiraling out of control. How did the health care system get into its current state of financial crisis?

Understanding the interesting history of the American health care system will help answer that question. The American health care system is remarkably good in many ways, and public confidence in the quality of health care in America is justified. However, the health care system also is extraordinarily complex. Much was said in the early 1990s concerning attempts at massive health care reform at the federal level, initiated under the leadership of President Clinton. However, attempts at government-sponsored reform had occurred long before that doomed effort. For example, President Franklin Roosevelt, as part of his New Deal, proposed that national health insurance be included in the Social Security legislation of 1935. However, it was never included because of lack of public backing and strong opposition from the American Medical Association (Ginzberg, 1994).

Although the development of the insurance industry was a factor that contributed to the growth of the American hospital industry, it also played a major part in the escalation of health care costs in several ways. In 1929, Blue Cross, a private, not-for-profit system, developed a plan to protect people from the high cost of hospitalization by offering a community-based prepayment plan. Blue Cross was very successful, and commercial for-profit insurance companies soon joined the ranks. However, the plans that the for-profits companies offered were "experience-based" and charged lower premiums for industries where the workforce was largely young and healthy and had a low frequency of illness or accidents. This became a more inviting model to employers, so Blue Cross shifted to the same model. The outcome was that health insurance became an established employee benefit. However, the elderly, high-risk persons, and the chronically ill were either not insured or had to pay for their own insurance (Ginzberg, 1994).

A mid-20th-century federal decision regarding taxes also played a significant role in the eventual escalation of health care costs. To control inflation during, and immediately after, World War II, the federal government had instituted wage, rent, and price controls. After the war, as the labor force grew, the power of unions grew along with it. The unions, always attempting to negotiate better financial and working conditions for their members, were able to bargain for health care benefits when the federal government agreed that receiving benefits would not be in violation of the existing freeze on wages. Furthermore, the federal government allowed employers to treat health insurance premiums as nontaxable business expenses. They also exempted employees from income-tax liability on health insurance premiums paid by their employers. Unions gained an important employee benefit for which to bargain, and neither employers nor employees had to pay any federal taxes on the money that was going into health insurance premiums. It seemed like everyone was winning. In effect, "this encouraged employers to provide health care to all workers and subsequently created a large pool of individual health care consumers who were unconcerned about the price of services" (Corder, Phoon, & Barter, 1996, p. 215).

Although these developments served employed Americans very well, it became apparent in the 1950s that the private health insurance industry, which was founded on employment, was not going to cover retired or disabled employees, those who needed the coverage the most. Once again, the federal government intervened by legislating **Medicare** and **Medicaid** in 1965. Medicare is a tax-based insurance system that provides health coverage for Americans over 65. Medicaid was set up to provide access to health care for the poor, especially women and children.

◼▶▶▶ CRITICALLY THINKING ABOUT . . .

Should Medicare and Medicaid pay all of a person's medical expenses? Why or why not?

Before Medicare and Medicaid were introduced, physicians and hospitals treated the poor for lower rates or for free. However, medical technology was advancing rapidly, hospitals were required to stay within their budgets, and free care for the poor cut into revenues. With the implementation of Medicare and Medicaid, money was no longer an issue. Hospitals could simply bill Medicare and Medicaid for services rendered and receive full reimbursement for their care of the elderly and the poor. Care to the elderly and poor no longer needed to be provided at the expense of the hospital. In fact, care to the elderly and indigent had become as profitable as care delivered to patients covered by private insurance plans. Money was now available not only for expansion of physical facilities, but also for acquisition of the high-tech equipment and services the American public had come to expect.

Another reason for the escalation of health care costs is that the funding for all health care services, including hospital care, traditionally was based on a **fee-for-service** model. After services were rendered, the cost of those services (plus an agreed-on percentage for overhead) was calculated, and the total bill was submitted to the third-party payer.

The result of health care legislation and the fee-for-service reimbursement structure was that "health care costs began climbing at increasing rates, which surpassed most other industries" (Corder, Phoon, & Barter, 1996, p. 215). The need for a complete reorientation of the American health care system was made clear in the 1995 Pew Health Professions Commission report:

> Feeding on an unlimited amount of public and private resources dedicated to health care, hospitals and other health care organizations have grown well beyond the needs of the current health care system and vastly beyond the needs of the system that is now emerging, which will use these resources far more judiciously. (Pew Health Professions Commission, 1995, p. 18)

Managed care is a major element in the emerging American health care system.

Elements of Managed Care

Managed care is a very general term that has a variety of meanings. One of the most useful definitions was offered by Elizabeth Hadley in her discussion of nursing in the political and economic marketplace: "any system that uses networks of providers to deliver coordinated care to a defined population for a prospectively determined payment" (Hadley, 1996, p. 8). **Prospective payment** is a key element in all **managed care organizations (MCOs)**. MCOs are business ventures, the primary purpose of which is to "deliver, finance, buy, and sell health care services as economically as possible" (Catalano, 1996, p. 220). As noted above, Peter Buerhaus (1997) identified the rapid growth of MCOs in the 1980s and 1990s as one of the primary economic pressures driving the current evolution of the American health care system.

In general, MCOs work to eliminate unnecessary and inappropriate health care services with **utilization review** programs, which can include:

- ◨ Requiring prior authorization for hospital admission (this role is often performed by nurses)
- ◨ Using primary care physicians or nurse practitioners as "gatekeepers"
- ◨ Requiring second opinions before proceeding with costly treatments and procedures.

MCOs also control costs by limiting enrollees' choice of providers. The MCO offers a network of providers from which enrollees may choose. Should the enrollee elect to see a provider outside the system (an "out-of-plan provider"), he or she would be responsible for all or most of the cost of the visit.

Health maintenance organizations (HMOs) are a familiar form of MCO. HMOs form contracts with employers (and individual subscribers as well) to provide basic and supplemental health maintenance and treatment at a predetermined price per patient. An HMO can be organized in two different ways. It may hire its own staff of health care providers and administrative personnel. Alternatively, it may serve as a "pass-through" organization, contracting with the employer for a given set of health services at a set price per enrollee, and then contracting with a medical group that actually provides the services.

The primary purpose of an HMO is to limit costs in several ways. In general, there are decreased referrals to specialists (whose services typically are expensive), limits are set on extensive diagnostic studies, and there are decreased days of hospitalization for enrollees.

HMOs have both advantages and disadvantages. After the premium is paid, services are free or require only a small copayment (assuming the client uses a provider who is in the system). Overall expenses are kept down by implementing cost-containment incentives. Paperwork for enrollees is minimized. However, if the HMO has a limited number of providers under contract, client options for care may be restricted, and going outside the system for treatment can be costly (Catalano, 1996).

Another form of managed care that emerged in the 1980s is the **preferred provider organization (PPO)**. In PPOs, contracts are established with a limited number of health care facilities and health care professionals who are willing to discount the price of their services. Providers usually are required to adhere to PPO utilization guidelines. In return for these concessions, more clients use the services of the provider. In PPO systems, physicians are reimbursed on a **fee-for-service** basis and members are charged each time service is provided; thus, care may actually be more costly in PPOs than in HMOs. However, clients have a wider range of choices among providers in PPOs than they may have in an HMO, and Americans have traditionally valued their freedom to choose their health care providers (Buerhaus, 1997; Catalano, 1996).

The public sector has given a big boost to the growth of MCOs. In the middle to late 1990s, state and federal governments started new programs to encourage Medicare beneficiaries and Medicaid recipients to enroll in MCOs. In 1995, about 25% of Medicare beneficiaries were enrolled in MCOs, and enrollments are expected to rise sharply as legislation is enacted that offers new incentives for older Americans to enroll. In Ohio, enrollment in the Medicare HMO jumped more than 50% in just 8 months, from about 65,000 in June 1996 to about 110,000 in February 1997 (Peer Review Organization for Ohio, 1997). This state is particularly active in helping older adults learn about and manage their Medicare choices (Ohio Department of Insurance, 1997).

In addition, the federal government has modified the management of Medicaid by providing block grants to states and encouraging each state to develop its own plan for Medicaid that maximizes efficiency. States are rapidly moving their Medicaid recipients into MCOs of various kinds.

All these systems are still evolving and are in a state of flux, but there is no doubt that MCOs are the future as the American health care system advances into the 21st century. MCOs will become more refined, and there will be increased competition among them as the demand for low-priced, high-quality health care delivery systems

---

Box 10-1

Changing Nature of Health Care Systems

From	To
▶ An illness and critical events management model	▶ A health and life processes management model
▶ A specialty care model	▶ A primary care model
▶ A privatized fee-for-service model	▶ A capitated cost-managed model
▶ A single organization or institution model	▶ An integrated network and health systems model

(Reprinted with permission from O'Malley J, Cummings S, King CS [1996]. The politics of advanced practice in nursing. *Admin Qtr, 20,* 62–72. Originally in O'Malley J [1995]. The editors page: Practice, challenges, and opportunities in advanced practice. *Nurs Qtr, 1,* iv–v.)

---

increases in both the private and public sectors. Box 10-1 compares the old health care system with the emerging one.

 CRITICALLY THINKING ABOUT . . .

Do you or anyone you know belong to an HMO or a PPO? Has the experience been a positive or a negative one?

The Managed Care Environment and Nursing

In January 1994, when it seemed that President Clinton's proposed health care reform measures would pass, Peter Buerhaus issued the following "friendly warning" to nursing:

> The near-term outlook for many hospitals and the nurses they employ is likely to be difficult and fraught with disappointments and anxiety. As the economic activity of healthcare becomes organized by the principles of managed competition over the next several years, the survival of some hospitals will be at risk. . . . Such institutions will be under great pressure to restrain the growth in nurse wages, accelerate substitution of professional nurses by unlicensed and nonprofessional personnel, initiate layoffs or voluntary termination of RNs, and possibly take other steps to lower the costs associated with providing nursing care. Consequently, given these conditions and the political and economic turmoil that reforming the system is sure to unleash, there is a great risk that nurses will be distracted during the next several years from doing the hard work of defining the value of nursing, when this is the very activity that will assure their long-term interests. (Buerhaus, 1994, pp. 25–26)

Contrary to Buerhaus's expectations in 1994, President Clinton's government-driven program did not come to pass, but everything else he foretold for nursing has occurred as health care reform has unfolded, driven by market forces operating within the private sector.

The most obvious targets in the war that is being waged on escalating health care costs in America are the hospitals, and logically so: the most expensive of all health care is provided in hospitals. Within hospitals, the most common targets are the nursing staffs. Some would say that because nurses make up the largest single employee group in hospitals, this target also is a logical one. Nurses obviously disagree. In a recent book, Suzanne Gordon, an investigative reporter who has been consistently "pro-nurse" for many years, argued that the dollars spent on salaries of qualified experienced nurses are not the primary source of financial stress in hospital and health care systems (Box 10-2):

> Nurses' salaries seem particularly paltry when compared with some of the most egregious waste in the system—the incomes of the CEOs of for-profit HMOs . . . Nurses are clearly not the cost escalators in the system. Quite the contrary. Their care saves not only lives but money. (Gordon, 1997, p. 14)

What Has Happened in Nursing Practice?

Despite support from those outside nursing, and through the efforts of the ANA, hospitals have generally responded to adverse economic pressures by downsizing and restructuring in ways that have significantly reduced the numbers of RNs engaged in

---

Box 10-2

Salary Comparison Between Nurses, Physicians, and Hospital Chief Executive Officers (CEOs)

Nurses

(1996 approximate average annual salaries)

▶ Staff nurse—$37,000
▶ Clinical nurse specialist—$41,000
▶ Nurse practitioner—$49,000.

Physicians

(1996 approximate average annual salaries)

▶ Internist—$135,755
▶ Family practitioner—$128,096
▶ Anesthesiologist—$193,242
▶ Oncologist—$164,621
▶ General surgeon—$199,342.

Hospital CEOs

(1995 average base salaries and total cash compensations)

▶ CEO of small or medium nonprofit hospital—$188,500
▶ CEO of large nonprofit hospital—$280,900
▶ CEO of Columbia/HCA Healthcare Corporation (for-profit)—$2,093,844.

(Farrell JP & Pagoaga, JA [1995]; Freudenheim, M [1995])

direct patient care. This has prompted widespread concern that the quality of patient care will be seriously compromised.

This concern prompted the *American Journal of Nursing (AJN)* to publish a **patient care survey** in its March 1996 issue. The results were published in the November 1996 issue. The *AJN* study was the largest survey ever conducted of nurses' views on health care and nursing practice. Of the 7560 nurse respondents, 41% had a diploma or an associate degree, 41% had a baccalaureate degree, and 18% had a master's degrees or higher. Figure 10-1 shows that more educated nurses responded at a higher rate than the nurses with diplomas and associate degrees (higher rates of response among more educated persons is common in surveys such as this). The responding nurses were relatively experienced; the average number of years in practice was 17, and the average number of years in their current position was 7. Hospital nurses were overrepresented in the sample, and nurses engaged in home and community nursing were underrepresented. Hospital nurses made up 77% of the respondents (nationally, 66% of nurses practice in hospitals), and home and community nurses made up 7% of the respondents (nationally, 15% of nurses practice in home and community nursing). Less than 0.5% of the respondents were employed in MCOs.

Nurses reported that they were taking care of more patients, they had been cross-trained to take on a broader range of nursing responsibilities, and they had less time to provide all aspects of nursing care. Almost half the nurses reported that part-time or temporary RNs had been substituted for full-time RNs. Also, 40% reported that unlicensed assistive personnel (UAPs) had been substituted for RNs. The highest rates of substitution were reported in the Pacific region (Shindul-Rothschild, Berry, & Long-Middleton, 1996). (UAPs are discussed later in this chapter.)

Many nurses reported that their employers were initiating new construction and making renovations (66%) and were establishing or acquiring community-based ser-

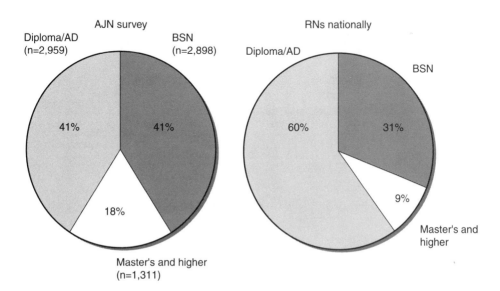

Figure 10-1. Education level of *AJN* study respondents compared to the education level of RNs nationally. (U.S. Department of Commerce, 1995.)

vices (43%). Almost half the respondents reported cuts in nurse managers, and well over two thirds of the respondents reported that a nurse executive had been lost in their institution and not replaced. A decrease in beds was a common hospital response to financial pressures; over half the nurses reported that their hospitals had downsized in this manner. Only 20% of the nurses reported that they actively participated in decision making regarding hiring, staffing, or budgets. Well under 20% felt that the introduction of UAPs had improved patient care. Less than half the nurses felt that the quality of care they provided met their own professional standards. Finally, more than a third of these nurses said they would not recommend their organization should a family member require care (Table 10-1).

In short, from a nursing perspective, these survey data do not present a pretty or encouraging picture. Indeed, the survey summary notes:

> Most health care economists agree that it's unlikely that every RN job lost in the hospital sector will be replaced. With half of all RNs over 40, many may find making a career transition a difficult and painful process. For new entrants into nursing, the uncertainty has left many wondering where, if at all, they fit in. It's important in this turbulent environment to avoid victim-blaming and characterizing some nurses as intransigent. Given what we know, nurses everywhere have every right to feel anxious about their jobs and their future. (Shindul-Rothschild, Berry, & Long-Middleton, 1996, p. 35)

In an article immediately following the *AJN* survey report, nursing leaders from all over the United States commented on the situation. Their commentary does little to lessen the atmosphere of doom cast by the survey summary. Norma Lang, then dean of nursing at the University of Pennsylvania, wrote:

> By repackaging and reconfiguring the nursing function and diluting the identity of nursing departments, hospital care is being jeopardized. This is an alarming trend for our profession, for the health care system at large, and most importantly for patients. (Lang, 1996, p. 40)

TABLE 10-1 CHANGING NATURE OF NURSING CARE		
Have you seen a change in the following?	Much Less/ Less (%)	More/ Much More (%)
Patient acuity	3.5	76.7
Unexpected readmissions of recently discharged patients	5.3	55.1
Length of stay	65.9	11.5
Continuity of care	55.2	10.9
Patient or family complaints	6.8	54.9
Teach patients and families	72.8	11.5
Comfort and talk to patients	73.5	9.9
Provide basic nursing care	68.5	7.2

(Shindul-Rothschild J, Berry D, Long-Middleton E [1996]. Where have all the nurses gone? *AJN, 96*[11], 27.)

Diane Sosne, president of a service employee union in Seattle, echoed Lang's concern:

> Health care is being transformed into a commodity, with diminishing regard for human life and dignity. This shift has profound implications for patients, nurses, and the whole community. . . . This untested approach amounts to a dangerous experiment with human subjects. (Sosne, 1996, pp. 41–42)

Patricia Benner, a leading educator and professor of nursing at the University of California—San Francisco, expressed serious concerns regarding the threat posed to continuity of patient care and even the ethical foundations of patient care:

> The health care business is based on the public's trust that those who deliver care will have a stronger ethos than the usual business ethos of just selling good products, that the provider will have the best interests of the patient as a top priority. Coaching patients or families to settle for less or to incur risk with delayed treatment or early discharge violates this basic trust. (Benner, 1996, p. 43)

Use of Unlicensed Assistive Personnel

The use of **unlicensed assistive personnel (UAPs)** has been of great concern to many nurses and nursing leaders. In 1964, Patricia Manuel and Kristine Alster argued that UAPs were "no cure for an ailing health system." When hospitals employ models of care that use UAPs, the RN's role is changed from providing patient care to delegating certain care tasks; the nurse develops the plan of care and selects certain activities to delegate to UAPs. The purpose of this model of patient care is to reduce costs by using less expensive employees and to improve nurse productivity in terms of numbers of patients for which one can care. Hospitals all across the country are adopting this model as a cost-saving measure. The data from the *AJN* patient care survey of nurses indicated that nurses were taking care of more patients than ever before, which is one of the goals of using UAPs. However, those nurses expressed a great deal of concern about issues of patient care quality and nursing practice associated with the UAP-based models of care (Shindul-Rothschild, Berry, & Long-Middleton, 1996).

Several assumptions underlie the use of UAPs, and Patricia Manuel and Kristine Alster (1994) have argued that these assumptions may be questionable. The first assumption is that using UAPs will improve care by freeing nurses from tasks that may no longer be appropriate for RNs: lower-level clinical tasks as well as tasks that are not clinical in nature. The ANA, addressing the appropriate use of UAPs, delineated two types of activities properly performed by UAPs: direct patient care activities (eg, feeding, toileting, and grooming) and indirect patient care activities (eg, housekeeping, transporting, and stocking supplies). Personnel that are properly trained and supervised can help nurses provide high-quality patient care when they are assigned appropriate tasks (ANA, 1993). However, the ANA also expressed concern that UAPs are being used to substitute for nursing care rather than supplement nursing care. This of course means that UAPs are acting outside the legal practice of nursing. Moreover, the time needed for RNs to supervise UAPs reduces the time available to provide care (Manuel & Alster, 1994).

The second questionable assumption relating to the use of UAPs has to do with the preparation of RNs to delegate tasks. Most nurses currently practicing have been educated to engage in primary nursing practice settings, and their education has not included content or practice in leadership and management. (Exceptions are older nurses who were in clinical practice before the large-scale implementation of primary nursing in the 1970s. Those nurses had experience in team nursing, an earlier care delivery model. A team was assigned to care for 12 to 15 patients and consisted of one or two RNs, possibly a licensed practical nurse, and two nurse's aides. The unit's nurse manager designated an RN as the team leader, and team leaders often changed on a daily basis. Thus, RNs had to provide leadership to the team and also had to be flexible. This model was largely supplanted by the primary care delivery model, in which each RN is responsible for the total care of a smaller number of patients.)

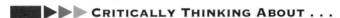 **CRITICALLY THINKING ABOUT . . .**

Is your nursing education preparing you to supervise UAPs in a clinical setting?

It is little wonder that these nurses, prepared for delivering patient care in a primary care model, find the shift in their responsibilities and scope of practice disturbing. Hospital staff development departments must be acutely aware of the needs of nurses educated in primary care models when those nurses take on the responsibility of providing care in a setting that uses UAPs. Kathleen Metcalf pointed out that the need for assistance in task delegation is particularly acute for newer nurses, who are still developing mastery of the tasks themselves. More experienced nurses, she contends, have less difficulty delegating. Ideally, more experienced nurses and clinical nurse specialists could help less experienced nurses in their learning. Unfortunately, these are the two groups of nurses who have been hit hardest in hospital downsizing (Metcalf, 1992; Gordon, 1993, Manuel & Alster, 1994).

The third questionable assumption addressed by Manuel and Alster is that adding UAPs to the staff mix will reduce patient care costs:

> It is tempting to suppose that the use of UAPs will save money for an institution, simply because unlicensed personnel can be paid lower salaries than those paid to RNs. However, as already noted, the implementation of care delivery models employing UAPs requires extensive preparation of the existing nursing staff. In addition, the UAPs themselves must be trained. Because no standard educational curriculum for UAPs exists, each institution must develop, implement, and evaluate its own training program. (Manuel & Alster, 1994, p. 19)

They cite studies conducted in the early 1990s that showed increased costs for RN overtime hours after the introduction of UAPs and found that UAPs had higher rates of absenteeism, creating workload problems for nurses as well as more RN overtime. They concluded their discussion of the perils of using large numbers of UAPs with the following warning and salient question:

> One danger of using UAPs for direct patient care is that RNs will not be freed to practice professional nursing, but, at a time when patient acuity is rising, will find themselves required to care for more patients, with the support of fewer professional colleagues. They will also have to assume the responsibility for supervising increasing

numbers of nonprofessionals. Will acute care facilities then find themselves in the position of long-term care facilities, struggling to attract nurses who may be reluctant to work in a setting where they feel isolated from colleagues and deprived of the stimulation of working with other nursing professionals? (Manuel & Alster, 1994, p. 21)

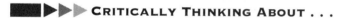 CRITICALLY THINKING ABOUT . . .

Do you foresee a time when UAPs supplant RNs as the central persons in patient caregiving?

The ANA's Report Card Study

The ANA's **report card study** of RN staffing in three states sheds some additional light on outcomes associated with RN staff reduction. According to this study, the ANA

is concerned both with the impact of nursing care on patient outcomes and the professional well-being of nurses. To affirm nursing's role in emerging health care systems and to advance knowledge in these areas, ANA commissioned and adopted a prototype for nursing report cards to measure nursing's impact on selected patient outcomes. (ANA, 1997, p. 1)

The data for this study were collected in 1992 and 1994 in California, Massachusetts, and New York. The primary goals were to test first the statistical relations between nurse staffing and selected patient outcome indicators and second the feasibility of "capturing the information necessary to develop specific nurse staffing and outcome measures for hospitals with acceptable degrees of reliability and validity" (ANA, 1997, p. 1).

The investigators quantified nurse staffing in the 502 hospitals used for the study. They also quantified "patient incidents" and length of stay for patients at the same hospitals. They then measured the relation between those two sets of variables. The patient incidents included were pressure ulcers, pneumonia (not community-acquired), urinary tract infections, and postoperative infections. All four of these untoward patient outcomes are generally recognized as being results of breakdown in the quality of nursing care. In addition to being highly undesirable for the patient, such an incident also becomes a financial burden for the hospital: it requires a longer hospital stay and more costly care above and beyond the costs associated with treating the admitting diagnosis and condition.

The findings from the study led to two very important conclusions. First, shorter lengths of stay were strongly related to higher nurse staffing. Second, preventable conditions (pressure ulcers, pneumonia, postoperative infections, and urinary tract infections) were inversely related to the proportion of RNs in the staffing mix. In short, nurses had a positive effect on patient outcomes.

Managed Care Environments and Advanced Nursing Practice

In 1994, at the same time Peter Buerhaus was issuing the warning regarding the short-term woes that would befall hospital nursing, he was also holding forth rosy predictions for the future of advanced practice nurses (APNs) in the managed care environment. Buerhaus noted that HMOs and other providers would face strong incentives to become more efficient, lower their costs, provide more primary and preventive care, and produce patient outcomes that purchasers value.

> APNs' comparative cost and quality advantages, combined with the shortage of primary care physicians, should result in prepaid health care plans employing more APNs as well as expanding their clinical roles and managerial responsibilities. (Buerhaus, 1994, p. 23)

However, Buerhaus also warned that the future was not entirely secure for APNs. He reasoned that because the success of APNs could come at the expense of physicians, physicians would try to pressure legislators to limit APN practice. These could include provisions that would:

1. Restrict nursing ventures by setting up certificate-of-need planning mechanisms
2. Define APNs who engaged in independent prepaid practice as illegally practicing medicine
3. Limit the number of APNs an HMO can hire
4. Enact federal legislation restricting APN practice that would override state nurse practice acts.

He concluded that:

> Although there is a good chance of obtaining fair employment opportunities and a level playing field for APNs in a future reformed health care system, APNs must bear in mind that Congress will be besieged by organized medicine (and every other provider group) who will spend a great deal of time and money to preserve their market positions. Therefore, APNs must be keenly aware of the efforts physicians are likely to take to influence legislators and be ready to counter them as necessary. (Buerhaus, 1994, p. 24)

 CRITICALLY THINKING ABOUT . . .

Is Buerhaus more pessimistic or optimistic about the future of nursing?

There is no doubt that the managed care environment will affect the practice of APNs, probably in both positive and negative ways. Linda Pearson, editor of *The Nurse Practitioner*, stated that one in five Americans was enrolled with an MCO by January 1996:

> Do patients really know what they are getting at these for-profit HMOs? Is this system good for patients or nurse practitioners? Is the rapid restructuring of the health care system to a managed-care system good or bad? . . . Well, that depends on who is doing the evaluating. Think of the analogy of two blindfolded people evaluating a soft and furry animal with a bushy tail. One may feel a sweet little head, the other may find the tail and discover the odiferous discharge from a skunk. (Pearson, 1996, p. 13)

Practitioners cite various advantages of working for a managed care system, such as:

1. HMOs support the theory behind preventive health care—a commitment that APNs share—and encourage clients to come in for well-patient visits that can offset or forestall potential health problems.
2. HMOs prevent the waste that is inherent to the fee-for-service system. This is a definite benefit to subscribers because it minimizes their costs.
3. The fight to obtain reimbursement from health insurance companies will be made easier because of an income guaranteed by the HMO.
4. A nurse practitioner's (NP) salary under a managed care system often includes generous benefits.
5. "If NPs can document their worth and cost-effectiveness within these managed-care systems, they will be in tremendous demand as HMOs look for ways to save money" (Pearson, 1996, p. 13).

However, NPs who have encountered the "tail of the skunk" have voiced three complaints about managed care systems. First, they object to the limits to quality of care and limits to patient services in the name of cost savings. Some NPs perceive that managed care is really a rationing system for delivering care at a fixed price, and the reality may be that providers put their income motives above concerns for their patients' health. Also, in managed care, it is often the insurer instead of the health care provider who decides what medicines, specialists, and hospitalizations will be covered.

Second, many NPs find it a problem that HMO subscribers have limited access to providers. If APNs are not listed on the provider panels of managed care organizations, patients, in effect, lose access to their services. Pearson stated that there had been many recent reports of discrimination against APNs being included on provider panels:

> APNs are used to fighting to be included in third-party reimbursement language. But when managed-care organizations take over fee-for-service reimbursement, NPs risk losing their jobs and being squeezed out of the system because third-party legislation does nothing to ensure a spot on provider panels. (Pearson, 1996, p. 14)

Finally, some NPs have found that they are accorded only a limited ability to perform their role. Pearson wrote that APNs may run a significant risk of having the HMO management dictate their practice in the name of cost savings. An important aspect of NP care delivery that distinguishes it from that of other providers is patient education. The average physician spends about 8 minutes per patient; an NP visit is more like 30 minutes because the NP takes more time for patient education. However, in the eyes of MCOs, spending a long time with patients is not good, because time equals money. Providers in an MCO who deviate too much from the time allotted for each patient will find their jobs threatened. "Cost analysis based on the patient encounter time presents a serious threat to NP professionalism and the NP role" (Pearson, 1996, p. 14).

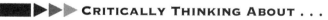 **CRITICALLY THINKING ABOUT . . .**

Should NPs and physicians charge the same for an office visit? Explain.

Thriving in the Managed Care Environment

Managed care, which is increasingly influencing the American health care system, has presented some problems for both patients and nurses. Rapid changes are occurring, and both providers and consumers have much to learn about how to make the system work in ways that at the same time are cost-efficient and produce high-quality health care. Some believe that many of the problems stem from the fact that private sector efforts to move to MCOs—especially those involving Medicaid recipients—have moved too fast and have had insufficient federal oversight (Fisher & Fein, 1995). Those who believe in a bright future for managed care believe that as the system continues to evolve, healthy competition and an open market for health care services will indeed produce a system superior to the fee-for-service model with which most American health care consumers are familiar. With the aging population and rising health care costs, Americans must receive better coordination of care (Fagin & Binder, 1997). All in all, MCOs probably offer the most promising solution to America's health care problems.

In theory, the philosophy behind managed care is in many respects consistent with the nursing model of care. Both emphasize the whole patient and coordination of care, and the goal of both is prevention and primary care for all clients. Moreover, most managed care environments emphasize collaboration between health professionals, which will move nurses further toward fully recognized professional status. As Clair Fagin and Leah Binder noted, "The convergence of the managed care philosophy with the professional belief system of nursing might suggest that nursing's moment has arrived. We believe that this is indeed the case" (Fagin & Binder, 1997, p. 445).

Despite the underlying philosophical similarities between nursing and managed care, however, in the short term—as we were warned by Peter Buerhaus in 1994—nurses appear to be increasingly marginalized by the emerging managed care systems. Hospitals are attempting to lower costs, but they seem to be doing so at the expense of nursing and the quality of patient care that nurses prize. At the same time, the future of APNs also is uncertain in the managed care market.

There is a paradox here: at the same time nurses are being devalued, the emerging model of health care delivery actually replicates the nursing model of care. There are at least three possible explanations for the paradox:

1. Nurses control their education but largely do not control their practice. This has resulted in nursing's inability to forge a completely independent professional identity within the health care practice setting.
2. Nurses' writings are not read by anyone but nurses—not other health practitioners and not the lay public.
3. When nurses bring up the fact that the organizations and ideas inherent in MCOs are what nursing has been and is about, and that these ideas were taught by nurses years ago, others in health care often dismiss their comments. Powerful groups involved in the creation of MCOs do not wish to hear a group without power say that it has invented that for which they are taking credit (Fagin & Binder, 1997).

■■■ ▶▶▶ CRITICALLY THINKING ABOUT . . .

Explain the meaning of "Nurses control their education but largely do not control their practice." Do you agree?

Nurses must act to contribute to the survival of nurses and to their thriving in a managed care environment. Many nurses have already demonstrated innovative strategies for developing cost-effective, high-quality nursing interventions that serve both the health care system and patients well. Some of these will be described in this section. This section also presents advice on how nurses can meet the challenges presented by the evolving health care environment in such a way that nursing will emerge as a stronger, more effective force in the health care industry. This advice has been provided to nurses by leaders in nursing and by knowledgeable observers of the health care scene who understand the important role of nurses in improving health care for all Americans.

What Nurses Are Doing

Home Health Care

Managed care has significant implications for **home health care**. Due to shorter hospital stays, there has been a substantial increase in the number of patients who require home health care, and patients are being discharged sicker. This has produced an ongoing debate in the home health environment focusing on issues of cost and quality of care. Carolyn Bonner and Barbara Boyd, nurse administrators associated with home care agencies in the Seattle area, have reported that a major obstacle to maintaining quality is the lack of documentation of clinical outcomes in home care. New tools for measuring and tracking outcomes are needed to reduce the number of visits per case.

Technology can play a large part in helping this larger group of home health care clients with more acute needs. The use of remote access and computer technology (especially laptop computers) makes it possible to make assessments and determine interventions wherever the patient is located.

Changes resulting from managed care also require a different approach to home care. The original approach was parental—goals were established and care was provided with minimal patient involvement. This approach must change to achieve positive clinical outcomes and lower costs. Patients must be involved in setting goals and must provide as much of the care themselves as possible (Bonner & Boyd, 1997).

To implement new models of home care, home health practitioners must function independently, apply critical decision-making skills, and provide patient teaching and coaching. They must be willing to work in a variety of interdisciplinary teams. Good communication skills are a must, as is computer literacy.

> A home health organization also has a role in providing a positive environment, culture and leadership to achieve and maintain quality services. . . . Leadership must encourage risk-taking behaviors, reinforce creative models and solutions, and promote systems thinking. (Bonner & Boyd, 1997, p. 5)

Perioperative Nursing

Hospital restructuring can mean significant role changes for nurses who practice in surgery. Until now, they have been identified as operating room (OR) nurses. That terminology—along with the nature of the job—is changing to **perioperative nurses**. As hospitals realign their cost structures, the OR skill mix is moving from being 80% to 100% RNs to only 50% RNs as technicians or licensed vocational nurses are given assignments and circulating in the OR. Although OR nurses may be reluctant to part with their traditional responsibilities, Mae Taylor Moss, a patient care executive consultant, has pointed out that this change actually allows RNs to participate in a broader range of care for the surgical patient, ranging from the initial office visit, where patient teaching can be initiated, on through the surgery itself, and finally into the home for postdischarge follow-up care.

In this expanded role, perioperative nurses will experience a shift in specialty from the place (OR or postanesthesia care unit) to the so-called "product line," such as cardiovascular surgery, orthopedic surgery, or OB/GYN surgery. The "product line" is simply a different area of specialty for the perioperative nurse. According to Moss, success will require three factors:

1. Nurses must obtain additional education to prepare for new roles and competence in new practice techniques.
2. Nurses must feel that change is a positive force.
3. New relationships must be forged within the OR, with supporting ancillary services, such as the laboratory and radiology, and with others involved in the preoperative, operative, and postoperative phases of patient care. Teamwork makes for better patient care and nursing practice that is holistic and rewarding (Moss, 1996).

With the trend toward managed care, perioperative nurses must address the challenge of instituting advanced technology in organizations with limited staffing and limited resources. Informatics systems can be a key factor in the smooth functioning of multidepartmental teams. New technology is not always welcome, so the implementation process must be designed so that it will achieve that goal. Williams, Sowell, and Smith reported four key elements that worked well in implementing an informatics system in one perioperative environment:

1. It must entail a collaborative planning process in which all divisions, departments, and personnel types are represented.
2. All staff members must be thoroughly educated regarding the systems design.
3. A timetable for implementation must be established, and everyone must agree that it is feasible.
4. Assessment of training requirements and the training itself must be done on an individual basis (Williams, Sowell, & Smith, 1997).

Other Practice Areas

The managed care environment also has spurred the development of alternative care delivery systems in a variety of other nursing specialty areas. For instance, new models of care rely less and less on inpatient psychiatric care; instead, psychiatric nurses, social workers, home health aides, and occupational therapists visit the patient at home. It is also now possible for all physicians, not only psychiatrists, to sign a Medicare psychiatric plan of care. This is consistent with the trend of primary care physicians treating psychiatric patients. Providing in-home interventions for psychiatric patients has resulted in significant reductions in hospitalization and recidivism rates. Once again, it is important for nurses to function effectively as part of a coordinated, interdisciplinary team (Biala, 1996).

CRITICALLY THINKING ABOUT . . .

Have you had psychiatric or mental health nursing experience yet? Inpatient or outpatient? What are the different challenges for nurses in these two environments?

Another example of the effect of managed care on psychiatric nursing is that a large percentage of nurses will shift from traditional inpatient care to work with patients in rehabilitation-oriented, community-based settings. As nurses increase their involvement in assessing patients and providing psychiatric rehabilitation in such settings, they will need information about rehabilitation for persons with serious mental illness (Furlong-Norman, Palmer-Erbs, & Jonikas, 1997).

In some cases, however, it is important for psychiatric nurses to document the need for continued inpatient care to achieve desired therapeutic ends. One such case is treatment in an inpatient chemical dependency unit, where patients often require lengthy treatment. Two nurses who worked on such a unit described how they modified and simplified charting to provide the data required by managed care plans rapidly and easily (Lavin & Enright, 1996). This change provided the managed care utilization review nurses with all the information they needed to justify patients' continued treatment. "This was the biggest payoff, since approval of benefits by the insurer gave patients the time that they needed to detoxify and complete their therapy programs—some of which lasted several months" (Lavin & Enright, 1996, p. 48).

Oncology nursing also has been affected by managed care: more and more patients receiving chemotherapy are being cared for at home. Thus, there is an increasing need for a system of assessment and intervention that is not based on face-to-face visits. Two oncology nurses described the use of "telephone triage" in the management of chemotherapy-related problems based on a combination of published articles, nursing texts, and their own experience. They concluded that with the use of established protocols for assessment and treatment, nurses can successfully manage many patient needs over the phone (Anastasia & Blevins, 1997).

What Nurses Should Be Doing

Documenting

Nursing leaders and those who value nursing have stated repeatedly that if nurses are to survive and indeed thrive in managed care environments, they must document. Elizabeth Harrison Hadley worked as a member of the group that staffed President Clinton's health care reform task force and later served as a senior policy fellow on health reform issues for the ANA. She argues that nurses must once again demonstrate that they provide cost-effective, high-quality care that can be measured (Hadley, 1996; Koerner, 1996). More than 100 years ago, Florence Nightingale recognized the importance of measuring health outcomes with good data. Good nursing care is essential for good patient outcomes, but the quality of that care must be measured and documented to be valued (Hadley, 1966). Part of the dilemma in which hospital clinical nurse specialists find themselves (see Chap. 9) is due to the lack of adequate documentation that clearly describes what they do and the resultant patient outcomes. Without these data, health care systems have no way of evaluating their actual contribution to care, much less their cost-effectiveness.

Everyone in the health care system faces the challenge of learning to live and work with accelerating change. Although many hospital nurses feel extremely distressed by cost-cutting measures, most health care systems are desperately seeking strategies to develop care delivery systems that are both efficient and of high quality. Nurses must assume responsibility for designing these strategies and conducting research to document how nursing interventions improve outcomes and advance patient safety and satisfaction. This includes forming collaborative relationships with other providers who share nursing's concerns (Luther, 1996; Patterson, 1996). In addition, nurses must take a hard look at the number of nurses being produced, how these nurses are prepared, and the skills they will need to function successfully and flexibly in the health care systems of the 21st century (Lang, 1996). Peter Buerhaus urges nurses to realize that the best way to ensure a strong future is to define and promote the value of nursing, which includes documenting and describing nursing interventions, determining their cost-effectiveness, relating them to patient satisfaction and measurable patient outcomes, and dispersing this information to all those involved in health care systems (Buerhaus, 1994).

Advancing the Case of Advanced Nursing Practice
Within Managed Care

APNs share many of the concerns of nurses in basic nursing practice. They must document their worth and cost-effectiveness, and to secure their future in the health care marketplace, they must show that they bring to the patient encounter a value-added component of both primary care skills and improved patient outcomes. APNs must identify the impact they can make in a managed care environment. Their challenge is to convey the importance of their role to the decision-makers in their organizations (Parr, 1996). To do this, they must learn to speak the language of health care administrators; they must learn to justify their services and prove that what they do is cost-effective. However, APNs must not become corrupted by the system and lose their holistic approach toward health care (Pearson, 1996).

APNs must also continue to insist on autonomy over their practice. Quite bluntly, they must insist that physicians stay out of the nurse practice acts; they must be totally regulated by the board of nursing (Pearson, 1996). APNs also must be vigilant about other impending threats to autonomy from within the managed care arrangement (eg, business and insurance laws that control health care structures).

To ensure nursing's advance toward professionalism into the 21st century, nurses should endeavor to assume a greater role in governance of the organizations and institutions of which they are a part. Governance means establishing and maintaining the social, political, and economic arrangements by which nurses control their practice, working conditions, and professional affairs. APNs are most experienced and best qualified to lead this endeavor.

Potential for Political Power

Nurses typically underestimate their potential for political power and often are characterized as having the collective mentality of an oppressed minority. That must change. Nurses as a group need to develop self-confidence and assume positions of leadership. They must believe that they can make a difference and must act collectively to accomplish this.

Nursing has great potential for political power. Nursing's notable strengths in the political arena include large numbers (about 2.2 million) and a tremendously positive public image. In the health care reform debates of the early 1990s, nurses were perceived as much less self-interested than other major stakeholders.

However, nursing has political weaknesses as well, primarily a lack of unity within the profession. Divisions have arisen due to the lack of uniform educational requirements and uniform title designations (Hadley, 1996). These divisions remain and still create problems for nursing, but nursing's best hope for realizing its potential political power is through a strong ANA.

Nurses must remain keenly attuned to politics and must not depend on the changing health care system to police itself. Nurses must form coalitions among themselves and with consumers to lobby for legal protections for nursing practice, patient rights, and patient care (Barry, 1996). Currently, health care in America is not a fundamental right; rather, it remains a privilege based on the patient's ability to pay for care. This is the nature of our capitalistic society:

> Unfortunately, many consumers continue to support the status quo by electing politicians who don't view health care as a right. It's up to us, as nurses, to galvanize the public into corrective political action. (Simpson, 1996, p. 44)

Nursing must exert political leadership to influence legislation that deals with health care delivery in a managed care environment. Nursing organizations need to unite with consumer and provider groups. By building a consensus on outcome measures and staffing, documenting quality indicators and collecting data, and educating the public and legislators on the value of nursing care, nursing can promote better regulation of all health care facilities. Nursing organizations have the opportunity and the responsibility to develop a broad political strategy that will ensure quality health care well into the 21st century (Harrington, 1996).

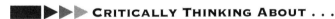 **CRITICALLY THINKING ABOUT . . .**

Do nurses have the mentality of an oppressed minority? What evidence is there for or against this assertion?

▶ **CHAPTER SUMMARY**

The last decade of the 20th century has been a turbulent one for nursing in America. In the early 1990s, nursing was emerging from yet another "nursing shortage" that was largely due to the sharp drop in enrollment in nursing education programs in the mid- to late 1980s. Moreover, nurses' salaries were rising, and more people—including more men—were finding nursing an attractive career prospect. In 1990, the prospects for the future demands for nurses seemed rosy indeed. *AJN* reported:

> By HHS arithmetic, the current FTE [full-time equivalent] requirements for RNs add up to a minimum of 1,614,200—199,400 more than are available. Demand is seen growing, at the most conservative guess, to 2,278,500 by 2020. Throughout the projection period, the requirements for FTE RNs exceed the supply, says the report. In fact, if this scenario comes true, the shortfalls will swell every year to a whopping 343,400 in 2000, 520,800 in 2010, and 874,900 in 2020. That kind of deficit could translate into vacancy rates of nearly 40% in 2020. (*AJN*, 1990, p. 97)

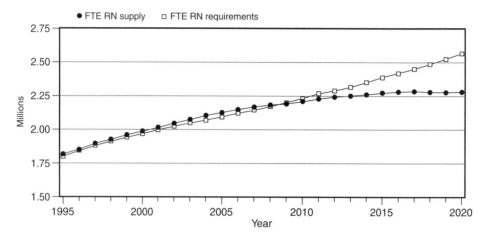

Figure 10-2. Projections of supply and requirements for full-time equivalent (FTE) RNs. (Division of Nursing, U.S. Department of Health & Human Services, 1996.)

However, by 1996, the projections of supply and demand for FTE RNs made by the same agency cited in *AJN* were not so wildly optimistic (Fig. 10-2). The curves show that by the year 2000, RN supply slightly exceeds demand. Between 2000 and 2007, supply is projected to exceed demand by about 30,000 nurses. The supply and demand curves cross at 2008 and then diverge, with supply remaining relatively steady and demand rising until 2020, when demand is projected to exceed supply by almost 300,000—about a third of the difference that was projected 6 years earlier (Division of Nursing, 1997).

What happened? Rapid private sector-driven implementation of managed care is the answer. Nurses were warned by Peter Buerhaus that the mid- to late 1990s would be chaotic, and that prediction has proven to be valid.

Will patient care in America be forever altered? Yes. Is nursing in America doomed? No. At all levels of American business, workers are being urged to work "smarter," and nurses are no exception. However, nurses have always been characterized (and have prided themselves) as being dedicated, hard-working, "can-do" people who creatively adapt things, situations, and themselves to provide the best possible care to their clients. Nursing will meet the challenges provided by the current changes in the health care system.

Proponents of a relatively recent systems theory known as chaos theory argue that chaos in an open, living system is required from time to time for that system to move to a new, higher level of functioning. Systems that never change simply die. Thus, as nurses we should view the current state of "chaos" as an opportunity to refashion ourselves and our whole practice to move to the next level of professionalization.

KEY POINTS

▶ 1 The American health care system is in a state of financial crisis due to the runaway escalation in health care costs that simply cannot continue. Factors that have contributed to the crisis include the availability of increasingly expensive care technology and techniques and the American public's demand for such care, regardless of its cost. Historical contributors to the current crisis include changes in the insurance industry and various federal legislative measures in the last half of the century, in combination with the fee-for-service model that has traditionally characterized the American health care system.

▶ 2 Managed care relies on networks of health care providers to deliver care to defined populations for a prospectively determined fee. Prospective payment and utilization review are key elements in all managed care organizations, which include health maintenance organizations, preferred provider organizations, and alternative models.

▶ 3 More than 7000 nurses who responded to *AJN*'s patient care survey (most of whom were practicing in hospitals) reported many changes in their practice between 1995 and 1996. Many nurses found these changes troublesome. The survey found that nurses were taking care of more patients, had been cross-trained for a greater range of responsibilities, and had less time to provide direct patient care; that part-time or temporary RNs had replaced full-time RNs; that unlicensed assistive personnel had been substituted for RNs; that hospitals are engaged in new construction and movement into community-based services; that the number of hospital beds has decreased; that patients are much sicker; that the length of stay is much shorter; and that continuity of care is compromised.

▶ 4 When hospitals employ models of care that use UAPs, the RN's role changes from that of providing patient care to that of delegating certain care tasks. Many RNs are concerned about the use of UAPs in hospitals for a number of reasons: (1) UAPs may be used to *substitute* for nurses in patient care rather than *supplement* nurses in patient care; (2) many currently practicing RNs do not have the knowledge and skills required for leadership and management of teams using UAPs; (3) the nurses who need assistance in learning leadership roles no longer have expert guidance from more experienced nurses and certified nurse specialists due to hospital downsizing and cost-containment; and (4) qualified nurses will be reluctant to practice in an environment where they have little or no support from other experienced nurses.

▶ 5 The managed care environment presents APNs with extraordinary opportunities as well as serious threats. If APNs can demonstrate that they can provide high-quality, cost-effective primary care within managed care systems, they will be highly prized and sought after. However, the success of APNs in a managed care environment probably will come at the expense of physicians. Should that happen, APNs must expect strong opposition from the highly organized, extremely well-funded medical community and be prepared to deal with it.

▶ 6 Different creative strategies can be used in different nursing care settings. In home care, nurses can use remote access and computer technology to make assessments and determine interventions anywhere the patient is located. In addition, a different approach can be implemented in home care, with the patient more involved in goal setting and providing his or her own care. In perioperative nursing, nurses can shift in their speciality from a place (eg, operating room, postanesthesia care unit) to a "product line" (eg, cardiovascular surgery, OB/GYN surgery). To do this, nurses need additional education, a positive attitude, and new relationships with supportive services (eg, laboratory, radiology). Another creative approach in perioperative nursing is the implementation of an informatics system.

Nurses in psychiatric nursing can help establish psychiatric home health care, which involves psychiatric nurses, social workers, home health aides, and occupational therapists. Another creative approach in psychiatric nursing is the development of rehabilitation-oriented community-based settings. In oncology nursing, the development of a telephone triage system for the management of chemotherapy-related problems for patients being cared for at home is another creative option for providing cost-effective, quality nursing care.

▶ 7 Nurses must document what they do. This involves writing down exactly what is done and the resultant patient outcomes, and passing along this information to those involved in the health care system. Nurses must also assume responsibility for designing and conducting research to document how nursing interventions improve outcomes and advance patient safety and satisfaction. APNs must communicate the impact of their work to decision-makers in their organizations. They must also justify their services and prove that their care is cost-effective, while holding on to their holistic approach to health care. APNs must also continue to insist on autonomy over their practice. Finally, nurses must become politically attuned by forming coalitions among themselves and with consumers to ensure legal protection for nursing practice, patient rights, and patient care.

REFERENCES

American Nurses Association (1993). *Position Statement on Registered Nurse Utilization of Assistive Personnel.* Washington DC: Author.

American Nurses Association (1997). *Implementing Nursing's Report Card: A Study of RN Staffing, Length of Stay and Patient Outcomes.* Washington DC: Author.

Anastasia PJ, Blevins MC (1997). Outpatient chemotherapy: Telephone triage for symptom management. *Oncology Nursing Forum, 24*(1, Suppl), 13–22.

Barry M (1996). Three areas for action. In: Survey reactions: A grim prognosis for health care? *AJN, 96*(11), 43–44.

Benner P (1996). Continuity of care is threatened. In: Survey reactions: A grim prognosis for health care? *AJN, 96*(11), 43.

Biala KY (1996). Beyond physical care. Psychiatric home care: The newest kid on the block. *Home Care Provider, 1,* 202–204.

Bonner C, Boyd B (January 6, 1997). Managed care: Threat or opportunity for home health? *Online Journal of Issues in Nursing* http://www.nursingworld.org/ojin/tpc25.htm.

Buerhaus PI (1994). Managed competition and critical issues facing nurses. *Nursing and Health Care, 15,* 22–26.

Buerhaus PI (1997). How changes in payment systems are affecting nurses. In McCloskey JC, Grace HK (Eds.), *Current Issues in Nursing* (5th ed.) St. Louis: Mosby.

Catalano JT (1996). *Contemporary Professional Nursing.* Philadelphia: FA Davis.

Congressional Budget Office (1995, February). *U.S. Congress, Health and Human Resource.* Washington DC: Author.

Corder KT, Phoon J, Barter M (1996). Managed care: Employers' influence on the health care system. *Nursing Economics, 14,* 213–217.

Division of Nursing (1997). *Report to American Association of Colleges of Nursing.* Washington DC: U.S. Department of Health & Human Services, Public Health Service, Health Resources and Services Administration, Bureau of Health Professions.

Farrell JP, Pagoaga JA (September 5, 1995). Making change pay. *Hospitals and Health Networks.*

Fagin C, Binder LF (1997). Dangerous liaisons: Nursing, consumers, and the managed care marketplace. In McCloskey JC, Grace HK (Eds.), *Current Issues in Nursing* (5th ed.). St. Louis: Mosby.

Fisher I, Fein EB (August 28, 1995). Forced marriage of Medicaid and managed care hits snags. *The New York Times,* p. B1.

Freudenheim M (April 11, 1995). Penny-pinching H.M.O.'s showed their generosity in executive paychecks. *New York Times.*

Furlong-Norman K, Palmer-Erbs VK, Jonikas J (1997). Exploring the field: Strengthening psychiatric rehabilitation nursing practice with new information and ideas. *J Psychosocial Nursing and Mental Health Services, 35,* 35–39.

Ginzberg E (1994). *The Road to Reform: The Future of Health Care in America.* New York: The Free Press.

Gordon S (1997). *Life support: Three nurses on the front lines.* Boston: Little, Brown.

Hadley EH (1996). Nursing in the political and economic marketplace: Challenges for the 21st century. *Nursing Outlook, 44,* 6–10.

Harrington C (1996). Nurse staffing: Developing a political action agenda for change. *Nursing Policy Forum, 2*(3), 14–27.

Koerner J (1996). Aspects of a broader truth. In: Survey reactions: A grim prognosis for health care? *AJN, 96*(11), 42–43.

Lang NM (1996). Hospital care in jeopardy. In: Survey reactions: A grim prognosis for health care? *AJN, 96*(11), 40–41.

Lavin J, Enright B (1996, August). Charting with managed care in mind. *RN,* 47–48.

Luther KM (1996). Data-driven interventions to improve patient satisfaction. *J Nursing Care Quality, 10*(4), 33–39.

Manuel P, Alster K (1994). Unlicensed personnel: No cure for an ailing health care system. *Nursing and Health Care, 15,* 18–21.

Metcalf K (1992). The helper model: Nine ways to make it work. *Nursing Management, 23*(12), 40–43.

Moss MT (1996). Perioperative nursing in the managed care era. *Nursing Economics, 14,* 252–253.

News (1990). *AJN, 97* (September), 97.

Ohio Department of Insurance (1997). *Ohio Shopper's Guide to Medicare Supplement Insurance: To Help You Patch the Holes in Medicare's Leaky Umbrella.* Columbus, OH: Author.

Parr MBE (1996). The changing role of advanced practice nursing in a managed care environment. *AACN Clinical Issues, 7,* 300–308.

Patterson C (1996). No prescribed staffing ratios. In: Survey reactions: A grim prognosis for health care? *AJN, 96*(11), 41.

Pearson LJ (1996). Annual update of how each state stands on legislative issues affecting advanced nursing practice. *The Nurse Practitioner: The American Journal of Primary Health Care, 21,* 10–16.

Peer Review Organization for Ohio (1997). *Healthtalk, 2*(1).

Pew Health Professions Commission (1995). *Critical Challenges: Revitalizing the Health Professions for the 21st Century.* San Francisco: UCSF Center for the Health Professions.

Shindul-Rothschild J, Berry D, Long-Middleton E (1996). Where have all the nurses gone? Final results of our patient care survey. *AJN, 96*(11), 25–39.

Simpson RL (1996). The realities of our time. In: Survey reactions: A grim prognosis for health care? *AJN, 96*(11), 44.

Sosne D (1996). Dangerous experiment with human subjects. In: Survey reactions: A grim prognosis for health care? *AJN, 96*(11), 41–42.

Williams PW, Sowell PM, Smith C (1997). Implementing an informatics system in a perioperative environment. *AORN Journal, 65,* 94–97.

RECOMMENDED READINGS

Astle S, Roth R (1987). HMO contracting: Know your costs. *Caring* (July), 23–24.

Butler RN, Sherman FT, Rhinehart E, Klein S, Rother JC (1996). Managed care: What to expect as Medicare–HMO enrollment grows. *Geriatrics, 51*(10), 35–42.

Cushing M (1986). How courts look at nurse practice acts. *AJN, 86,* 131–132.

Erlen JA, Mellors MP, Doren AM (1996). Ethical issues and the new staff mix. *Orthopaedic Nursing, 15*(2), 73–77.

Fields TT (1996). health care in the United States: Understanding the alphabet soup. *J Health Education, 27,* 365–369.

Johnson SH (1996). Teaching nursing delegation: Analyzing nurse practice acts. *J Continuing Education in Nursing, 27*(2), 52–58.

Ketter J (1994). Use of UAP on the rise in public health. *The American Nurse,* June, 4–20.

Michili AJ, Smith CE (1997). Unlicensed assistive personnel in the perioperative setting. *Nursing Clinics of North America, 32,* 201–213.

Mundt MH (1997). Books on health policy and health reform: How is nursing represented? *J Professional Nursing, 13,* 19–27.

Philbin P, Altman D (1990). HIV/AIDS: An HMO experience. *Caring* (August), 42–45.

PART V

Strategies to Enhance Professionalization in Nursing

11

Power, Politics, and Policy: Advancing Nursing's Professionalization

CHAPTER OUTLINE

Power: The Concept
Nursing and Politics
Policy to Further
   Professionalization

Chapter Summary
Key Points
References
Recommended Readings

LEARNING OBJECTIVES

▶ **1** Describe the nature of power, and explain the interaction between sources of power and power orientation.

▶ **2** Discuss the reasons many nurses have traditionally been considered powerless.

▶ **3** Describe strategies for increasing nursing's power.

▶ **4** Discuss the strategies the American Nurses Association developed and used in being a key player in the health care reform debates in 1993 and 1994.

▶ **5** Describe the roles nurses can play in politics.

▶ **6** Identify major policy issues that face American nurses as we enter the 21st century.

KEY TERMS

ANA-PAC	nurse politicians	power
latent power	1993 Nursing	powerlessness
networking	Summit	power orientation
nurse activists	policy	power sources
nurse citizens	politics	social policy statement

The only way nursing can become truly professionalized is by confronting and embracing the realities of power, politics, and policy. Nursing recognizes that it must have power if its professional status is to be advanced. Nursing leaders are seeking ways to obtain additional power for nurses, both collectively and individually. However, many nurses do not understand why nursing needs to build a strong power base among its practitioners. In fact, practicing nurses generally have given the concept of power serious consideration only within the last two decades. Practicing nurses must understand the nature and meaning of power and its importance in the professionalization process. They also must understand that obtaining power for nursing is not self-serving. When nursing has power, it also will have the freedom to act in the best interest of patients. Practicing nurses rarely ask questions such as, "Who are the power holders?", "How is power acquired?", and "How can I become a more powerful nurse?" Indeed, some nurses would say that these are unseemly questions for people in a helping profession to ask. This must change if we are to make progress in our growth toward full professional status.

Nurses have underestimated their power for too long. Nursing represents the largest group of health care workers in the country; there are about 3 million RNs. Nursing's greatest resource is people. If nurses as a group mobilized for patient advocacy, they could radically change health care delivery in the United States. That kind of change almost occurred in the mid-1990s with the health care reform proposal put forth by the Clinton administration, with the strong support of the American Nurses Association (ANA) and other nursing organizations. However, the effort fell short, and in the current political and economic climate, that kind of massive, federally based effort directed toward positive change is not likely to be seen again.

Instead, changes in the health care marketplace are being driven by very powerful players in the private sector. Not all these players share the same concerns for patient care and welfare that nurses have always had. Therefore, it is even more important that nurses be prepared to exert power adroitly and effectively to further the professional status of nursing in a dramatically changing environment. The effective use of power also enables nursing to take advantage of the opportunities offered in the rapidly changing health care environment to ensure better quality as well as increased efficiency and economy.

To affect policy at the federal, state, and local levels, people and organizations must be knowledgeable about, and adept at, the use of politics and the political process. Politics is a social institution, the purpose of which is to distribute power, set society's agenda, and make decisions (Macionis, 1997). Politics deals largely with social issues, which are moral matters that affect the well-being of most segments of the American public. Health care—one of the most important social issues in modern America—is a focus for much political action and decision making. Nursing's voice must be heard in political deliberations surrounding health care issues.

To be an effective political force, it is important to obtain and maintain access to the political figures who make key decisions. As the ANA matured in its ability to bring political power to bear, it recognized the need to be close to the political process and key decision-makers. The ANA's national headquarters had been in Kansas City for many years, but this is not where the primary political figures are, nor is it where national decisions about health care are made. The Governmental Affairs Office of the ANA has been located in Washington DC for more than 30 years and functioned as the lobbying arm of the organization. Primarily in the name of organizational efficiency, in 1992 the ANA moved its entire operations to Washington DC.

Since then, the ANA has become an increasingly significant political entity. In a speech to the ANA House of Delegates meeting in June 1997, First Lady Hillary Rodham Clinton

> credited the American Nurses Association with much of the progress made in the past few years in improving the quality of health care . . . Clinton attributed much of nursing's success in reaching the public to nurses' growing political activism. (Helmlinger, 1997, p. 1)

The objective of nursing's political action is to ensure beneficial public policy related to the American health care system. Public policy is the course of action taken by a government to deal with a matter of public concern (Hall-Long, 1995). The enactment of public policy results in the rules and regulations by which any enterprise is conducted. In the case of nursing, we must focus our political actions on the formulation of health care policy to ensure that these rules and regulations serve the interests of the American public.

To be effective, political activities by organizations such as the ANA must be integrated throughout the four stages of the policy-making process: agenda setting, adoption, implementation, and evaluation. These stages overlap and repeat, and the process of policy develop and implementation sometimes seems endless. Thus, vigilance and perseverance are required for organizations who would influence the development of policy (Hall-Long, 1995).

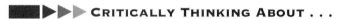 **CRITICALLY THINKING ABOUT . . .**

Do you think of nurses as being powerful or powerless?

Power: The Concept

To advance to full professional status, nursing must concentrate on getting its unique expertise recognized and valued by society; by doing so, nursing can gain a monopoly over services in which nurses alone possess expertise. Gaining such recognition and control is one way of acquiring a strong power base. However, the concept of power must be clearly understood and valued before nurses will be willing to exert their collective efforts toward acquiring and increasing power, both individually and as a group.

The Nature of Power

Sociologists and political scientists have attempted to define power for a long time. In its broadest context, **power** may be defined as the ability to influence and change the behavior of others, even if they do not desire the change. As one's power increases in a given situation, one's influence will be more effective. Power is the source of influence, although influence can be exerted by people who have little or no power. Several renowned scientists in history, for example, have greatly affected the thinking of others, and their findings have altered behavior, but they have had little or no personal power at all. Power implies the vigor or strength to control or command others. It is the ability to achieve ends despite resistance (Weber, 1947).

A slightly different view is that power is the ability of a person or an organization to achieve desired goals through the use of resources (Moore, 1997). In nursing, as in other developing professions, power is associated with autonomy, the control of practice, and organizational influence within the sphere of the health care system.

Power is an interactive phenomenon; one has power only if it is accorded to him or her by others. Power is not given. It must be taken, because when one person gives power to another, he or she diminishes his or her own power. Nurses, by virtue of their very large numbers, already have **latent power** (power that is untapped and underused). To convert nursing's latent power into actual power, nurses must want power, they must take power, and they must use power. Using power is a hallmark of political activity, which is discussed later in this chapter.

Nursing may achieve and maintain power in a different way than medicine has obtained its powerful position in the world of health care, simply because until recently the vast majority of physicians have been men and most nurses have been women. In general, there are differences in the ways men and women obtain and use power. The traditional male model of power has been described as "power grabbing" (hoarding power and control, taking power from others, or wielding it over others). Women are more likely to use "power sharing" (equalizing resources, knowledge, or control). One strategy is not necessarily superior to the other; in fact, people and organizations who use power most effectively are adept at using both (Chitty, 1997).

Sources of Power

People and groups derive power from specific **power sources**. The following list of power bases has been derived from the work of many authors:

- ◨ *Reward power*—implies the use of rewards such as recognition, money, opportunities for travel, and greater visibility; involves the perception that there are possible rewards or favors if one honors the wishes of a powerful person
- ◨ *Coercive power*—ability to inflict punishment or withhold rewards for nonacquiescent behavior; involves the real or perceived fear of one person by another
- ◨ *Legitimate power*—power derived from an organizational position rather than any personal qualities or actions
- ◨ *Referent power*—based on the basic attractiveness of the person that others identify with and aim to please; power flows from admiration or personal charisma; may be rooted in similarity of backgrounds or some other mutual identification
- ◨ *Informational power*—arises from the ability to gain and share information; one has exclusive access to information needed by others
- ◨ *Expert power*—arises from knowledge or special talents or skills that one possesses
- ◨ *Reputational power*—one is known as being an influential person
- ◨ *Connection power*—originates from privileged connections with powerful people or organizations
- ◨ *Collective power*—ability to mobilize a critical mass of people or a system to work on one's behalf.

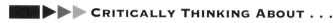 **CRITICALLY THINKING ABOUT . . .**

What examples can you give for the various sources of nursing power?

People and organizations derive their power from one or (usually) more of these power bases. But a power base that is not used does not itself constitute power. To be a leader by using one's power base, one operates with a particular **power orientation** (how a person perceives or uses power).

Power Orientations

Regardless of the source of power, one may see power in several ways:

- *Power is good.* Power is natural and desirable and is used in an open and honest manner. This orientation would probably build on expert, reward, and legitimate power bases.
- *Power is resource-dependent.* This is the perception that power depends on possession of things, including information, property, and wealth. This could be associated with withholding patterns of behavior when one has an information power base.
- *Power is an instinctive drive.* Power is viewed as a personality attribute. This is usually is associated with a referent power base.
- *Power is charisma.* This orientation involves the influence over people through personal magnetism.
- *Power is political.* This orientation draws heavily on referent, connection, and collective power bases. With this orientation, power is perceived as being linked to the ability to negotiate the system.
- *Power is control and autonomy.* The power broker is always in control, operating from a base of coercion, information, and connection (Ferguson, 1993).

Together, the concepts of power base (the source of one's power) and power orientation (one's perception or use of power) have a great deal of utility in managing organizations and political systems.

The power base of people in combination with their power orientation allows prediction of how they will function and provides you with a model to identify your own capacity and style. It can also provide direction for what people expect before they will *give* power. (Kelly & Joel, 1996, p. 288)

An Alternative View of Nursing Power

Patricia Benner, a highly respected nursing leader, has argued that nurses also derive power from the art and science of nursing practice as well as the fact that nurses are the health providers the public most respects and supports. Benner based her argument on her landmark study of the development of excellence in clinical nursing practice conducted in the early 1980s. Benner expressed the concern she feels when she hears nurses say that the very qualities essential to their caring role are the source of their powerlessness in the male-dominated hospital hierarchy. Such a statement disparages feminine qualities and elevates the masculine view of power, one that emphasizes competitiveness, domination, and control. (Benner, 1984, p. 207)

She believes that defining either power or nursing exclusively in traditional masculine or feminine terms is a mistake because this disparagement of women's perspectives on power is based on the misguided assumption that it is feminine values that have kept women and nursing subservient. Actually, she argued, society's devaluing and discrimination against women have been the sources of the problem. She claimed that this was a case of blaming the victim. Implicit in the underlying misguided assumption is the promise that "discrimination will stop when women abandon what they value and learn to play the power games like men do" (Benner, 1984, pp. 207–208). Benner identified six qualities of power that are associated with excellence in nursing care (Box 11-1).

 CRITICALLY THINKING ABOUT . . .

Do you agree or disagree that there are feminine and masculine concepts of power? Discuss.

Powerlessness in Nursing

The origins of nurses' perceived **powerlessness** have been both external and internal. The external forces that have silenced "nurses' voice" (the unique perspectives and contributions that nurses bring to patient care), and thus rendered them largely powerless, include the historical role of nurse as handmaiden and the hierarchical structure of health care organizations. Other factors have been the perceived authority and directives of physicians, hospital directives, and the threat of disciplinary or legal action. Currently, the simple fear of losing one's job due to health care restruc-

---

Box 11-1

Qualities of Power Associated With Excellence in Nursing Care

Transformational—Ability to help clients transform their self-image
Integrative—Ability to help clients return to normal lives
Advocacy—Ability to remove obstacles
Healing—Ability to create a healing climate and nurse–client relationship
Participative/Affirmative—Ability to draw strength from a caring interaction with a client
Problem Solving—Ability, through caring, to be sensitive to cues and search for solutions to problems.

(Huber D [1996]. *Leadership and Nursing Care Management.* Philadelphia: WB Saunders, p. 395.)

turing has proven to be a powerful "silencer of nurses' voice" (Pike, 1997, p. 532). It is little wonder that many nurses perceive themselves as powerless.

Forces that silence nurses' voice are not all external; powerful internal forces also constrain full expression of nurses' identity and power. These include role confusion, lack of professional confidence, timidity, fear, and insecurity or a sense of inferiority. These characteristics often lead nurses to choose silence and accept powerlessness. Adele Pike, a clinical nurse with the Visiting Nurse Association in Boston, observed that a

> poor professional self-concept sabotages any possibility of collaboration between nurses and other care providers because it identifies nurses as embattled victims and customarily marks physicians as their antagonists . . . [The] stance of victimization is very seductive; and there are many incentives for maintaining this role. Victims are perceived as innocent; they avoid responsibility; and they are spared the stress of change because in the matrix of victimization, it is the oppressor who must change for the victim's condition to improve. (Pike, 1997, p. 533)

Thus, in attempting to achieve power, one must forgo the "safety" of the victim role, taking risks and refusing to have one's voice silenced. Some maintain that the lack of self-confidence and willingness to assume the victim role is the fundamental cause for nurses' apparent lack of interest in—or even fear of—gaining power. However, they should remember that

> both the powerful and the powerless tend to take existing social systems for granted and rarely recognize that it is not talent, but rather laws, customs, policies and institutions that, in reality, keep the powerless . . . powerless. (Lipman-Blumen, 1984)

Increasing Power in Nursing

Unity

The best way nurses can gain power in all areas is through unity. Unfortunately, groups within nursing often act like separate classes competing with each other for status in the system. A collective class consciousness on the part of the total nursing community is largely noticeable by its absence. As a result, collective action on any national scale is almost unheard of, and the powers of the several groups are scattered in many diverse directions. A notable exception to the lack of collective action among groups of nurses was demonstrated when the ANA and other nursing groups allied in strong support of President Clinton's health care reform bill in 1994.

For the most part, nurses' potential power has been negated by internal power struggles. However, as evidenced by 1994's events, there is considerable potential for power in nursing, and this should make nurses willing to unite to exercise it to the fullest extent. To move nursing closer to professionalism or to effect any significant changes in health care delivery, nurses must use their power to reach agreement on such goals.

Nursing derives its greatest power source from a dynamic professional association that is substantially supported by its members. Although many nurses agree with this statement, the ANA's actual membership is less than 7% of the total number of RNs (ANA membership office, personal communication, July 31, 1997). The power of a professional association to effect change is in direct proportion to the size of its membership. Such a low percentage of membership significantly dilutes this important source of power.

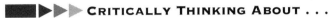

CRITICALLY THINKING ABOUT . . .

If only a small percentage of nurses belong to the ANA, how has it managed to achieve such important goals?

Despite its low membership, the ANA has contributed substantially to improving economic security among all nurses, not just its members. For decades, the ANA has worked tirelessly toward upgrading nursing education to a collegiate level. The ANA has contributed toward professionalism by defining nursing in its **social policy statements** of 1985 and 1995. Establishing standards for nursing practice is another significant contribution the ANA has made toward the professionalization of the discipline.

Bowman and Culpepper noted in 1974 that the ANA established positions on many important issues but rarely took follow-up action. This is still true. Substantial organizational power is needed to translate these positions from words into actions. Without actions, written standards and definitions become meaningless. However, it is very difficult for any organization to enact change if it cannot say that it truly represents the whole of its constituency. Thus, the ANA simply must have more members if it is to make its voice heard more often and more widely. Nurses who want to contribute to the movement of nursing toward true professionalism must meet this challenge and participate in their primary professional organization as well as any specialty nursing organizations that serve their needs.

> If nursing is to have the full autonomy of a profession, there must be unity of purpose and action on major issues. Leadership is vital, but grassroots nurses must be a part of the final decision, or achievement of the goals will continue to be an uphill struggle. (Kelly & Joel, 1996, p. 297)

Networking

Nursing can gain power by establishing support networks, much like the well-established "good old boy" system that remains alive and well in many organizations (eg, universities, governmental systems, and businesses). A network is an informal web of relationships that provides advice, information, guidance, contacts, and protection to those within the group. **Networking** provides many benefits to the members of the network. Younger members are offered encouragement, support, and nurturing, enabling them to move up through the ranks into positions of leadership. Members of a network do not criticize each other publicly, even though they may have private disagreements (in fact, they probably do). In short, networks operate on the basis of offering mutual support and avoiding destructive competition and in-fighting (Catalano, 1996; Kelly & Joel, 1996).

Joseph Catalano (1996) has proposed that the reason nurses have had difficulty establishing a support network is that only recently have significant numbers of nurses held high-level positions in the health care system. Thus, few nurses had sufficient power to provide less experienced colleagues with the benefits networking can offer.

Networking works well when members agree that the following points are important:

- One must learn how to ask questions.
- One should give as much as he or she gets.
- Contacts are important. Good networkers follow up on contacts, keep in touch with contacts, and report back to contacts.
- One should be businesslike when networking.
- One should never pass up opportunities to participate in networking and expand one's networks (Kelly & Joel, 1996; Puetz, 1991).

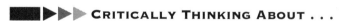 **CRITICALLY THINKING ABOUT . . .**

Have you seen networking in action? Discuss. Some people belong to more than one network. What are the implications of that?

Nursing and Politics

Politics is generally understood to be the art or science of guiding or influencing government policy. Politics also can mean political actions, practices, and policies. "Politics focuses on the acquisition of power, resources, or influence that results in attaining desired outcomes in a situation" (O'Malley, Cummings, & King, 1996, p. 68). Nurses and their practice have always been affected by actions in the political arena, but only recently have nurses entered politics in an active way. Florence Nightingale was politically astute and knew how to use the power of her wealthy, influential Victorian family. She was accustomed to dealing with government leaders at the highest levels and was a brilliant, determined player in the political scene of her day. It was precisely because of her political acumen that she could have such a tremendous impact on her society and advance the cause of modern nursing.

The call for nurses to become politically active has appeared frequently in nursing literature since the 1970s (eg, Ashley, 1976; Kalisch & Kalisch, 1982; Powell, 1976; Archer & Goehner, 1982, O'Malley, Cummings, & King, 1996; Blanchfield & Biordi, 1996; Betts, 1996; Helms, Anderson, & Hanson, 1996). For nursing to increase its power and have its interests represented, it must emerge as a political force. To accomplish this goal, nurses are learning to use their power and are becoming more politically active. In the past, nursing tended to isolate itself from policy-making groups and did not assert its views. Until the early 1990s, nursing's contribution in discussions aimed at solving the nation's health care problems was noticeably lacking, except for a few nurse leaders who served on boards of directors and national interdisciplinary health teams. Another problem already mentioned—that nursing's internal strife gave it an image of conflict—often prevented nursing from having any serious impact on health policy decisions.

CRITICALLY THINKING ABOUT . . .

Do ordinary nurses need to become politically active, or should they leave politics to nursing leaders? Discuss.

Why has nursing in 20th-century America been largely uninvolved in politics? Many of the factors discussed earlier have no doubt contributed—the predominance of women in nursing; poor self-image and occupational image; lack of confidence, interest, and assertiveness; and fear of confronting other health professionals. Unfortunately, for many years nursing allowed other health care disciplines to shape national and local health policies. However, as the focus in health care gradually changes from illness to wellness, nurses are moving to the forefront in shaping health policies for the future. Shaping such policies occurs through the use of political power, which allows people, organizations, and associations to make sure their concerns are addressed.

Nurses have several good bases for exercising their political power. First, they have numbers—very large numbers. Political decision-makers are impressed by large numbers of voters who can get them in office and keep them in office. Through the ANA and other professional organizations, nurses have organizational structures in place that contain all the elements necessary to yield influence. Finally, most nurses are informed, active, and dedicated people, but they should become better informed about proposed and existing legislation affecting health care issues. In 1978, Madeline Leininger stated that "the nurse of tomorrow must understand the nature of power and politics . . . [and] will need to know about political behavior, political processes, and their consequences" (Leininger, 1978, p. 3). Since that time, many nurses and nursing leaders have taken up that challenge. Nursing is more politically active today than it has ever been.

The ANA: Using Nursing's Political Power

Nursing is well represented at the national level by ANA nurse lobbyists in Washington DC. By active and intense lobbying efforts, several bills vital to nursing have been passed. For example, nurse practitioners who can convince members of Congress that they are well prepared to provide primary care in underserved areas can be eligible to receive third-party reimbursement directly. Changes in nurse practice acts throughout the country and continuation of the Nurse Training Act over several years have been the result of nursing's visibility and skillful use of political strategies.

The early 1990s was a time when nursing began to be a key player in the national health care agenda. In the end, nursing did not get what it wanted, but it learned a lot about politics and policy in the process. Virginia Trotter Betts, the ANA president at that time, gave an eloquent account of the active participation and leadership by the ANA in the health care reform debates from 1991 to 1994:

> In that debate the nursing profession achieved high visibility and recognition for the cogency of its policy positions and for its united voice through the leadership of the ANA . . . While healthcare reform failed to pass the 103rd Congress, nursing and nurses gained much in the process of their participation. (Betts, 1996, p. 1)

 CRITICALLY THINKING ABOUT . . .

What percentage of the annual ANA membership fee should go to political action? Why?

Identification of Problems in the Health Care System

By the end of the 1980s, it was clear to everyone that the American health care system was in a state of crisis, and that drastic measures of some kind must be taken. The ANA determined that it was well within the scope of its mission of improving the health care of the American public to play a leading role in health care reform. In June 1989, the ANA's board of directors formed a task force charged with identifying creative solutions to the health care crisis and developing the positions the ANA should take and the public policy agenda it should formulate.

The task force's first challenge was to get a clear picture of the nature and scope of the problem:

> That first step (assessment) . . . was (and is) critical to success in any public policy undertaking. Without a full and accurate diagnosis, governmental solutions have only a happenstance of 'curing' their ill-defined problems. (Betts, 1996, p. 2)

By studying documents developed by the ANA staff and consultants, the task force identified four broad problem areas:

1. *Access to health care.* Access was greatly limited because many Americans had insufficient financial coverage (35 million uninsured in 1991). Access also was a problem due to the geographically and socioeconomically uneven dispersion of services and providers.
2. *Escalating costs* (see Chap. 10). Health care costs had been rising at two to three times the consumer price index for more than 20 years. This was a cause for great concern among government, businesses, and citizens.
3. *Uneven, unpredictable, and often unproven health care quality.* Many countries that spent much less on health care surpassed the United States in indicators such as length and quality of life and simple health measures such as infant mortality and immunizations.
4. *An illness-model delivery system.* Fully 94% of every health care dollar was being spent on illness care in tertiary and secondary care settings. Only 6% was going toward services aimed at prevention and primary care. "This upside-down approach as a national delivery system overemphasized illness, acute and late interventions, cure and technology and devalued health, prevention and primary care" (Betts, 1996, p. 2). This upside-down system is depicted in Figure 11-1.

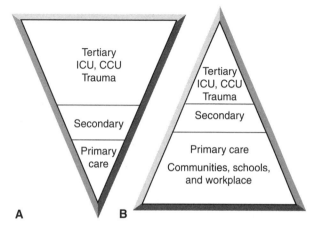

Figure 11-1. (A) What's wrong with the U.S. health care delivery system. **(B)** Suggested restructuring. (Reprinted with permission from *Nursing Administration Quarterly* Spring 1996:3–4. Copyright 1996, Aspen Publishers Inc.)

Tertiary
ICU, CCU
Trauma

Secondary

Primary care

Tertiary
ICU, CCU
Trauma

Secondary

Primary care

Communities, schools, and workplace

A   **B**

Moreover, the task force determined that the concerns of physicians, hospitals, third-party payers, pharmaceutical companies, and medical suppliers received considerably more attention in the system that did the needs of patients, families, and communities. Finally, the inclusion of alternative providers (such as advanced practice nurses [APNs]) and multiple care settings beyond the hospital were severely limited.

The conclusion was that the solution to the myriad problems within the American health care system in the early 1990s was to search for public policy solutions rather than solutions directed toward interpersonal actions, clinical approaches, or even the development of new facilities (Betts, 1996).

Nursing's Agenda for Health Care Reform

After 2 years of diligent effort, *Nursing's Agenda for Health Care Reform* was published in June 1991 (Box 11-2). This agenda was succinct (23 pages), was written in understandable language, and included helpful pictures. It was eventually endorsed by 76 nursing and health care organizations. It provided nursing's description of the health care crisis along with nursing's proposal for public policy resolution. One reason that the agenda had such broad appeal was that it focused simultaneously on access, quality, and cost. The goal that was set forth was a health care system that was health-oriented, equitable, and just, not simply one with a single-minded focus on cost-containment (Keepnews & Marullo, 1996).

Betts called the document a radical proposal because it called for an entirely new paradigm in U.S. health care. It called for a delivery system based on

> a community and health model, a patient-focused system of care, patient self-determination with informed consent, a balance of health and illness services, a value on care and caring, and an expanded health care work force with direct consumer accessibility to professional nurses. (Betts, 1996, p. 4)

In effect, implementation of *Nursing's Agenda for Health Care Reform* would have turned Figure 11-1*A* into Figure 11-1*B*.

Box 11-2
Nursing's Agenda for Health Care Reform

1. A federal standard of a uniform basic benefits package for
2. All U.S. citizens and residents
3. Financed through a public–private partnership
4. Delivering a continuum of services
5. In convenient, accessible sites by a
6. Variety of qualified providers whose activities would
7. Balance services for health and illness while
8. Improving quality of care, which would be measured and openly reported.

(Betts VT [1996]. Nursing's agenda for health care reform: Policy, politics, and power through professional leadership. *Nursing Administration Quarterly, 20*(3), 4.)

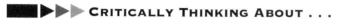 **CRITICALLY THINKING ABOUT . . .**

> Do you agree with Betts that *Nursing's Agenda for Health Care Re-form* was a radical proposal?

The ANA as a National Political Force

By the time the 1992 election cycle began, the ANA was in a strong position to be an influential player in the health care reform debates that would follow. The ANA had developed a highly credible political action committee (**ANA-PAC**). The purpose of ANA-PAC was to identify federal candidates who would support the agenda and the legislation necessary to implement it. Acceptable candidates received financial contributions from ANA-PAC and received assistance from nurses in their campaigns. Thus, a very effective political network was forged through one-on-one working relationships with members of Congress. "This network gave ANA and politically-oriented nurses access to members of Congress and was so effective that many members of Congress called their nurse coordinators for health policy advice" (Betts, 1996, p. 5). The network also was used to distribute *Nursing's Agenda for Health Care Reform* to all members of the 102nd Congress, and nurse members participated in more than 200 town meetings with members of Congress throughout 1991 and 1992.

At this point, it became very clear that fundamental health care reform could not be accomplished without the leadership of the president. Therefore, in March 1992, ANA-PAC started the presidential endorsement process. They asked the three major presidential candidates (Bill Clinton, George Bush, and Ross Perot) many health care questions and sent them copies of *Nursing's Agenda for Health Care Reform*. The ANA president, Virginia Trotter Betts, attended both the Democratic and Republican conventions. On August 15, ANA-PAC announced its endorsement of Bill Clinton at a huge outdoor rally in Pittsburgh, California, thus becoming the first health professional organization to endorse what would become the winning ticket.

The active political involvement of the ANA and nurses all across the country yielded dividends. Of the 260 congressional candidates endorsed by the ANA, 76% were elected.

In August 1993, the **1993 Nursing Summit** was held. Betts has referred to that meeting as a "benchmark in professional maturity and pragmatism. Leaders of 63 major nursing organizations demonstrated a recommitment to unity, leadership, colleagueship, and followership and a willingness to speak with one strong voice of activism to make health reform a reality" (Betts, 1996, p. 6). The task of the summit was to reach a consensus regarding nursing's fundamental issues related to health care reform:

1. Universal benefits
2. Removal of barriers to nursing care
3. A nursing workforce transition plan to provide money and opportunities for hospital nurses requiring retraining and re-employment in the restructured health care system
4. A graduate nursing education fund
5. Inclusion of nurses on federal, state, and local policy boards (Betts, 1996, p. 6).

Items 2, 4, and 5 would have had a particularly significant impact on the professionalization of nursing and are discussed in more detail in the following section. Through much hard work by the ANA and many nurses, nursing's fundamental issues made it into the president's plan for health care reform.

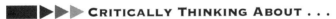 **CRITICALLY THINKING ABOUT . . .**

Should nurses "block-vote" in matters of health care? Why or why not?

Unfortunately, when the president's proposal, the Health Security Act (HSA) of 1993, went to Congress, it failed to pass, as did any of its amended versions. "Debate of the HSA was ended in September 1994, and gone was this nation's best change to ensure health care to all its citizens" (Betts, 1996, p. 7). However, due to the tremendous growth in nursing's political sophistication that came out of that struggle, nursing, power, and politics will never be the same. Many of the nursing-specific promises contained in the HSA continued to have strong bipartisan support in the next congressional session. Lobbying and grassroots efforts served to educate the administration, Congress, key opinion leaders, and the public about the value of nurses and nursing. Nurses gained unprecedented visibility in the press. Media coverage of nursing increased by 300% from 1992 to 1993, and 95% of that coverage was positive. ANA leaders became regarded as sources of expert opinion on health care and health care policy issues. Finally, the public came to know that nurses stand with them as their advocates for high-quality, accessible, and affordable health care (Betts, 1996).

Advanced Practice Nursing: A Critical Arena for Political Action

As noted in several earlier chapters, the increasing number of APNs helps nursing make strides toward full professional status in many ways. However, to realize their full potential, APNs must work toward reducing the barriers to their practice. Some of these barriers are internal, such as whether to merge the clinical nurse specialist and nurse practitioner role and the current inconsistency of educational requirements. However, other barriers are external and are, therefore, subject to change through diligent and astute use of power in the political environment. External barriers to expanding the role of APNs in the emerging health care system that require attention include the multiple legal and regulatory inconsistencies that exist between the various APN roles and even within the same role, depending on the state where an APN practices, as well as the related issue of licensing requirements (also highly variable). There is also state-to-state variation in who actually regulates the practice of APNs—the board of nursing, the board of medicine, the board of pharmacy, the board of medical examiners, or some combination. The lack of resolutions mandating hospital admitting privileges is an additional impediment to the full use of APNs in emerging health care models (O'Malley, Cummings, & King, 1996).

APNs (and other nurses as well) must raise their level of political participation. Political participation is considered electoral when it focuses on activities such as campaigning and voting and nonelectoral when it involves activities such as letter writing, personally contacting officials on important issues, and working to solve community problems. It is also important to understand the legislative process. One must know how to reach legislators, how to write to them, and how to visit them. State nursing associations typically have materials that can be very helpful in learning these important political practices. Giving public testimony in legislative hearings is an excellent way to gain visibility and be proactive in the legislative and regulatory processes (O'Malley, Cummings, & King, 1996).

 **CRITICALLY THINKING ABOUT . . .**

> In matters related to health care, would you: (1) write letters to po-
> litical leaders? (2) personally contact public officials? (3) contribute
> to political action bodies? (4) run for office? (5) seek appointment
> to a health care board? Explain.

In short, if APNs are to have a say in shaping the practice environment in which their knowledge, skills, and talents can be put to the best use, they must take an active part in the political process. They must be visible, and they must give clear messages to stakeholders in the emerging health care systems about the importance of APNs. APNs must know the opposition and have at hand information that will support their position. Because many people—including decision-makers—are unclear about APNs' roles, one should be prepared to provide basic definitions. APNs must lobby legislators to eliminate statutory requirements for required physician supervision and mandated practice agreements.

To achieve the full practice authority for which they are prepared, APNs also must communicate with the state board and state and federal legislators to reduce barriers that limit the use of APNs. For instance, APNs should support the granting of admitting privileges and prescriptive authority. APNs need to work with third-party payers, both public and private, to ensure that covered services can be provided by APNs. It is also important for APNs to work with government agencies to facilitate direct reimbursement by third-party payers of all kinds. Finally, APNs must lobby for additional funding for graduate nursing education for advanced nursing practice in all specialty areas.

This is a large order indeed, but a lot is at stake for APNs in the next two decades. They would do well to focus immediately on the political realities that are bound to shape their futures.

Nursing Power, Politics, and the Media

Nurses, for many years, have observed the power plays that the medical profession engages in to increase its power and resources. The medical profession continues relentlessly to validate its public image by acquainting the public with new techniques, new equipment, and research efforts that will improve the nation's health and keep physicians in great demand. For example, the press regularly and eagerly reports on findings published in *The New England Journal of Medicine* and the *Journal of the American Medical Association*. Rarely does one see or hear a quote from the *American Journal of Nursing, Image*, or *Nursing Research*. Consequently, through the media, the public continues to believe that the medical profession safeguards their most precious commodity—health.

Earlier in this section, we noted Virginia Trotter Betts's observation that one great benefit derived from the ANA's vigorous participation in the health care reform debates and related political action was significantly increased media coverage of nurses and nursing. Through this media coverage, people came to understand that nurses really are the public's best advocates for good health care. It was demonstrated time and time again that nurses were the least self-serving of all the parties who had a stake in the legislative decision making. However, use of the media during the 1993–94 debates on health care reform also had a definite downside from the perspective of nurses. It is generally agreed that one of the most significant factors contributing to the downfall of President Clinton's proposed health care reform measures was the series of "Harry and Louise" advertisements sponsored by the health insurance industry. Harry and Louise were, ostensibly, a sincere middle-class American couple struggling to understand the nature of the proposed health care changes and the implications those changes would have for them, their family, and their community. In the final analysis, all the implications turned out to be bad, and the whole ad campaign had the effect of creating a climate of fear and distrust about legislating health care (Leavitt, Betts, & Peterson, 1997).

More recently, nursing has been using the media as a powerful political tool in its attempt to curtail the potential for disastrous cuts in nursing personnel in the wake of the hospital mergers and restructuring that have occurred since 1995. The ANA launched the multimedia public awareness campaign, "Every patient deserves a nurse" to raise awareness of the need for adequate numbers of RNs to provide safe patient care. The goal of the campaign was to support legislative and regulatory measures to ensure patient safety while at the same time providing job security for RNs. Using the media is a powerful way for nurses to communicate their messages to influence the public at large and in turn legislators (Leavitt, Betts, & Peterson, 1997).

▶▶▶ CRITICALLY THINKING ABOUT . . .

What type of promotional spot would you make to encourage the public to have a more positive image of nursing? Describe it, and explain your rationale.

Nurses "Doing Politics"

Nurses are becoming more politically active as they become increasingly aware of how the political process at all levels affects their lives and their practice. Effective use of the political process is key in the efforts to enhance the professional status of nursing. Nurses can be politically effective at different levels. Leavitt, Betts, and Peterson (1997) have identified these as nurse citizens, nurse activists, and nurse politicians.

Nurse citizens vote regularly, participate in public forums that are relevant to health and human services, and are active in community activities. They bring their perspectives of health care to all these activities, and act in such a manner as to serve as health care advocates for their fellow citizens. Nurse citizens stay informed about health care issues and speak out when services or conditions are not contributing to a healthy environment. They know who their local, state, and federal elected officials are, and they join nursing organizations that are politically active. When community organizations need health experts, nurse citizens volunteer to serve.

Nurse citizens also know how to bring influence to bear by communicating with policy makers from their home districts. Decision-makers generally welcome the input of concerned nurses on matters related to health care. Effective communication is a key to influencing the political process. Some advice for writing to legislators has been provided by Leavitt, Betts, and Peterson (1997):

1. Use your own stationery rather than your employer's or generic stationery.
2. Tell them you are both a voter and an RN.
3. In a concise and positive manner, tell them where you stand on the issue and why.
4. State clearly what action you want the policy maker to take.
5. Be persistent. Follow up with calls, letters, or personal visits.

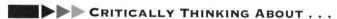 CRITICALLY THINKING ABOUT . . .

> Compose a letter to the president about a health care concern of yours. Explain how you have used each of these five tips.

Nurse activists, as the name would suggest, take a more active role in the political process than do nurse citizens. Nurse activists work directly to effect changes in practices and legislation. Among the ways nurse activists work to make changes are many of the same activities of nurse citizens. They also may register people to vote, contribute money to a political campaign, and work in campaigns of potentially "nursing-friendly" officials. Nurse activists also may write letters to the local newspaper, hold a media event to publicize an issue, or provide testimony in board meetings or legislative hearings (Leavitt, Betts, & Peterson, 1997).

Nurse politicians become intrigued with the political process and the things that can be achieved in nursing through the power of political action. The nurse politician is no longer satisfied simply to influence legislation that supports the goals of nursing; he or she wants to develop the legislation.

> Nurse politicians use their knowledge about people, their expertise about health, their ability to communicate effectively, and their superb organizational skills in running for office. Because the public places a high value on nurses, nurse politicians are trusted. If nurses know how to run a campaign and can raise money, they stand a good chance of being elected. (Leavitt, Betts, & Peterson, 1997, p. 458)

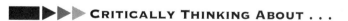 CRITICALLY THINKING ABOUT . . .

> Bernadine Healy, a physician, was the secretary of the Department of Health and Human Services. Can you foresee a day when a nurse will hold a similar position?

Policy to Further Professionalization

Policy is "a purposive course of action followed by an actor or set of actors in dealing with a problem or matter of concern" (Anderson J, as cited in Helms, Anderson, & Hanson, 1996). Policy governs action that is directed toward a given end. Policies may take the form of laws, regulations, or guidelines that govern behavior in various settings. Policy often is considered the product resulting from the application of politics, which is the process.

Nursing practice is affected significantly by policy. One's ability to provide care is affected by innumerable public policy decisions. The definition of the legal scope of nursing practice is, of course, one of the most important of these policies.

Policies change over time as the needs of society change. Thus, nursing must keep a close eye on many aspects of health care policy. Nursing must also be an active participant in the formation of health care policy through vigilant political action.

David Keepnews and Geri Marullo, both with the ANA, have observed that the health policy environment facing nursing in the last half of the 1990s is dramatically different from that in the early 1990s. In fact, they say, it is "virtually unrecognizable" (Keepnews & Marullo, 1996, p. 19). Earlier, nursing had taken the "high ground" with *Nursing's Agenda for Health Care Reform* and was working closely with the new political leadership in Washington who had promised sweeping health care reforms. Those reforms included some of nursing's most cherished goals:

- ▶ A system based on universal access
- ▶ Equity
- ▶ Primary care
- ▶ Prevention and wellness
- ▶ Recognition and fuller use of nursing's role both in health care delivery and in shaping a dynamic new health care system (Keepnews & Marullo, 1996).

◼◼◼▶▶▶ **CRITICALLY THINKING ABOUT . . .**

What are the crucial elements of any federal health care program?

The defeat of the comprehensive health care plan and a very different political environment in Washington and many state capitals have resulted in a very different health care industry. Rather than taking the proactive stance that was characteristic of nursing leadership in the early 1990s, nursing now must expend a great deal of energy on simply defending past gains and protecting patient safety and nursing practice. The political environment is increasingly hostile toward government regulation, preferring market-based approaches in which all eyes stay firmly fixed on the bottom line (Keepnews & Marullo, 1996).

The failure to pass the proposed health care reform legislation also dealt a powerful blow to one of the best opportunities nursing has ever had in its progress toward full professional status. Had the reforms been passed, they would have included four significant nursing-supportive measures, three of which had direct ramifications for enhancing the professionalism of nursing:

1. There was language in the federal bill to override the restrictions on nursing's scope of practice contained in the licensure laws of many states.
2. The Social Security Act was to have been amended to permit direct reimbursement under Medicare and Medicaid for all nurse practitioners and clinical nurse specialists, regardless of where they practice.
3. It would have been possible to obtain funding for graduate nursing education (Hadley, 1996).

These goals remain important targets in nursing's policy agenda. However, as Keepnews and Marullo noted, times are different, and nursing's policy goals must be ordered accordingly. Health care safety and quality must remain the highest priority. Many nurses are concerned that patient safety is being severely compromised in the single-minded drive to cut costs. Nursing is appropriately most concerned about the health care industry's efforts to reduce the use of RNs, replacing them with lower-paid nonskilled staff (discussed earlier in this book). There is indeed reason for concern:

> Until recently, the assumption that hospitals and health facilities would, with rare exception, staff at safe levels and would prioritize patient care needs may have appeared to be a safe one. In an era when a restructuring health care system stresses cost and revenue as its central priorities, the assumption no longer appears so safe. (Keepnews & Marullo, 1996, p. 24)

Strategies that nursing can use to address issues related to patient care safety and quality are reflected in many of the broad initiatives the ANA has taken up. One of these initiatives is the development and testing of the nursing "report card" for acute care discussed in the previous chapter. Using specific, proven indicators of the quality of nursing care (eg, skin integrity, patient satisfaction, nosocomial infections, and patient injury rates), the level of care provided by acute care hospitals can be evaluated. Moreover, strategies must be developed and set in place to ensure that these data are kept current and are easily available to potential patients, their families, and all members of the health care community.

Nursing also can merge its quality measurement efforts with those of other groups who are also interested in measuring and ensuring quality of care. These include organizations such as the National Coalition for Quality Assurance, the Foundations for Accountability, the federal government's Health Care Financing Administration, and the California Public Employees Retirement Board (Keepnews & Marullo, 1996).

The second primary policy matter that must receive nursing's unflagging attention is breaking down the many barriers to nursing practice and payment for nursing services to maximize the use of nurses in the emerging managed care environment. At the federal level, nursing must continue to push for Medicare and Medicaid payment for all APNs, regardless of where they practice or what their specialty is. Developing policy that ensures the inclusion of APNs on care provider panels is especially important. This will not be easy; in general, nursing faces strong opposition from the medical community in this regard. In the 1995 House of Delegates meeting of the American Medical Association, the delegates supported giving more assistance to state medical associations to oppose the removal of barriers to nursing practice (Keepnews & Marullo, 1996). Continued professional unity, such as that so well demonstrated in the 1993–1994 health care reform debates, must remain a high priority if nursing is to attain these critical policy goals.

▶CHAPTER SUMMARY

Nursing's power base and potential for increased power are substantial. It must continue to grow to advance the goal of professionalism. But to date the ability of nurse leaders, national professional nursing associations, and the collectivity of nursing to achieve unity and consensus on issues involving education, autonomous practice, and monopoly over practice is not as we would have it.

Sen. Daniel Inouye of Hawaii, in writing the Foreword to *Politics of Nursing*, raised four pertinent questions that nurses should consider. These questions were posed in the early 1980s but remain salient almost two decades later:

1. Why haven't enough professional nurses been promoted to nonclinical leadership positions—for example, in the area of developing health policy on both the state and federal levels?
2. Why hasn't the nursing profession used its potential political power?
3. Do our nation's nurses really want to be true professionals? In other words, are they willing to accept and, if necessary, to demand both the responsibility and prerogatives of power and authority?
4. Is there any serious institutional support for the development of a true cadre of professional nurses? (Inouye, 1982).

Individually, nurses can evaluate themselves in light of these four questions. Their answers would undoubtedly enlighten those interested in the professionalization process. Nurses must convert into action their beliefs about what nursing is and what, ideally, it must become to mobilize and empower nurses to reach their full potential in this evolving, powerful profession.

Nurses must decide what they should focus on to leverage their effectiveness even further. We must use both power and political strategies to our advantage to continue to effect change. We must overcome ignorance and political inertia to maximize our work in the health care environment. Being proactive rather than reactive is the only alternative if we are to expect success.

> Nursing leaders have the obligation and responsibility to guide the less experienced through the maze of political realities, give them a fundamental appreciation of politics, and assist them to learn to use political behaviors astutely and to their advantage. (O'Malley, Cummings, & King, 1996, p. 67)

Nursing has come a very long way in terms of developing and exercising its political awareness, its political savvy, and its political power in the last third of the 20th century. Nursing has learned how to be a key player in the health care policy arena. What we have learned can be used fully in the continuing drive toward full professional status. Nursing must keep up the momentum.

KEY POINTS

▶ 1 It is very important for nursing to enhance its power to move toward the status of a fully recognized profession. Power is the ability of a person or organization to influence and change the behavior of others, even if they do not desire the change. There are different sources of power, and people have different power orientations (how power is perceived or used). The combination of power source and power orientation allows one to predict how a power-holder will function.

▶ 2 Powerlessness in nursing has traditionally come from sources that are both internal and external. Internal sources include role confusion, lack of professional confidence, timidity, fear, insecurity, or a sense of inferiority. External sources of powerlessness have included the historical role of the nurse as handmaiden, the hierarchical structure of health care organizations, the authority and directives of physicians, hospital directives, and the threat of legal or disciplinary action.

▶ 3 Two primary strategies that nurses can use to increase their power, both individually and collectively, are maintaining unity among all nurses and using networking to form active coalitions. The potential for power in nursing—due to the large numbers of nurses—is considerable and should make nurses willing to unite to exercise it to the fullest extent. Networking provides many benefits to all members of the network, such as encouragement, support, and nurturing to the younger members of the network that enable them to move up into positions of leadership. Networks operate on the understanding of providing mutual support and avoiding destructive competition and infighting.

▶ 4 The ANA became a major player in the debates on health care reform in the early 1990s. It did so by acting in a carefully thought-out, proactive manner. It first identified the major problems in the current American health care system, then identified its own vision of what the health care system should be. This was described in *Nursing's Agenda for Health Care Reform*. By the use of its political action committee, the ANA established a network of "nurse- and health-friendly" potential legislators and helped them get elected. The ANA achieved a high degree of national nursing unity through the 1993 Nursing Summit. Although the goal of these actions—the passage of health care reform legislation—failed, nursing learned much about how to amass and use power and the political process.

▶ 5 Nurses can play many roles effectively as part of enhancing nursing's political power. Nurse citizens register to vote and vote regularly, participate in public forums relevant to health and human services, and engage in community activities, bringing to all of these their perspectives on health care. Nurse activists work directly to effect changes in practice and legislation by registering people to vote, contributing money to political campaigns, working in campaigns for nurse-friendly politicians, and even providing testimony in legislative hearings. Nurse politicians run for office, seek appointments to regulatory agencies and boards, and work in developing legislation that supports quality health care.

▶ 6 Major policy issues that face nursing into the 21st century include protection and improvement of health care safety and quality. This includes measures to ensure that the health care industry does not drastically cut RN staff and replace them with lower-paid nonskilled staff to the point where patient safety is compromised. A second major policy focus must be to break down the many barriers to nursing practice and payment for nursing services to maximize the use of nurses in the emerging managed care environment.

REFERENCES

Archer S, Goehner P (1982). *Nurses: A Political Force.* North Scituate, MA: Wadsworth Health Sciences Division.

Ashley J (1976). *Hospitals, Paternalism, and the Role of the Nurse.* New York: Teacher's College, Columbia University Press.

Benner P (1984). *From Novice to Expert: Excellence and Power in Clinical Nursing Practice.* Menlo Park, CA: Addison-Wesley.

Betts VT (1996). Nursing's agenda for health care reform: Policy, politics, and power through professional leadership. *Nursing Administration Quarterly, 20*(3), 1–8.

Blanchfield KC, Biordi DL (1996). Power in practice: A study of nursing authority and autonomy. *Nursing Administration Quarterly, 20*(3), 42–49.

Bowman, R. and Culpepper, R. (1974). Power: Rx for change. *American Journal of Nursing, 74*(6), 1056.

Catalano JT (1996). *Contemporary Professional Nursing.* Philadelphia: FA Davis.

Chitty KK (1997). *Professional nursing: concepts and challenges* (2nd ed.). Philadelphia: W.B. Saunders Company.

Ferguson VD (1993). Perspectives on power. In Mason DJ (Ed.), *Power, Politics and Policy in Nursing.* New York: Springer, pp. 118–128.

Hadley EH (1996). Nursing in the political and economic marketplace: Challenges for the 21st century. *Nursing Outlook, 44*(1), 6–10.

Hall-Long B (1995). Nursing education at the crossroads: Political passages. *J Professional Nursing, 11,* 139–146.

Helmlinger C (1997, July–August). First lady praises ANA for work on patients' behalf. *The American Nurse, 1,* 13.

Helms LB, Anderson MA, Hanson K (1996). "Doin' politics": Linking policy and politics in nursing. *Nursing Administration Quarterly, 20*(3), 32–41.

Inouye D. Foreword in B. Kalisch and P. Kalisch, *Politics of nursing.* Philadelphia: J.B. Lippincott.

Kalisch B, Kalisch P (1982). *Politics of Nursing.* Philadelphia: JB Lippincott.

Keepnews D, Marullo G (1996). Policy imperatives for nursing in an era of health care restructuring. *Nursing Administration Quarterly, 20*(3), 19–31.

Kelly LY, Joel LA (1996). *The Nursing Experience: Trends, Challenges, and Transitions* (3rd ed.). New York: McGraw-Hill.

Leavitt JK, Betts VT, Peterson C (1997). Nurses and political action. In Chitty KK (Ed.), *Professional Nursing: Concepts and Challenges* (2nd ed.). Philadelphia: WB Saunders.

Leininger M (1978). Political nursing: Essential for health service and education systems of tomorrow. *Nursing Administration Quarterly, 2*(2), 2–3.

Macionis JJ (1997). *Sociology* (6th ed.). Upper Saddle River, NJ: Prentice-Hall.

Moore K (1997). Leadership in nursing. In Oermann MH (Ed.), *Professional Nursing Practice.* Stamford, CT: Appleton & Lange, pp. 255–272.

O'Malley J, Cummings S, King CS (1996). The politics of advanced practice. *Nursing Administration Quarterly, 20*(3), 62–72.

Pike AW (1997). Entering collegial relationships: The demise of nurse as victim. In McCloskey JC, Grace HK (Eds.), *Current Issues in Nursing* (5th ed.). pp. 532–536. St. Louis: Mosby.

Powell J (1976). Nursing and politics: The struggle outside nursing's body politic. *Nursing Forum, 15,* 341–362.

Puetz BE (1991). Networking: Making it work for you. *Healthcare Trends Trans, 3,* 20–28.

Sweeney S (1990). Traditions, transitions, and transformation of power in nursing. In McCloskey JC, Grace HK (Eds.), *Current Issues in Nursing* (3rd ed.). St. Louis: Mosby, pp. 460–464.

Weber M (1947). *Theory of Social and Political Organization.* Translated by Henderson AM, Parsons T. New York: Oxford University Press.

RECOMMENDED READINGS

Hagedorn S (1995). The politics of caring: The role of activism in primary care. *Advances in Nursing Science, 17*(4), 1–11.

Rafael AR (1996). Politics and caring: A dialectic in nursing. *Advances in Nursing Science, 19,* 3–17.

White KR, Begun JW (1996). Profession building in the new health care system. *Nursing Administration Quarterly, 20*(3), 79–85.

12

Nursing, Ethics, and the Law

CHAPTER OUTLINE

Ethics and Codes of Ethics
Biotechnology and Nursing Ethics
Research Ethics and Human Subjects
The Law and Nursing
    Professionalization

Chapter Summary
Key Points
References
Recommended Readings

LEARNING OBJECTIVES

▶ **1** Explain the nature of ethics and describe the five general social values on which most Western codes of ethics are built.

▶ **2** Describe how ethical conflicts can arise, especially for health care workers.

▶ **3** Identify the 10 steps in a general model for bioethical decision making.

▶ **4** Describe the impact of acquired immunodeficiency syndrome (AIDS) and why it has ethical implications.

▶ **5** Explain why it is important to have codes of ethics specifically related to the rights of human subjects in research studies and why it is important for nurses to understand the processes involved in protecting the rights of human subjects in nursing and medical research.

▶ **6** Differentiate the types of law and explain how nurses are involved in the legal system.

▶ **7** Explain how law, codes of ethics, and professionalization are related.

KEY TERMS

accountability

advocacy

anonymity

autonomy

Belmont report

beneficence

bioethics

civil law

code of ethics

common law

confidentiality

criminal law

Declaration of Helsinki

diminished autonomy

ethics

euthanasia

everyday ethics

fidelity

informed consent

justice

laws

negligence

Nuremberg Code

practice acts

statutory law

stigma

technical ethics

tort law

Tuskeegee study

veracity

One of the primary defining characteristics of a profession is that it has a code of ethics to which all practitioners must closely adhere in their practice. Violations of the code of ethics carry severe sanctions from both the profession and society at large. Professionals bear significant ethical responsibilities in their delivery of services to the public. To behave in a manner that is inconsistent with the ethics of one's profession violates the professional covenant between the profession and those it has vowed to serve. Although nursing does not have all the characteristics of a fully recognized profession, nurses have long had a strong commitment to maintaining ethical practice at the highest level to ensure the health and well-being of those entrusted to our care.

Nursing practice also is regulated by law. The law grants nursing licensure, thereby permitting a nurse to practice within the scope of activities defined by the state to ensure the safety of its citizens.

This chapter discusses ethics and ethical decision making and how they play out in nursing practice. The relation between the societal and personal impact of biotechnology and nursing ethics is also addressed, as are ethical practices involving subjects in nursing or medical research. Finally, the relation between the law and the continuing process of professionalization is addressed.

Ethics and Codes of Ethics

Throughout the last 50 years, health care technology has progressed greatly. Today there are many more options than ever before for the diagnosis and treatment of health problems. In addition to technological change, there has been a shift in the moral evaluation of these options. According to Janet E. Smith, a professor of moral philosophy at the University of Dallas, technological advancement combined with a change in society's moral climate has led some health care practitioners to be "involved in practices that some decades ago would have been unthinkable" (Smith, 1997, p. 182). She cites as examples Dr. Kevorkian's "death machine"; the birth of a baby to a 61-year-old women, the baby having been conceived in a Petri dish with the ovum of another woman; the creation of embryos solely for experimental purposes; the use of vital organs taken from living anencephalic infants; and the millions of abortions each year. To this list must be added the potential for cloning humans.

Only a few decades ago, all these procedures would have shocked and angered most people. There was a consensus within society at that time that these procedures were wrong or immoral. Some people would say that such activities violate the laws of God or nature. Others would say that the procedures violate the dignity of the person, and some would question the motivations of the practitioners. Some would see the practitioners as evil persons working their will on a naïve society or as amoral fiends grasping for financial gain at the expense of moral virtue. Today, however, rather than being seen as bad or immoral *per se*, these practices, and others like them, have become the focus of ethical analysis within the health care community and within society at large. A principal goal of such analysis is to help society determine what is fundamentally right and fundamentally wrong in today's high-tech, culturally diverse society.

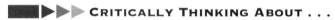 **CRITICALLY THINKING ABOUT . . .**

> Consider the issues of euthanasia, assisted suicide, abortion, gene splicing, organ transplantation, and acquired immunodeficiency syndrome (AIDS). Do you find them to be moral or immoral?

A Matter of Ethics

People are continually confronted with situations that they evaluate as good or bad, right or wrong. People make moral judgments all the time, about work, home, and family, as well as about local and world political and economic events. This tells us that for most things in life, there is a moral dimension, and this moral dimension is the realm of ethics. **Ethics** means "a declaration of what is right or wrong, and of what ought to be" (Catalano, 1996, p. 92). In effect, ethics can be considered as a system of morals used by people to evaluate their experiences and plan their courses of action.

Ethics may exist on several levels. People may construct their own moral code based on their religious beliefs or philosophical orientations, their socialization to society's values, and their daily experiences. Ethics also may exist on the community or society level, where the group's shared experiences help clarify what most members think should be done in a variety of situations.

Organizations and professions also develop ethics that help them make decisions about courses of action in their practice or operation. Often the moral values of a profession are enshrined in a **code of ethics**, such as that of the American Nurses Association (ANA) (Box 12-1). The code of ethics provides a framework for professional practice and, if done well, contributes to the day-to-day decision making that professionals face (Catalano, 1996). Codes of ethics cannot be taken lightly; they are the final arbiters of what is considered professional or nonprofessional behavior (see Chap. 1). Codes of ethics reflect a great deal of time and effort spent by the profession in reaching an agreement as to what is and what is not good professional behavior. They represent the fundamental consensus about standards of practice. People who violate a profession's code of ethics face strong sanctions by the profession's governing body or even expulsion from the profession.

Box 12-1
Code for Nurses

1. The nurse provides services with respect for human dignity and the uniqueness of the client, unrestricted by considerations of social or economic status, personal attributes, or the nature of health problems.
2. The nurse safeguards the client's right to privacy by judiciously protecting information of a confidential nature.
3. The nurse acts to safeguard the client and the public when health care and safety are affected by the incompetent, unethical, or illegal practice of any person.
4. The nurse assumes responsibility and accountability for individual nursing judgments and actions.
5. The nurse maintains competence in nursing.
6. The nurse exercises informed judgment and uses individual competence and qualifications as criteria in seeking consultation, accepting responsibility, and delegating nursing activities to others.
7. The nurse participates in activities that contribute to the ongoing development of the profession's body of knowledge.
8. The nurse participates in the profession's efforts to implement and improve standards of nursing.
9. The nurse participates in the profession's efforts to establish and maintain conditions of employment conducive to high-quality nursing care.
10. The nurse participates in the profession's efforts to protect the public from misinformation and misrepresentation and to maintain the integrity of nursing.
11. The nurse collaborates with members of the health professions and other citizens in promoting community and national efforts to meet the health needs of the public.

(American Nurses Association [1985]. *Code for Nurses with Interpretive Statements.* Kansas City, MO: Author.)

It is hard to change professional codes once they are in place because underlying the codes is a political process that attempts to resolve conflicting points of view among the members on a wide variety of issues. In effect, the professional code is a "moral balance point" that reflects the consensus of the day. However, as new situations arise, the profession may need to rethink its stance about what is right and wrong for existing situations and bring into the code moral judgments about the new situations. For example, health care professionals currently are grappling with the morality of euthanasia and assisted suicide. Nathan I. Cherny (1996) has argued that euthanasia and assisted suicide fall outside the boundaries of the Hippocratic code when other options are available to relieve suffering. He argues that health care professionals must develop ethics about right and wrong in these situations based on medical, psychological, social, and financial variables that describe the totality of the patient's situation.

The issue of **euthanasia** has received much attention from health professionals. The Supreme Court of the Netherlands recently listed the following conditions as ones that would absolve a health professional from criminal prosecution in cases of euthanasia:

1. Unbearable suffering on the part of the patient
2. Verbal or written request on the part of the patient for euthanasia
3. Lack of therapeutic alternatives
4. Consultation with more than one other doctor
5. A doctor's diary describing the course of the disease and the decisions made along the way (Hessing, Blad & Pieterman, 1996).

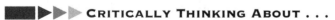 **CRITICALLY THINKING ABOUT . . .**

Should these criteria be adopted in the United States?

American health care ethics are not yet to a point where the Dutch solution would be a consensus position. In fact, in American society there are several large religious groups, including the Roman Catholic church, who are unalterably opposed to any attempt to establish euthanasia as an acceptable health care activity. The Catholic position is that human life is a "seamless cloth" not to be terminated willfully. Any attempt to rend that cloth by abortion, euthanasia, or assisted suicide violates the church's ethical standards. Although the church accepts the position that no extraordinary attempts need to be made to save life (eg, multiple resuscitations), it takes a firm line against activities purposely aimed at ending life. Without the agreement of Catholics and the fundamentalist religious groups that share this position, it is not likely that the Dutch model could be included today in American health care ethics.

Values and Codes of Ethics

Codes of ethics in general, and in nursing in particular, share the social values of justice, autonomy, fidelity, accountability, beneficence, veracity, and advocacy.

Justice is the professional obligation to be fair to all people. All people have the right to be treated equally, no matter what their age, sex, social class, or religious beliefs. This value is reflected in the nursing code of ethics: "The nurse provides services with respect for human dignity and the uniqueness of the client unrestricted by considerations of social or economic status, personal attributes, or the nature of health problems" (ANA, 1976).

Autonomy is the right to independence and personal freedom, which leads to the primacy of self-determination. In the health care setting, this means that it is the patient, not the doctor, nurse, or the patient's family, who has the sole right to make health care decisions affecting the patient. The health care professional may disagree with the patient's decision, but this does not matter: persons are sovereign in their own affairs. They may or may not rely on the advice of others, and they have the final say.

Fidelity is a person's obligation to keep the commitments he or she has made. It means keeping one's word without exception. Therefore, if one subscribes to a professional code of ethics, fidelity is behaving consistent with the code. This fidelity might be reflected in a nurse's close adherence to a basic component of the *International Council of Nurses' Code for Nurses* (International Council of Nurses, 1973). This code states that the fundamental responsibilities of the nurse are to promote health, to prevent illness, to restore health, and to alleviate suffering.

Accountability, closely related to fidelity, means that one is ultimately responsible for one's acts and is liable to be judged on them by others. Fidelity and accountability have become the ultimate standards by which a professional's actions are judged in uncertain or unclear situations.

Beneficence means doing only things that are good. Beneficence also requires the prevention of harm or evil, the removal of harm or evil, and the promotion of doing good by oneself and others (Frankena, 1988; Hadjistavropoulos, 1996). Sometimes in the health care setting beneficence comes into conflict with autonomy. Health professionals prescribe and carry out procedures that they are convinced are good for the patient, but the patient may want no part of them. For instance, a cancer patient may decide, after completing 10 of 14 prescribed chemotherapy treatments, that "enough is enough" and may decline further treatment.

Veracity is truthfulness. This value requires the health care provider to tell the truth to every patient and to make sure that the patient fully understands the message. Some argue that there a limit to veracity, such as when the truth would harm the patient's prognosis for recovery. Others disagree, arguing that such a view is simply the old paternalistic view that "doctor knows best." Because people are autonomous, they have the right to full information about their situation.

Advocacy gets to the heart of today's nursing practice. Advocacy has been defined as active assistance by the nurse to aid patients in their self-determination concerning health care alternatives. It involves three steps:

1. Helping patients understand what they want in a given situation
2. Helping patients discern and clarify their values in the context of the current situation
3. Helping patients examine options in light of those values.

In actuality, these steps do not play out in a simple 1-2-3 order. There is much revisiting and reconsideration of each step because these decisions are usually so difficult. It is hard for a nurse to engage in advocacy when patients have short hospital stays and when there is a changing complement of nurses and a predetermined course of treatment.

Types of Ethics

People who study ethics often distinguish between "everyday ethics" and "technical ethics." **Everyday ethics** involve our more intuitive, spontaneous reactions to events (Seedhouse, 1988). Everyday ethics are based on a simple set of principles; these principles may or may not be internally consistent with each other, but they provide a framework for a response to life. Examples of everyday ethics codes are, "Sex before marriage is wrong," "It is wrong to be underhanded and deceitful to others," "People should look out for number one," "Adultery is acceptable so long as the adulterers are happy and no one is hurt," or "You shouldn't break your back for low wages."

 CRITICALLY THINKING ABOUT . . .

List your four most important everyday ethics. Do you think your fellow students would agree with them?

Technical ethics attempt to overcome the inconsistencies often found in our everyday ethics. They do so by developing a set of ethical beliefs that speak to the highest state of morality possible and that are maximally consistent with each other. Technical ethics usually are the domain of moral philosophers. Although there are analysis problems with contemporary ethical systems, these problems are identifiable and, presumably, fixable.

When professions develop their own codes of ethics, they are faced with the task of marrying everyday ethics to technical ethics. Professions must identify the commonly held everyday ethics of their members as based on their experience in practice. These ethical beliefs must then be woven together into a consistent and maximally moral set of statements that are general enough to state the goals of the profession and specific enough to assist the practitioner in daily decision making on the job. A profession's technical ethics must be both understandable and useful to the everyday practitioner as well as to the profession's moral philosophers.

Ethics in Conflict

In small-scale, nonindustrial, traditional societies, almost all members of society share the same moral code and the same system of ethics. However, in large-scale, nontraditional, industrial societies, that is not the case. A defining trait of industrial societies is social diversity (see Chap. 13). Although members of such societies share certain core values such as freedom, individualism, and social mobility, there are still major differences in values among major social groups. Such differences arise out of the original cultures of the groups, their experience of the society in which they live, and the highly specialized and limited part of the world they confront on a daily basis. Making things even more difficult in large-scale societies is the fact that the society is at the cutting edge; new technologies appear, develop, and demand application. Members of society must either apply their existing code of ethics to these new technologies or develop new ethical standards.

Ethics and Health Care Workers

In the past, most health care workers have not had the opportunity to study the links between moral philosophy and health. This is so, according to David Seedhouse (1988), for several reasons. First, with few exceptions health care workers receive little formal training in ethics, even though their everyday practice activities involve direct and many times crucial interventions into other people's lives. Second, health care workers usually have a crowded schedule, filled with urgent practical jobs to be accomplished in a short period of time. Under such conditions, there is little time for reflective thought regarding connections between general ethical principles and specific actions. Third, most discussions of these topics use language that is much too dense, vague, and removed from everyday affairs for the more practically oriented health care professional.

Biotechnology and Nursing Ethics

Ethics are an important foundation for a profession. In nursing, they serve as a framework within which professional decisions may be made in a consistent manner that is beneficial to the patient. Today, the rate of technological change is astounding, and there is even more change ahead. Life will never be the same as it was in the past. This is true for the public in general and is especially true for health care professionals, who must practice and make decisions about this new technology in ways consistent with their codes of ethics.

For health professionals, developments in biotechnology have created many new situations requiring the clarification and expansion of codes of ethics—for instance, abortion, the use of fetal tissue for research, genetic research, organ transplantation, assisted suicide, euthanasia, and AIDS. **Bioethics,** the name given to issues of this type, is the application of society's moral code to issues of life, illness, and death. Although these bioethical concerns cover a wide range, and each has unique issues, many argue that nurses should use a common model to address all of them.

In discussing the complexity of bioethical issues, neurologist Robert E. Cranford wrote:

> We are beginning to realize that our wonderful medical advances enable us to prolong the dying process. The first question is, Should we? And then come all the others. Who lives? Who dies? How do you decide? . . . Who decides? . . . Machines give us more choices. But the more choices there are, the more dilemmas there are. (quoted in Kornblum & Julian, 1995, p. 44)

 CRITICALLY THINKING ABOUT . . .

Do you agree or disagree with Dr. Cranford's assessment of the results of biotechnology?

A Model for Bioethical Decision Making

Shake Ketefian (1997) has developed a 10-step model for bioethical decision making (Box 12-2) that focuses on the behavior of the nurse in the decision-making process. The model was originally developed by Thompson and Thompson (1985) and has served well the nurses who have been guided by it.

Box 12-2

Ketefian's Ten-Step Basic Model for Bioethical Decision Making

1. Review of the total situation to determine health problems, key people in addition to the patient, the decisions that need to be made, and the ethical aspects of those decisions
2. Gathering of additional information to clarify the situation to a point where ethical determinations may be made
3. Identification of the ethical issues in the situation that need consideration
4. Definition of the personal and professional moral positions involved
5. Identification of the moral and ethical positions of all the key people involved
6. Identification of the moral and ethical conflicts that exist
7. Determination of who should make the decisions about these issues and how the decisions should be made
8. Identification of the full range of actions possible in the situation and the likely outcomes of each
9. Decisions about the courses of actions required, and implementation of them
10. Review and evaluation of the results of the actions taken as well as the decision-making process.

(Ketefian S [1997]. Moral and ethical dimensions of nursing practice. In Oermann MH (Ed.), *Professional Nursing Practice*. Stamford, CT: Appleton & Lange.)

Other models of bioethical decision making have been developed (Bandman & Bandman, 1985), but common threads run through them (Ketefian, 1997):

1. Clarity and relative certainty about the facts of the situation
2. Identification of the questions that need to be answered in the decision-making process
3. The underlying ethical principles and theories of the situation
4. The collaborative nature of the decision-making process in which patient, family, and health care practitioners participate as fully as possible.

In reality, the use of any model is the goal. In actual practice, however, both the time constraints under which decisions must be made and the total patient load of the health care professional severely limits the extent to which a model may be used. Nevertheless, such models do provide sound frameworks for bioethical considerations.

Bioethics: The Case of AIDS

The Nature of AIDS

AIDS begins with exposure to the human immunodeficiency virus (HIV). The virus attacks certain white blood cells, called T cells, and weakens the body's immune system. AIDS occurs when an HIV-infected person develops a life-threatening condition (eg, cancer, infections) or when the number of disease-fighting T cells becomes dangerously low.

Common forms of illness produced by HIV are:

- *Pneumocystis carinii* pneumonia: a form of pneumonia that is a major killer of people with HIV
- Kaposi's sarcoma: a rare form of malignant skin cancer and organ tumors
- Infections of the nervous system that damage the brain and spinal cord
- Opportunistic infections that attack all parts of the body, such as fungal, parasitic, and bacterial infections (eg, tuberculosis).

According to American Pharmaceutical Research Companies (1997), a person with HIV/AIDS can be infected for many years and not show any symptoms. It is impossible to tell if someone is infected by the way he or she looks, feels, or acts. When symptoms appear, they usually include:

- Painful, swollen lymph glands
- Recurring fever or night sweats
- Rapid weight loss for no apparent reason
- Constant fatigue
- Persistent diarrhea
- Persistent skin problems
- Sores in the mouth
- Dry cough or shortness of breath
- Recurring vaginal yeast infections.

It is only when the symptoms are well advanced that the presence of AIDS can be detected by the public.

AIDS: A Serious Public Health Problem

HIV/AIDS has become one of the worst public health problems ever faced by this country, but there are some signs of improvement. The Centers for Disease Control and Prevention announced on July 14, 1997, that the AIDS death rate had declined 19% for the first 9 months of 1996, compared to what it had been a year earlier. However, the number of deaths was still high (30,700 for the period; 37,900 for the same period in 1995) (CDC, 1997). The current estimates are that in the United States, 513,485 AIDS cases were reported by 1995; 319,849 of them have already died. Even though AIDS is now classified by many as a "chronic disease" because the life expectancy of AIDS patients is getting longer, AIDS carries a near-100% fatality rate and is the leading cause of death among American men aged 25 to 44 years.

AIDS trends differ with demographic categories. African-Americans now account for the largest proportion of AIDS cases (41%). AIDS cases are increasing more rapidly among women than they are among men, particularly minority women. Heterosexual AIDS cases are increasing at a rate of 15% to 20% a year, compared to an increase of 5% or less among gay men. On the whole, the people most likely to contract AIDS are:

- Men (86%) rather than women (14%)
- Adults (99%) rather than children (1%)
- Homosexual or bisexual males (51%) rather than heterosexual males (49%)
- Intravenous drug users (25%).

AIDS experts attribute the decline in deaths of AIDS victims to a drop in the number of new AIDS cases—the fewer that get it, the fewer die of it—and to powerful new treatments that help people with AIDS to live longer. The high cost of the new drugs, estimated to be $10,000 to $15,000 per year, keeps them out of the hands of many who need them.

HIV spreads through contact. It is transmitted through:

- Bodily fluids, including blood, semen, and vaginal secretions during unprotected oral, vaginal, or anal sex with an HIV-infected person
- Needle sharing among injection drug users, or sharing a needle for tattooing, ear piercing, or other procedures
- Mothers with HIV/AIDS transmitting it to their babies during pregnancy, birth, or breast-feeding
- Transfusions of infected blood or blood products before 1985 (today all blood donors and blood products are screened for HIV/AIDS)
- Contact with open sores or wounds of an infected person.

Researchers and public health officials around the world are concerned that within the next 10 to 20 years, AIDS will reach the level of a worldwide plague (Kornblum & Julian, 1995). They expect it to be even more serious than the plague of the Middle Ages, which in the years 1347 to 1350 killed one third to one half of Europe's population.

Stigmatization and AIDS: A Changing Ethical Perspective

The first people diagnosed with AIDS in the United States were stigmatized because of their homosexuality. A **stigma** is a social marker that defines a group as deviant, beyond society's mainstream, and subject to sanctions because of their deviant status. The stigma brings shame to those who bear it. Stigmatized people are often shunned by others, including some who share the stigma. Many times stigmatized persons incorporate the stigma into their self-concept. This leads them to use the stigma as a guide for their behavior and as a focus of their life. Homosexuality was considered deviant behavior; therefore, AIDS became associated in people's minds as the disease of homosexuals. Many people even viewed AIDS as retribution from God for engaging in homosexual relations.

As a result, AIDS became a stigmatized disease. Early in the development of the AIDS epidemic in the United States, some heterosexuals unfortunate enough to contract AIDS hid the fact because they did not want to be stigmatized, nor did they want their families to bear the shame that would come with their stigmatization. For example, Arthur Ashe, one of the 20th century's greatest tennis players, contracted AIDS from a blood transfusion and kept the fact from the public until the illness was well advanced.

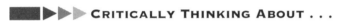 **CRITICALLY THINKING ABOUT . . .**

How do you feel about AIDS?

The early and rapid stigmatization of AIDS in the United States resulted in a general lack of public sympathy for AIDS victims. Consequently, there was little motivation for research and treatment because of the widely held attitude that they (the HIV victims) were engaging in immoral behavior and deserved what they got.

HIV/AIDS presented an early challenge to the ethics of health care practitioners. As members of society, health care professionals had their own views of the morality or immorality of those infected with AIDS. However, the value of beneficence so fundamental to their ethical codes demanded that, in the role of health care professional, they should be guided by compassion and do their best for the patient. Even so, some practitioners refused to work with AIDS patients despite the code of their profession.

As time has passed, it has become clear that AIDS can strike anyone. As a result, AIDS is no longer seen by most people as the "homosexual disease" or the disease of the immoral; it is now the disease that anyone can contract. Consequently, the stigma of AIDS has decreased greatly. This has permitted society to develop an aggressive research and treatment program that simply was not possible in earlier years. This change represents a fundamental reorientation of ethics in regard to a serious health problem.

AIDS serves as an example of the "tug-of-war" between a health practitioner's personal ethics and values and those reflected in his or her professional code of ethics. This occurs in many matters, including suicide, euthanasia, and abortion. When faced with a conflict between personal ethics and professional ethics, many health care professionals resolve the dilemma in favor of their personal ethics. Such ethical dilemmas contribute to the difficulty of developing ethical codes for new bioethical issues.

CRITICALLY THINKING ABOUT . . .

Do you know anyone who is HIV positive or has AIDS? How would you describe his or her life?

Research Ethics and Human Subjects

Chapters 1 through 3 pointed out that one of the most important elements in enhancing the professional status of nursing is the development of a nursing-specific knowledge base using sound scientific principles. Thus, expanding the scope and volume of nursing research is vital to the continuing professionalization of nursing. Most nursing research has and will continue to be conducted using human subjects, and many of those subjects will be patients in the care of nurses. Patients are also likely to be the subjects of medical research. It is medical research that has brought us the sophisticated technology now available for the treatment of disease and injury. To meet their obligations for advocacy for their patients, nurses must understand the ethics involving the use of human subjects in research.

Broadening the Participation of Patients in Research

Until recently, most medical research was conducted in teaching hospitals affiliated with research universities. However, actions taken by the National Institutes of Health (NIH) in the mid-1990s are likely to result in a broader base of human subjects being used in medical research in many other care settings.

Traditionally, subjects in clinical trials that test the safety and efficacy of experimental drugs, treatments, and devices—particularly drugs—were young to middle-aged white males. Women were commonly excluded from drug trials for at least two reasons. The first was that there was a possibility of pregnancy, either at the outset or during the clinical trial. This raised the concern that the fetus could be harmed or even aborted as a side effect of the treatment. The second reason was that many researchers believed that the variability in hormone levels across the menstrual cycle was a threat to the scientific validity of their findings. Racial minorities also were rarely subjects in clinical trials, but for different reasons. The primary problem was the difficulty of recruiting enough minority persons into clinical trials to form a subsample large enough to generate valid, reliable statistical results.

In the early 1990s, the virtual exclusion of women and minorities from clinical trials was challenged. The argument was that most of the data regarding the efficacy and safety of experimental drugs and treatments had been established for white males, and there was still little known about the efficacy and safety for excluded subjects. Some argued that excluding women from clinical trials on the basis of "potential pregnancy" was sexist, paternalistic, and inconsistent with a woman's right to self-determination, and therefore was an unacceptable stance in contemporary America.

As a result of these concerns, NIH now has requirements regarding the proportions of the samples for clinical trials (as well as other research it funds). The result usually is a considerably larger, much more diverse sample than had been used earlier. This requirement for a broader base of subjects means that researchers will have to reach far beyond the walls of university-affiliated teaching hospitals to obtain sufficient subjects. Thus, many nurses who work in settings where they rarely, if ever, needed to deal with issues of human participation in research may now have to do so.

Rights of Human Subjects

The rights of human subjects in research have not always been zealously guarded. During the 1930s and 1940s, the Nazis used prisoners of war and other imprisoned racial and ethnic "enemies," such as Jews and Gypsies, as subjects in experiments to test the limits of human endurance and to study human reactions to intentionally inflicted diseases and physical wounds (Polit & Hungler, 1997). Many of these experiments resulted in the death and permanent maiming of thousands of victims. The horrors of those medical experiments were brought to the world's attention only after World War II was over. The Nazi atrocities were revealed in the Nuremberg trials, and one outcome was the establishment of the **Nuremberg Code**, one of the first sets of ethical standards to be internationally recognized.

In the United States, the **Tuskegee study** was another dark chapter in human research. In this 40-year-long study funded by the U.S. Public Health Department, poor, black, unschooled men from rural Alabama were used—without their knowledge—to track the natural progression of syphilis. The men who survived remained as untreated subjects in the study for years, even after an effective cure for syphilis had been discovered. It was only in 1997 that the federal government offered apologies and a modest financial reparation to the few survivors, who are now in their 90s.

 CRITICALLY THINKING ABOUT . . .

Could what happened in the Tuskegee study happen in another study today?

Since the Nuremberg Code was established, other international standards for the protection of human subjects have emerged. The most important was the World Medical Assembly's **Declaration of Helsinki**, adopted in 1964 and revised in 1975 (Levine, 1986). This declaration differentiated between therapeutic and nontherapeutic research. In the first, patients have the opportunity to receive an experimental treatment that may benefit them; in the second, although the research may benefit future patients in some way, the actual subjects generally do not stand to benefit. The declaration went on to state that:

- Greater care should be exercised to protect subjects from harm in nontherapeutic research.
- Strong, independent justification is required for exposing a healthy volunteer to substantial risk or harm just to gain new scientific information.
- The investigator must protect the life and health of the research subject (Burns & Grove, 1995).

The Belmont Report

During the 1970s, the federal government turned its attention to the need for nationally mandated protection for the rights of human subjects. The National Commission for the Protection of Human Subjects of Biomedical and Behavioral Research was established by the National Research Act (Public Law 93-348). In 1978, the Commission issued the **Belmont report**, which served as the basis for regulations regarding research sponsored by the federal government. This has also become the norm for researchers who are not funded by the government. The Belmont report set forth three principles that must underlie the conduct of biomedical or behavioral research involving human beings: beneficence, respect for persons, and justice.

BENEFICENCE

Beneficence as a principle in research means the obligation to do no harm, paralleling the general ethical principle discussed earlier. There are several dimensions of beneficence in a research context. Freedom from harm means that intentionally exposing subjects to serious or permanent harm is unacceptable. Should such a situation emerge during the conduct of a study, the study must be terminated immediately. Researchers must also be sensitive to the fact that not all harm is clearly evident. In some cases, participation in a study may have psychologically adverse effects that, although more subtle, nonetheless have the potential for harm to the subject. Where possible, researchers must minimize the risks and maximize the benefits of the research to subjects. A person's decisions must be respected, and participation or nonparticipation in the study and any information they provide must not be used against him or her. (There is one exception to the last condition: when a person reveals that he or she has engaged in illegal behavior that is reportable by law. However, if a researcher believes that information of that kind could possibly emerge, that warning should be made very clear in the statement of informed consent the subject reads, understands, and signs.)

RESPECT FOR PERSONS

Respect for persons—the respect for the human dignity of participants—means that everyone has the right of self-determination. A person may participate in the research or not; it is his or her choice. The decision to participate or not carries no penalties or prejudicial treatment. Participants also have the right to discontinue participation in the research anytime they choose, also without penalty or prejudice. This issue is of particular importance when the person conducting the research is the same person caring for the potential subject. The caregiver-researcher must be particularly sensitive to the perceived (and real) vulnerability these patients experience. Therefore, caregiver-researchers must take great care to avoid any form of behavior, either verbal or nonverbal, that could be construed as coercive in any way.

Respect for persons also entails the right of full disclosure. The researcher or a designee must fully describe the study to the potential subject, carefully adhering to the process of obtaining **informed consent**. Informed consent has been defined as:

> The knowing consent of an individual or his or her legally authorized representative, under circumstances that provide the prospective subject or representative sufficient opportunity to consider whether or not to participate without undue inducement or any element of force, fraud, deceit, duress, or other forms of constraint or coercion. (Code of Federal Regulations, 1983, pp. 9–10)

Investigators are not permitted to enter a subject into a study before informed consent is received. Moreover, potential subjects should be given sufficient time to make a considered judgment in the matter. Box 12-3 outlines the minimum content of a statement of informed consent; some institutions require additional elements. The language in the statement of informed consent must be understandable to each potential subject. If the subject cannot understand the language of the statement, he or she may be giving consent to participate, but it is not informed consent. Therefore, the researcher must give careful consideration to the reading level, vocabulary comprehension, and probable level of understanding that characterizes the potential subjects. Medical, nursing, and technical jargon should be avoided whenever possi-

> ## Box 12-3
> ### Elements of Informed Consent
>
> 1. A statement that the study involves research.
> 2. An explanation of the purposes of the research, delineating the expected duration of the subject's participation.
> 3. A description of the procedures to be followed, and identification of any procedures which are experimental.
> 4. A description of any reasonably foreseeable risks or discomforts to the subject.
> 5. A description of any benefits to the subject or to others that may reasonably be expected from the research.
> 6. A disclosure of appropriate alternative procedures or course of treatment, if any, that might be advantageous to the subject.
> 7. A statement describing the extent to which anonymity and confidentiality of the records identifying the subject will be maintained.
> 8. For research involving more than minimal risk, an explanation as to whether any medical treatments are available if injury occurs and, if so, what they consist of, or where further information may be obtained.
> 9. An explanation about who to contact for answers to questions about the research and researcher subjects' rights, and who to contact in the event of a research-related injury to the subject.
> 10. A statement that participation is voluntary, that refusal to participate will not involve any penalty or less benefit to which the subject is otherwise entitled, and that the subject may discontinue participation at any time without penalty or loss of otherwise entitled benefits.
>
> ("Protection of Human Subjects" in *Code of Federal Regulations, OPRR Reports,* March 8, 1983.)

ble. Additional aspects of obtaining informed consent will be addressed later in the consideration of the nurse's responsibility to protect the rights of human subjects who are also patients.

 CRITICALLY THINKING ABOUT . . .

> Have you ever been a subject in a research study? Were you adequately informed about the nature of the study? Did you give consent? Written or verbal? Describe your experience.

Some potential subjects have **diminished autonomy**; in other words, they are limited in exercising their rights to self-determination by virtue of age, disability, physical debilitation, terminal illness, or confinement to an institution. The principle of self-determination means that these people are entitled to protection, because their decreased ability or inability to give informed consent is limited. People with diminished autonomy are considered "vulnerable populations." Another group of people defined as a vulnerable population is that of pregnant women. Stringent guidelines have been developed by the federal government regulating research with pregnant women, reflecting a significant societal concern for the well-being of both the pregnant woman and her fetus, who certainly cannot give informed consent.

Researchers who want to include these vulnerable people in a study must present a convincing rationale. They must be explicit in their plan for protecting the rights of those who are less able to or unable to protect their own rights.

Justice is the third fundamental principle set forth in the Belmont report. Once again, this parallels the same overall principle of ethics in general. Justice means that human subjects must be treated fairly before, during, and after their participation in the research process. Participants should be selected in such a way that any risks or benefits will be shared equally. They must not be denied benefits to which they are entitled, nor should they carry an unreasonable burden of responsibility. The researcher has the responsibility to select subjects appropriately and to assign them to treatment groups fairly. The researcher must honor all agreements made with the participants before the study, including the payment of any promised stipends. Participants must be assured access to appropriate professional assistance should any untoward physical or psychological damage occur. Justice also involve sensitivity to and respect for lifestyles as well as courteous, considerate treatment at all times.

A significant component of justice is careful consideration of a participant's right to privacy. Investigators must be sensitive to the fact that "virtually all research with humans constitutes some type of intrusion into their personal lives." Participants in any research "have the right to expect that any data collected during the course of a study will be kept in strictest confidence" (Polit & Hungler, 1997, p. 137). This can be done using a research design that assures participants either anonymity or confidentiality. **Anonymity** means that there is no way of connecting the identity of the participant with the information he or she provided, not even by the researcher (Burns & Grove, 1995). A stack of questionnaires left in a hospital waiting area accompanied by a poster inviting people to complete one (unsigned, of course) and drop it into a slotted box would afford anonymity to participants.

However, in most health care research, the investigator must know the identity of the participants to meet the research goals. Thus, it is far more common to devise research designs and methods in which the identity of the participant is known to the investigator, but the identity is held in confidence. To provide **confidentiality**, participants are promised that their participation will not be reported publicly and that their participation and information about them will be known to members of the research team alone. Providing confidentiality sometimes requires elaborate schemes and great creativity on the part of researchers. However, the importance of a participant's right to privacy makes it an essential component of ethical research.

Nurses' Responsibilities in the Conduct of Ethical Research in Health Care Settings

Although it is truly unfortunate and should never happen, egregious violations of the rights of human subjects sometimes occur in research in health care settings. Nurses, as part of their role as patient advocates, have a responsibility to ensure that patients' rights as research subjects are carefully guarded. This is a hallmark of a nurse who is carrying out practice in a truly professional manner. If the nurse is the researcher or part of a research team, concern for the rights of human subjects entails designing and conducting the study in such as manner as to maximize the protection of subjects in the study.

The most common involvement of nurses working in clinical settings where research is conducted centers around obtaining informed consent from potential research subjects. It is not uncommon for a nurse to be assigned the task of obtaining a patient's signature on a statement of informed consent. Unless the nurse is part of the research team or has a thorough knowledge of the study, this is an inappropriate assignment, and the nurse should not comply. Admittedly, this can pose a significant workplace dilemma for the nurse. However, being a patient advocate means that the nurse should participate in the process in such a way as to be sure that the patient has, in fact, given consent that is informed, and that proper ethical procedures were followed. This may seem presumptuous on the part of a "mere" staff nurse, but it is part of the ethical obligation of professional nursing practice.

The nurse must be aware of the studies that are going on in the unit into which his or her patients may be entered. The nurse also should know of and report to researchers any cognitive, language, or cultural factors that may compromise a patient's ability to understand the nature of the research in which he or she is agreeing to participate. Although a nurse should not be the agent for obtaining a signature on an informed consent document related to a study with which he or she is unfamiliar, a very appropriate role for the nurse is to serve as a witness to the process of obtaining informed consent.

The Law and Nursing Professionalization

Each society establishes laws that are binding on all citizens. Nurses are subject to society's laws, just as are other people, in their daily personal and professional lives. **Laws** are the rules that are enforced and sanctioned by government authority (Brinkerhoff, White, & Riedmann, 1997). Laws generally fulfill three major functions in society:

1. Laws provide formal sanctions for certain behaviors to encourage conformity with society's core values, thereby discouraging deviance and disorder.
2. Laws help settle disputes that otherwise would never be resolved or would be resolved through violence.
3. Laws can be instruments for social change—as laws are changed, behavior in society is changed as well.

Some social theorists argue that laws and the legal system were designed and run by the politically powerful in society in a way that permits the elites to dominate the lower and middle classes (Brinkerhoff, White, & Riedmann, 1997). The law both helps maintain social order within a society and protects the rights of most citizens—especially those with the largest amount of social, economic, and political power.

Types of Law

There are several types of laws. **Statutory law** is law written and enacted by governing bodies, such as the U.S. Congress, state legislatures, and local communities. The laws that govern health care professionals in the performance of their professional duties are statutory laws. Most of the laws governing professions are enacted by state legislatures because professional licensure is a state-level function. Each state's nurse practice act is an example of a statutory law. The nurse practice act is the law that establishes a state board of nursing, defines its functions, specifies its scope of operation, and grants it power to perform its mandated tasks, the purpose of which is to protect the safety of the citizens of that state.

Common law is not specifically enacted by a government body; rather, it emerges from the judgments and decrees handed down by courts in adjudication of specific cases. The development of common law has resulted from the widely held legal principle of "stares decisis." This principle holds that a judge presiding over a current case must make a decision similar to those handed down in similar previous cases. Each case in the American legal system has a potential for being a precedent-setting case if existing common laws do not or cannot apply.

Another distinction is that between criminal law and civil law. **Criminal law** consists of laws governing behaviors that a legal body, such as the state legislature, thinks threaten society as a whole and not just the people in a specific situation. For example, murder is considered unlawful not only because a life is taken but also because uncontrolled murder threatens the long-term stability and existence of society itself. Criminal law distinguishes between misdemeanors (minor criminal offenses) and felonies (major criminal offenses). In criminal cases, the court is the arena where the state argues for the conviction and punishment of the accused.

Sometimes nurses become enmeshed in criminal law matters when they are accused of murdering a patient or being part of a conspiracy to unlawfully terminate a patient's life (eg, in assisted suicide or euthanasia), diverting hospital narcotics for personal use or financial gain, and failing to be licensed. Practicing without a license is considered a very serious matter by all states and can be punished by incarceration in a state prison.

■■▶▶▶ **CRITICALLY THINKING ABOUT . . .**

Using your school's library, can you find examples of nurses who have been charged under the criminal code?

Civil law deals with violations of one person's rights by another person or set of persons, such as in an organization. A lawsuit by a person against tobacco companies is an example of a civil suit. Disputes over contracts and claims for monetary damages for injuries received make up much of civil litigation. In civil lawsuits, the court is the place where the plaintiff (the person bringing the matter before the court) and the defendant (the person against whom the complaint is directed) present their sides of the situation and ask for a resolution of their dispute by an impartial body. That body might be a judge, a panel of judges, or a jury.

There are several categories of civil law, including contract law, tax law, and tort law. **Tort law** is very important for health professionals because the resolution of malpractice suits involves tort law. Tort law deals with wrongful acts committed against another person in which the other suffers injury and personal damages. There is a distinction in tort law between unintentional and intentional torts. Unintentional torts are usually caused by **negligence**, the omission of an act in a situation that a reasonable and prudent person would perform or an act that a reasonable person would not do in that situation (Louisell & Williams, 1990). Intentional tort law deals with acts that are willful and in violation of another person's rights or property.

Intentional torts are distinguished from unintentional torts by three characteristics. In intentional torts, the defendant:

1. Must intend to harm the victim
2. Must intend to interfere with the victim and the victim's property
3. Must act in such a way that the act is a significant factor in bringing on the injury experienced by the plaintiff (Catalano, 1996).

Nurses may become involved in civil law actions in a number of ways. Examples could include leaving a surgical instrument inside a patient, failing to assess accurately a patient's condition or failing to report that condition to the attending physician or the physician's designee, failing to report to the appropriate person or office another health care worker's incompetence, and failing to take action to provide for a patient's safety. In today's legal climate, nurses must carry adequate malpractice insurance.

 CRITICALLY THINKING ABOUT . . .

Should student nurses be required to carry malpractice insurance? Why or why not?

Codes of Ethics and Laws

As we have seen, nurses are subject to laws regulating the behavior of all citizens and to laws regulating their professional behavior. Earlier in this chapter, we discussed the purpose of the professional code of ethics and how such codes are developed. Certainly, professionals are responsible to society and the law to fulfill those codes. Society also formalizes what it expects of its professionals in **practice acts**. Practice acts are passed by state legislatures and combine what the profession defines as its domain of action with the concerns of the state for the well-being of its residents. Sometimes these acts may be controversial. For example, advanced practice nurses (APNs) in a given state might want in their practice act the right to prescribe medications. This would be seen by physicians as a great infringement on their professional rights. The physicians would wage a major battle with the legislature to block such a move on the part of nurses. The possibility of "turf battles" such as this is one reason why interrelated professions scrutinize very carefully each others' practice acts.

Practice acts vary considerably from state to state, but they do have common core features:

- They define the nature of nursing practice within the state.
- They set the requirements for licensure for practice.
- They set the educational and other qualifications required for practice.
- They determine the legal titles and abbreviations that may be used by nurses.
- They provide for disciplinary action for certain specific causes (Chitty, 1997; Aiken, 1994).

Practice acts are not set in stone. They are revised from time to time through the political process. Such revisions attempt to achieve two things. First, the intent is to make the practice act reflect the expanded nature of professional practice (eg, by including regulations for APNs). Second, changes are made to include society's views on health, health care, and the role of nursing. For example, one of the major reasons that nurse practice acts have been updated to include recognition of APNs is because people who have had experience with them have found them to be a valuable asset in the health care system. Thus, the changing law reflects public opinion and acceptance. In effect, practice acts join the profession's code of ethics with the demands that society places on the profession.

It is useful to think of ethics, professional codes of ethics, and state practice acts as a continuum. As discussed earlier, professional ethics grow out of professional practice, and personal ethics grow out of the practitioner. As the practitioner's work becomes professionalized, a code of ethics is developed as a framework for thinking about and acting in the name of the profession. As professionalization continues, the state comes to recognize the independence and importance of the profession's contribution to the well-being of its citizens. At that point, the state enacts a practice act that, in addition to regulating professional behavior, also incorporates the concerns of the public with the standards of care delivered by the profession. In a sense, the development of a practice act indicates that the area of practice has arrived at advanced professional status. Nursing practice acts in all states tell us that in the public's eye, at least, nursing is one of the basic human professions.

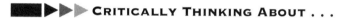 **CRITICALLY THINKING ABOUT . . .**

> Have you read your state's practice act? If not, when should a nurse read it? Why? How do you think your state's nurse practice act should be modified?

▶ CHAPTER SUMMARY

Since its origins in the early religious communities of western Europe, modern nursing has consistently demonstrated a strong commitment to ethical standards of the highest quality. These ethical standards have been firmly instilled in generation after generation of nurses as part of the process of nursing education. The commitment to high ethical standards of practice and conduct has always been made clear in statements from the ANA, nursing's preeminent professional organization. In this regard, nursing has established and maintained its professional stature at the highest level.

Advances in medical science and biotechnology within the past half-century have presented moral challenges and ethical dilemmas that no one has faced before. Nurses and the patients for whom they care and for whom they must be ardent advocates are at the center of this moral and ethical maelstrom. Nurses must remain committed to the distinguished level of ethical principles and practice that have always characterized our discipline. Moreover, their actions must be consistent with their commitment. Such a commitment is an essential component of nursing's continuing progress toward recognition as a fully developed profession.

KEY POINTS

▶ 1 Ethics is a system of morals used by people to evaluate their experiences and plan their courses of action. Most codes of ethics in Western societies are based on six broad social values: justice (the obligation to be fair to all people), autonomy (the right to make one's own decisions), fidelity (the obligation to keep one's commitments), beneficence (doing no harm), veracity (truthfulness), and advocacy (helping others to maintain and exercise their rights to self-determination).

▶ 2 The United States is a socially diverse society and represents a wide range of values among major social groups. Moreover, rapidly changing health care technology means that the ethical dilemmas faced by nurses become increasingly complex; older ethical systems may no longer apply.

▶ 3 Ketefian has described a ten-step model for bioethical decision making: review the total situation; gather additional data to clarify the situation; identify specific ethical issues; define possible moral positions involved; identify key persons' moral and ethical positions; identify moral and ethical conflicts that exist; determine who should make the decision; identify the range of possible actions; decide on a course of action and how to implement it; and review and evaluate the outcomes.

▶ 4 HIV and AIDS have had a powerful impact on our society, and they pose a serious public health threat globally. When first recognized in the United States, AIDS was found primarily in groups that were already stigmatized: homosexuals and intravenous drug users. Thus, the disease itself became associated with "immoral" behavior, and many viewed AIDS as retribution from God. Even many health professionals experienced conflicts between their personal and professional ethics and values.

▶ 5 Increasing numbers of clients are likely to be potential subjects in the expanding arena of nursing and medical research. A very important part of the nurse's role as patient advocate is to have a clear understanding of the rights of human subjects in research. Nurses also must be very clear as to what constitutes informed consent and must work actively to ensure that every patient's rights are protected.

▶ 6 Laws are society's rules that are enforced and sanctioned by government authority. Statutory laws are those written and enacted by governing bodies. Common law emerges from the judgments handed down by courts in judging specific cases. Criminal law consists of laws governing behaviors that could threaten society as a whole. Civil law deals with the violation of one person's rights by another person. Nurses are most often involved in tort law because the resolution of malpractice suits involves tort law.

▶ 7 The practice of nursing is regulated internally by nursing's code of professional ethics. It is also regulated by the state, which enacts laws in the form of nurse practice acts. Nurse practice acts spell out the scope of activities that constitute the legal practice of nursing in each state. Existence of a practice act is evidence that the public at large recognizes nursing as a practice separate from medicine and recognizes nursing's contribution to the well-being of the citizens of the state.

REFERENCES

Aiken TD (1994). *Legal, Ethical and Political Issues in Nursing*. Philadelphia: FA Davis.

American Nurses Association (1976). *Code for Nurses With Interpretive Statements*. Kansas City: Author.

American Pharmaceutical Companies (1997). *HIV/AIDS*. Washington DC: Author.

Bandman E, Bandman B (1985). *Nursing ethics in the lifespan*. Norwalk, CT: Appleton-Century-Crofts.

Brinkerhoff DB, White L, Riedmann AC (1997). *Sociology*, 4th ed. Belmont, CA: Wadsworth Publishing Co.

Burns N, Grove SK (1995). *Understanding Nursing Research*. Philadelphia: WB Saunders.

Catalano J (1996). *Contemporary Professional Nursing*. Philadelphia: FA Davis.

Centers for Disease Control and Prevention (1997). *National HIV Seroprevalence Summary*. Atlanta: U.S. Department of Health and Human Services, Public Health Services, Centers for Disease Control.

Cherny NI (1996). The problem of inadequately relieving suffering. *J Social Issues, 52*, 13–38.

Chitty KK (1997). *Professional Nursing: Concepts and Challenges*. Philadelphia: WB Saunders.

Code of Federal Regulations, 45 CFR 46, Protection of Human Subjects. *OPRR Reports*, revised March 8, 1983.

Frankena WK (1988). *Ethics* (2nd ed.). Englewood Cliffs, NJ: Prentice-Hall.

Hadjistavropoulos T (1996). The systematic application of ethical codes in the counseling of persons who are considering euthanasia. *J Social Issues, 52*, 169–188.

Hessing DJ, Blad JR, Pieterman R (1996). Practical reasons and reasonable practice: The case of euthanasia in the Netherlands. *J Social Issues, 52*, 149–168.

International Council of Nurses (1973). *International Council of Nurses' Code for Nurses*. Geneva, Switzerland: Author.

Ketefian S (1997). Moral and ethical dimensions of nursing practice. In Oermann MH (Ed), *Professional Nursing Practice*. Stamford, CT: Appleton & Lange.

Kornblum W, Julian J (1995). *Social Problems* (8th ed.). Englewood Cliffs, NJ: Prentice-Hall.

Levine RJ (1986). *Ethics and Regulation of Clinical Research* (2nd ed.). Baltimore-Munich: Urban, Schwarzenberg.

Louisell D, Williams H (1990). *Medical Malpractice*. New York: Matthew Bender.

Polit DF, Hungler BP (1997). *Essentials of Nursing Research: Methods, Appraisal, and Utilization*. Philadelphia: Lippincott-Raven.

Seedhouse D (1988). *Ethics: The Heart of Health Care*. New York: John Wiley & Sons.

Smith JE (1977). The pre-eminence of autonomy in bioethics. In Oderberg DS, Lang JA, eds. *Human Lives: Critical Essays on Consequentialist Bioethics*. New York: St. Martin's Press.

Thompson JB, Thompson HO (1985). *Bioethical Decision Making for Nurses*. Norwalk, CT: Appleton-Century-Crofts.

RECOMMENDED READINGS

Ellner LR (1997). What Grandma Clara wanted. *AJN, 97*(8), 51.

Goodhall L (1997). Tube feeding dilemmas: Can artificial nutrition and hydration be legally or ethically withheld or withdrawn? *J Advanced Nursing, 25*, 217–222.

Ivy SS (1996). Ethical considerations in resuscitation decisions: A nursing ethics perspective. *J Cardiovascular Nursing, 10*(4), 47–58.

Kirkpatrick MK (1997). Storytelling: An approach to client-centered care. *Nurse Educator, 22*(2), 38–40.

Lisanti P, Zwolski K (1997). Understanding the devastation of AIDS. *AJN, 97*(7), 26–35.

Matzo ML (1997). The search to end suffering. *J Gerontological Nursing, 23*(3), 11–17.

Melix G (1995). Nora's world . . . the right to die in a humane way. *AJN, 95*(1), 80.

Omery A, Henneman E, Billet B, Luna-Raines M (1995). Ethical issues in hospital-based nursing practice. *J Cardiovascular Nursing, 9*(3), 43–53.

Pyne R, Booth B (1995). The euthanasia debate: How NT readers view the issue. *Nursing Times, 91*(35), 36–38.

Volker DL (1995). Assisted suicide and the terminally ill: Is there a right to self-determination? *J Nursing Law, 2*(4), 37–48.

Zimbleman J (1994). Good life, good death, and the right to die: Ethical considerations for decisions at the end of life. *J Professional Nursing, 10*, 22–37.

13

Nursing for the Future: 2000 and Beyond

CHAPTER OUTLINE

The Great Social Transformation
Nursing and the Great Social
   Transformation
Chapter Summary

Key Points
References
Recommended Readings

LEARNING OBJECTIVES

▶ **1** Describe the nature of the great social transformation that is occurring worldwide and the changes it engenders in society.

▶ **2** Discuss the five social forces that drive the great social transformation and the changes they engender in society.

▶ **3** Explain the relations among bureaucratization, the growth of the managed care environment, and nursing roles in the emerging health care system.

▶ **4** Discuss how the impact of industrialization and postindustrialization relates to technological advances in nursing and to the practice of nursing in the community.

▶ **5** Describe the impact of urbanization, and its resulting social diversity and multiculturalism, on nursing education and nursing practice.

▶ **6** Discuss the relations among globalization, health, and nursing.

▶ **7** Explain how the force of rationalization within the great social transformation contributes to the professionalization of nursing.

KEY TERMS

associational
  societies
bureaucratization
communal societies

ComputerLink
computerized nursing
  taxonomies
core nations

critical thinking
culturally
  competent care

(continued)

cultural nursing
assessment

culture values

expert systems

globalization

great social
transformation
(GST)

HELP

industrialization

infectious parasitic
diseases (IPDs)

interactive planning

International Council
of Nurses (ICN)

multiculturalism

nursing informatics

nursing information
systems

periphery nations

postindustrialization

rationalization

semiperiphery
nations

sick-role orientation

social diversity

transitional societies

urbanization

Nursing has been and always will be played out in the context of the society of which it is a part. Thus, nurses must understand the broader societal context in which they will practice in the 21st century. It is a society characterized by complex, multidimensional change, change that has a profound impact on the population at large, on the clients for whom nurses care, on the systems in which nurses work, and on nurses themselves.

This chapter discusses the sociologic concept of the great social transformation that is occurring globally. This is then used as a framework for discussing the current and future changes and challenges in nursing.

The Great Social Transformation

To understand the broad social forces that are shaping the social, political, and economic conditions in which nursing operates today, we must understand the fundamental processes of societal change that are underway in most societies, including the United States. According to sociologists, a **great social transformation (GST)** is occurring. Societies the world over are being totally reconstructed from organization around families, clans (groupings of related families), and villages to organization around large-scale, impersonal social units, which include formal organizations, bureaucracies, and corporations (Curry, Jiobu, & Schwirian, 1997). Social units such as the family and community are not disappearing from modern life but are losing their centrality in society as larger organizations increasingly become society's primary "movers and shakers."

From Communal to Associational Societies

Communal and **associational societies** are societies that are in the early and later stages, respectively, of this GST. **Transitional societies** are in between the communal and associational stages.

Communal societies, those based on family, clan, and village, are characterized by:

1. Relationships that are rich and highly personalized
2. A limited division of labor in common activities, usually along sex and age and skill lines

3. An economy based on commodities in the nearby habitat
4. An overall low level of technology, although some specific handicraft skills such as weaving or ceramics may be highly developed
5. A nonbureaucratic political organization—those in power are directly accessible to society's members
6. A limited system of social classes because there is little wealth or surplus to divide among members
7. A rich ceremonial life, with religious beliefs and practices infusing most areas of life
8. Limited contact with other societies; the resulting isolation helps preserve the traditional way of life
9. A great value on traditional beliefs and ways of doing things.

In contrast, associational societies—those based on large-scale organizations, bureaucracies, and corporations—are characterized by:

1. Relationships that are formalized, transitory, and less personal
2. A complex division of labor in all activities
3. An economy based on manufacturing and related activities
4. Technology at a high level, with constant attempts by social units to improve it. Technology is an important key to future developments in all areas, including the economy, service delivery, education, and health care.
5. Political institutions that are complex and bureaucratic, with political leaders remote from ordinary citizens
6. Complex social stratification, with a small upper class, a large middle class, and a small lower class
7. High value placed on rational thought, which serves to diminish the role of religion in the daily life of the average citizen
8. The society exists as part of a global network of societies through which people, goods and services, and information flow.
9. Devaluing of traditional beliefs and practices, which are replaced with critical thinking in decision-making processes.

Given these social characteristics, sociologists find that life in mainly communal societies, such as in South Asia's Ganges Valley, is less complex, less diverse, more traditional, and more personal than in the mainly associational societies such as the United States, Germany, or Canada. Few societies are either totally communal or totally associational; most fall somewhere in between. However, economically advanced countries are mainly associational, while economically dependent countries are mainly communal.

■■■▶▶▶ **CRITICALLY THINKING ABOUT . . .**

What characteristics of our society reflect associational influences?
What characteristics reflect communal influences?

Transitional societies comprise a very large percentage of the world's population and are struggling to improve their position in the global economy. Their people suffer the stresses and the social, economic, and political dislocations brought on by dealing with the conflicting communal and associational elements of their changing life. Within associational societies, pockets of communal relationships may still be found in some regions, some families, some organizations, and some communities. These pockets can help blunt the negative, depersonalized consequences of life in an associational society.

Sources of Uniqueness in the Transformation

Each society experiences the GST in a unique way, and no two associational societies become exactly alike in their social structure. For example, the United States and Japan are both experiencing the GST and are similar in many ways because of their associational features. Nevertheless, they are culturally distinct and will probably never become identical.

Countries develop in different ways because they have different traditional cultural and economic bases at the outset of the GST. The pace at which change proceeds also varies between nations; the process may occur over years or over centuries. Another difference is whether the country has a central or a peripheral position in the world. How recently the GST started also varies from one society to another. Other factors affecting the course of the GST are the nature of the economic and political leadership and the willingness of citizens to join social movements to improve their lives. Other catalysts for change include revolution and war, natural catastrophes, technological breakthroughs, and cultural processes such as:

- ◘ Invention—combining known cultural elements in a novel way
- ◘ Discovery—something that has not been noticed before becomes noticed and put to use
- ◘ Diffusion—transmission of a cultural element from one group or society to another.

Not all members of society welcome the changes that come with the GST. In fact, societies commonly experience social, political, and economic turmoil as people and groups vie for control of the processes of change. Some people resist change because they doubt its legitimacy. Without a critical mass of people giving legitimacy to a potential change, the likelihood of the change occurring is diminished. People also resist change when—rightly or wrongly—they believe they stand to lose something of value if the change occurs. There is also social inertia in resistance to change. People resist change because they are comfortable with things as they are; something new is seen as personally disturbing and, therefore, to be avoided if possible.

 CRITICALLY THINKING ABOUT . . .

If your school added 1 more year of education as a requirement for your degree, how would you feel? Would you welcome it or would you resist? Discuss in terms of the usual reasons people resist change.

Forces of Change

Accompanying the GST are several forces that act to restructure society from the communal form to the associational form: industrialization, bureaucratization, urbanization, globalization, and rationalization.

Industrialization

Industrialization is the force that brings about the reorganization of the society's economic base so that it becomes built on:

- ☐ Assembly line, mass production
- ☐ Production in large factories employing extensive power machinery
- ☐ A workforce characterized by a highly specialized division of labor in production and administration
- ☐ Highly mechanized methods of transportation and communication (Hoult, 1969).

In contrast, the preindustrial economies of communal societies are characterized by:

- ☐ Handicraft production units consisting of only a few workers who work in small, scattered villages
- ☐ Sources of energy are human and animal power, supplemented by limited tools, such as the water wheel.
- ☐ Primary production, which is the extraction of raw materials from the local environment by means such as farming, fishing, hunting, and mining
- ☐ Close integration of work with the rest of life because the typical work group contains family members, lifelong friends, and acquaintances (Brinkerhoff, White, & Riedmann 1997).

Industrialization changes all these characteristics and, in effect, forces the conversion of highly skilled artisans into assembly line workers. The shift from handicraft to factory production has increased efficiency and productivity. Negative consequences include a loss of control over one's work and feelings of alienation from the factory and from society as a whole.

Sociologists argue that societies that are well into the GST are moving from industrialization to **postindustrialization**. These include countries such as the United States, Germany, and Canada. In postindustrial societies, the economy once again shifts its base, from the production of manufactured goods to the production of services. Occupations that specialize in services become more prominent in postindustrial societies. These occupations include hospital workers, schoolteachers, police and fire personnel, information specialists, banking and finance employees, and government workers. These occupations are characterized by the type of service they provide to people rather than the goods they produce.

Bureaucratization

Bureaucratization is the process in which human organizations increase the number of tasks they perform and the number of workers they employ. They develop a complex division of labor, which is manifested in a high degree of specialization in the performance of tasks, and create a multilevel power and decision-making structure. Bureaucracies also develop explicit written rules for worker performance, develop a reward system for workers based on their job performance rather than social connections, and create an extensive system of written and electronically stored records on worker and organization performance that constitutes a major paper flow in the organization.

In theory, a bureaucracy is a well-oiled machine that performs its tasks with maximal efficiency. However, most bureaucracies don't live up to this ideal. Several negative aspects of bureaucracies are:

1. "Service without a smile"—employees of bureaucracies, because of growing alienation caused by their work conditions, respond minimally or even negatively to clients and coworkers.
2. "Rules are rules"—employees of bureaucracies come to follow the organization's rules mechanically rather than using their imagination to solve problems and better serve their clients.
3. "Goal displacement"—the concern of employees shifts from doing a good job to maintaining the job at all costs.
4. "Work expands to fill available time"—the tendency of workers to produce "busy work" when their normal work activities require only part of their time
5. "Bureaucrats rise to their level of incompetence"—people who are good at their tasks are often promoted to the next level of administration, for which they are unprepared; as a result, they perform poorly (Curry, Jiobu, & Schwirian, 1997).

Although bureaucracies are plagued by organizational problems, they remain the most productive and cost-effective way society has found to complete a large amount of work in a short period of time.

 CRITICALLY THINKING ABOUT . . .

What negative features of bureaucracy have you experienced in your degree program, your school, or your job? Have you been guilty of one or more of the negative activities listed?

Urbanization

Urbanization is the process through which, over time, an increasingly larger percentage of the population lives in cities. In the United States, this figure currently exceeds 75%. Rural-to-urban migration has been a major factor in the growth of cities. People migrate to cities from nonurban areas primarily because they think economic opportunities in the city will be better than in the countryside. If the perceived gap between city and rural opportunities is large enough, concerns such as family attachments at home will not prevent migration to the city.

The diversity of American cities today reflects the history of immigration to this country. The first city populations came from northern and western Europe—Britain, Germany, and Scandinavia. The second wave of immigrants—in the late 19th and early 20th century—was made up of people from southern and eastern Europe—Italians, Greeks, and Poles. In a third wave of immigration, at the turn of the 20th century African-Americans left the rural poverty of the South for what they thought would be an improved life in the northern industrial centers. Latins—Mexicans, Cubans, and Puerto Ricans—make up the fourth immigrant wave, which peaked in the middle and latter part of the 20th century. Like the Europeans before them, Asians also have come to this country in two different waves. The first wave came during the early years of city building, when they worked on the railroads and related activities. These immigrants were from China and Japan. More recently, especially since the end of the Vietnam war, there has been a wave of immigrants from Cambodia, Vietnam, and Laos.

The effect of these waves of newcomers was a very heterogeneous population and a highly differentiated mosaic of subcultures. For most of the 20th century, cities have been complex mosaics of ethnic and racial groups held together by city government, service institutions, and economic opportunity. At times the competition among the groups for jobs, housing, and services has turned to conflict, riots, and violence.

City growth today is characterized by two processes. The first process is urbanization itself, in which people are attracted to cities. The second process is suburbanization, the redistribution of people, jobs, shopping, and entertainment from the city to the surrounding suburbs. At the edge of many older and larger cities are other growing cities ("edge cities") that compete with the old downtowns for economic activities.

One negative consequence of the urbanization and suburbanization processes has been a migration of affluent persons to the suburbs and the containment of economically disadvantaged populations in the city. Many inner-city neighborhoods have become seriously distressed, with high unemployment rates, high poverty rates, low average family income, crowded dwellings, crime, violent gangs, broken families, and personal pathologies such as alcohol and drug addiction. Many of these people are handicapped in their attempt to succeed in mainstream society by limited language skills, poor education, limited access to transportation to the jobs in suburbia, and racial or ethnic discrimination, which results in their being excluded from consideration for employment opportunities.

Globalization

Globalization is the process by which people and societies become knit together through economic and political ties. A global society engages in trade with other societies, holds memberships in regional and worldwide political pacts, and exchanges people and goods with many countries. A nonglobal society is isolated, inward-looking, and largely excluded from the world's mainstream. The United States is a global society; Tibet is a nonglobal society. Global societies are primarily associational societies, and nonglobal societies are primarily communal societies.

The network of relations among societies in the global system today—called the world system—has at its center the **core nations** (Curry, Jiobu, & Schwirian, 1997; Wallerstein, 1979). These nations are highly industrial and powerful in both economic and political matters. The United States and Germany are examples of core nations. Core nations, through their economic and political might, set the general conditions under which other nations' economies function. **Periphery nations** in the world system are economically dependent on the core nations and often export raw materials to manufacturing and processing operations in the core nations. Typically, periphery nations have a low level of technological development, a high level of poverty, political instability, and little prospect for improving their position in the world system. Madagascar and Somalia are examples of periphery countries. **Semiperiphery nations**, such as Puerto Rico and the Bahamas, have benefited economically and politically from their close ties to the core nations and thereby receive more benefits from the world system than do periphery nations.

Rationalization

Rationalization means that society's members place an emphasis on rational thought rather than tradition in understanding the world, in identifying problems to be solved, and in planning actions to be undertaken. Rationalization includes a heavy emphasis on "deliberate calculation, efficiency, self-control and effectiveness in the accomplishment of explicit goals" (Curry, Jiobu, & Schwirian, 1997). In a society that prizes rationalization, tradition is no longer accepted as the yardstick by which things are measured. Rationalization has given us science, technology, and greater efficiency in the production of goods and services. However, it also has left us with a tendency to replace warm, communal social relationships in productive activities with cold calculation, and to view other humans as inanimate inputs into the production, distribution, military, and governing processes.

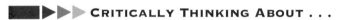 CRITICALLY THINKING ABOUT . . .

> As you think about nursing, how do your thoughts reflect rationalization? How do they reflect tradition?

Nursing and the Great Social Transformation

The GST is not a one-time-only change; it is a continuing process that will shape our lives for centuries. The GST and the forces that drive it have shaped nursing in the past and will continue to do so far into the future. Having established the societal context within which nursing will enter the 21st century, the remainder of the chapter will address major trends, challenges, and opportunities that are having, and will continue to have, a significant effect on nursing's potential for realizing full professional status.

Industrialization and Nursing

The shift from the industrial to the postindustrial phase of the GST is in full swing in the United States. It affects every aspect of society, and the health care industry in general and nursing in particular are no exceptions.

Two fundamental characteristics of industrialization are the factory production system and technological development. In the factory production system, work is done in a large-scale, labor-intensive, single-site environment. Technological development is the ever-expanding use of knowledge and tools in the production of new and improved goods in an increasingly efficient manner. Technological development is the process by which scientific principles and derived knowledge are converted into materials, tools, and information that can be used to achieve human ends.

The industrial society gave us the hospital industry as we have known it (large-scale, high-tech, and physically centralized)—hospital as factory, so to speak. Our associational society is moving from the industrial into the postindustrial period. Among the consequences of this change for nursing is the nucleation of the health care service delivery system, which means the tendency for the activities of the single-site service delivery system (the factory/hospital) to be redistributed to multiple satellite sites. Another highly significant consequence of the shift to the postindustrial society is the increasing importance of high-tech communication methods, which are needed to link the nucleated units.

Thus, as nursing enters the 21st century, nurses must be prepared to deliver care in the new, reconfigured structures that characterize the American postindustrial health care system. The delivery of care in the community will gain increasingly greater importance, as will the role of nursing information technologies. Both of these trends are inextricably linked, and they are addressed in the following section.

Nursing Care in the Community

Beverly Malone, president of the American Nurses Association, noted in 1995 that by the year 2010, the proportion of nurses working in hospitals and those working in community settings (currently two thirds and one third) will have flip-flopped (Schardin, 1995). Not everyone may agree with the high degree of change Malone predicted, but the shift will occur. The hospital is the most labor-intensive, and thus the most expensive, environment in which to deliver care. As noted in the previous section, existing ambulatory and community-based alternatives must be expanded and new forms developed to provide a more cost-effective structure of care while still maintaining quality of care.

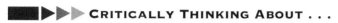 **CRITICALLY THINKING ABOUT . . .**

Do you agree with Malone's prediction? Why or why not?

Do nurses who provide care in the community need to be prepared to do things differently than nurses do in the hospital? The scope of community health practice is very broad, and the ability to conceptualize this scope and breadth is crucial for nurses in the community. Nurses need to be able to see the whole of the practice environment and bring to bear a well-developed systems perspective. Nurses caring for patients and families in the community must understand the overall health care system, its services, the client base, and the range of resources available to them and their clients. A nurse who works in the community must encourage clients' "ownership" of their own health care needs and must always remember that nursing means working with clients rather than for them (Bramadat, Chalmers, & Andrusyszyn, 1996).

Nurses who practice in the community need "process skills" that may be different than those needed by hospital nurses. Like all nurses, they must have a firm grasp of the nursing process. Assessment skills for a wide range of patients must be especially keen; this includes skills in functional assessment as well as overall health assessment. Assessment skills are particularly important in working with older adults, who make up a very large segment of patients cared for in the community. The effectiveness of nurses practicing in the community also depends a great deal on their communication and counseling skills. The role of teaching and counseling has always been an important aspect of community health nursing practice, and it is likely that it will become even more important as the number of community-based patients increases, and the health problems they are managing become more complex. Nurses in the community often are a part of groups that work toward solving community health problems, so they must also be skilled at group process (Bramadat, Chalmers, & Andrusyszyn, 1996).

Clinical decision making is the basis for all aspects of practice. Effective practice in the community requires finely honed critical thinking and problem-solving skills, because in community health practice there are often no quick and easy answers to a care dilemma (Kuennen & Moss, 1995). Community health nurses also require considerable management and leadership skills, including the ability to delegate tasks and supervise nonprofessional staff. On top of all these important skills, the community health nurse needs strong technical skills and the ability to adapt those skills to the clinic and home setting. Nurses working in the community usually operate without the expert back-up systems available in hospitals.

Nurses who practice in the community must have a broader knowledge base than that afforded by experience limited to the medical or surgical environment. The focus must be on caring for specific client groups. Community nurses must be able to look beyond the individual patient to see "health issues from a broader family and community perspective." Reproductive health and the care of young families is important for community health nurses, and they must be prepared to work with "a variety of family issues and structures, such as single-parent or blended families, high-risk and dysfunctional families, and families in crisis or abusive situations" (Bramadat, Chalmers, & Andrusyszyn, 1996, p. 1229). Thus, family assessment and problem solving are an important part of the community nurse's tool kit. Community nurses also must be prepared to care for geriatric clients and their caregivers (Bramadat, Chalmers, & Andrusyszyn, 1996).

Much more "illness care" will be moving into the community; there is concern that unless current reimbursement policies are changed, illness care will continue to be most profitable and adequate support for programs that promote health and healthy lifestyles will not be forthcoming (Baldwin, 1995). Therefore, the traditional focus of community health nursing on wellness and health promotion must not be forsaken.

> As a nation, we have made certain that health promotion strategies have been included in the latest national health objectives, *Healthy People 2000* [Public Health Service, 1990] . . . It is clear that the present and future paradigm for health care is demanding that nursing's focus move toward, or at least begin to recognize the importance of, community health promotion if we are to forge ahead toward a health-promoting and wellness-achieving nation. (Baldwin, 1995, p. 159–162)

Baldwin's assertion should serve as a beacon to nurses as care in the community becomes increasingly important.

Information Technology

Computers have had a significant impact on all organizations, including hospitals (Fondiller & Nerone, 1996). The first information management systems to be used in hospitals were financial systems, coming on the scene in the early 1980s. Data management systems for such ancillary systems as pharmacy, radiology, dietetics, and admission and discharge soon proliferated. In their initial stages, these information management systems were basically stand-alone systems that had very little in common with each other. They functioned using entirely disparate computer languages and thus had no common means of communication or data sharing. In effect, this agglomeration of hospital hardware and software was a "nonsystem." However, it had one common characteristic—it all came to rest on the nurse's desk and it all had to be interpreted and applied by nurses.

Missing in the early configuration of information management systems in most hospitals was any kind of data management system to support nurses, their patient care, and their documentation requirements. Advanced information technology enables nurses and other clinicians to perform their duties more accurately, quickly, and sensitively (hence the term 'enabling technology'). The point-of-care system that frees nurses from tedious manual documentation activities is an example of enabling technology. The clinical data repository for clinical backup and decision making is another example. (Simpson, 1995, p. 88)

Conditions in many hospitals have improved considerably, but a marketing study conducted in 1995 by HBO & Company revealed that "of 400 hospitals with more than 100 beds, 99% had financial management systems in place . . . only 24% had nurse documentation systems; 14% had point-of-care documentation systems, and a paltry 9% had a clinical data repository." (Simpson, 1995, p. 88)

Among the reasons that the development of clinical data systems have bogged down is the lack of a universally accepted Nursing Minimum Data Set, one form of a taxonomy to support patient care.

COMPUTERIZED NURSING TAXONOMIES

Thompson (1996) stressed the importance of using informatics research to further the development of nursing taxonomies such as those discussed in Chapter 4. These include the North American Nursing Diagnosis Association taxonomy, the Nursing Minimum Data Set, the Iowa Intervention Project taxonomy, Susan Grobe's taxonomy for the classification of nursing interventions, and the home health care taxonomies developed by Virginia Saba and by the Omaha Visiting Nurses' Association.

Taxonomies are necessary if nursing is to participate productively in the evolving health care system. They can be used to standardize nursing language, to predict the use of nurses and other resources, and to increase nurses' understandings of their discipline and the relations among concepts. In other words, taxonomies can enhance quality, cost-effective care and further nursing science at the same time (Thompson, 1996).

As patients are cared for in an increasingly complex, multi-unit, multilevel environment, it is vital to maintain a longitudinal patient record. An integrated computer information system can help achieve that end. Thus, patient information must be standardized to facilitate its movement across computerized networks and to collate it into a meaningful record of care; all systems must use the same language in the same way. The use of nursing taxonomies provides a method for formalizing a lexicon that contains both consistent definitions and a common understanding of relations among concepts (Thompson, 1996).

The manner in which **nursing information systems** are structured will affect our understanding of nursing as a discipline and a practice. Although the ideas underlying **nursing informatics** (the use of computers in nursing clinical practice, administration, research, and education) and computer-based patient information systems may seem incongruent with the nursing ideal of holistic care for patients, many argue that this is not so. Rather, nursing informatics will allow us even broader options for the capture, storage, and retrieval of information that are entirely different than we have had before (Turley, 1996).

◼▶▶▶ **CRITICALLY THINKING ABOUT . . .**

In your college educational experiences, have you had experiences with computerized nursing information systems? What web sites useful to nurses can you find on the Internet? Describe and download something you find especially interesting.

EXPERT SYSTEMS FOR NURSING

Another area in which nursing informatics must move forward is the development of **expert systems**. Expert systems, a branch of applied artificial intelligence, has become possible through the use of powerful computers. Expert systems combine "human knowledge and heuristics (rule-of-thumb reasoning) to emulate the problem-solving behavior of human experts" (McFarland, 1995, p. 32). A limited number of expert systems have been developed in nursing. They have focused on nursing diagnosis, care planning, and patient assessment. Expert systems have proven very useful in other industries, but their development in nursing has been very slow. One major barrier is that no consensus has been reached concerning what constitutes "expertness" in diagnostic reasoning processes in nursing, so it is impossible to select expert nurses to serve as system models. A second barrier to the timely development of expert systems has been that nursing in general has been slow to support computerized technology (McFarland, 1995; Woolery, 1990; Ozbolt, 1988; Johnson, 1992).

NURSING INFORMATION SYSTEMS IN HOSPITAL-BASED HEALTH CARE

As the American health care system changes, so does nursing. "Changes in health care delivery include support for managed care, case management, quality improvement initiatives, and clinical outcomes management . . . The ideal information system will support these changes in nursing practice" (Willson & Neiswanger, 1996, p. 84).

One excellent example of how a well-designed information system supports nursing care in a multi-unit, multilevel health care system is the Intermountain Health Care (IHC) system, based in Salt Lake City, which provides medical and health care services to 2 million people in Utah, Idaho, and Wyoming. IHC is an integrated, not-for-profit system composed of three major groups—hospitals, physicians, and IHC health plans. IHC offers subscribers a choice among several different health care plans. The total network consists of 23 hospitals, 33 rural and urban clinics, 16 home health agencies, and many other ancillary agencies. IHC employs more than 225 physicians, who see patients in the hospitals and the neighborhood clinics.

The major hospitals in this system have installed a comprehensive hospital information system, Health Evaluation through Logical Processing (**HELP**) (Box 13-1). The HELP system (now marketed by 3M Corp.) is a fully integrated system: all parts of the system communicate with each other using a common patient data file. HELP interfaces with a logic database, providing the ability to generate alerts and to help in decision support.

On nursing units where HELP is fully installed, almost all nursing documentation is done entirely on the computer. By using the HELP system, nurses can achieve four primary goals that help them to meet the increasing demands of the changing health care environment:

1. This type of system can streamline the process of documentation. This is a significant contribution, because studies routinely show that nurses spend one third to one half of their time doing clerical work. "If health care reform is to accomplish anything, it should be the enhancement of the work of health care professionals so that an increasing percentage of professional time is spent on patient care and a decreasing percentage spent on paper care" (Korpman, 1994, p. 18).

Box 13-1

Clinical Applications Supported by the Health Evaluation through Logical Processing (HELP) Hospital Information System

Admission/discharge/transfer
Order entry
Results review
Respiratory therapy
Radiology-dictated results
Physician-dictated admission
 and discharge summary
Blood gas interpretations
Cardiac output interpretations
Infectious disease monitoring

*Medication scheduling
*Medication charting
*Medication teaching
*Patient documentation (intake, output, vital signs, physical assessment, activities, treatments, patient teaching)
*Problem or event documentation

*Applications used primarily by nurses (From Willson & Neiswanger, 1996)

2. Systems such as HELP can help nurses move toward a practice that is based on standards. "Competent professional care can be specified by the creation of standards that define who does what, when, where, and how" (Willson & Neiswanger, 1996, p. 89). Such standards include diagnosis-based standards of care, which are basically standard care plans for patients who fit into a particular diagnostic category.

3. Use of the HELP system at IHC hospitals also has facilitated nurses' access to standards and other reference information they need in making good clinical decisions. Graves and Corcoran (1988) reported that nurses spend a great deal of time searching for information such as patient-specific information, institutional policies, domain knowledge, and procedures. A good information system provides clinicians with direct online access to this kind of vital information in an efficient and timely manner.

4. A good information system can give clinicians access to data and information to support clinical and management decisions for which they are responsible. One advantage of an integrated information system is that data need to be entered only once, but they can be reported many times, either alone or in combination with associated data needed by different practitioners.

In hospitals where nurses have been designated as care managers, they need access not only to extensive patient data but also to data and information that will facilitate their management of the health care team for whom they bear responsibility. Nurses have a huge information management responsibility. The amount of information confronting nurses, who must make decisions about the care of individual patients and must coordinate the care of many patients as leaders of a health care team, is vast indeed. Those demands far exceed the limits of human capabilities for information processing. The role, therefore, of information systems is to assist nurses in selecting, acquiring, and managing data. The information system also must serve as a tool to assist in making inferences based on these data (Willson & Neiswanger, 1996, p. 94).

COMPUTERIZED INFORMATION SYSTEMS AND NURSING CARE IN THE COMMUNITY

Increasingly, computerized nursing information systems are being used to support the care of patients in ambulatory care settings and in their own homes. Patricia Brennan, a nurse who holds a doctoral degree in computer and information science engineering, has described how electronic computer networks can help nurses "initiate, facilitate, and sustain interpersonal contact with patients . . . Computer networks are electronic links between remote sites and as such provide a pathway for communication between nurses and patients" (Brennan, 1996, p. 97).

Brennan described an innovative project known as **ComputerLink**, an electronic network whose purpose is to provide home care support to patients with complex health problems and their family caregivers. A computer terminal is placed in the patient's home, and the patient and family members can use it whenever convenient. ComputerLink has three components: a communications module, an information module, and a decision support module. Using the communications module, users can gain access to private electronic mail; a bulletin board service (the Forum) where they can post and read messages; a question-and-answer section where users can post messages anonymously for response by a registered nurse moderator; and a private mail system. The role of the nurse moderator is to "facilitate communication through judicious observation and comments in the Forum discussion" (Brennan, 1996, p. 99). The information module, called the electronic encyclopedia, provides more than 200 indexed screens containing information about home care, selected illnesses, and descriptions of social services. The decision support module helps users make decisions by means of an analysis process that uses their own words and their own preferences. This helps people make choices consistent with their own values.

Brennan described two experiments evaluating the feasibility of ComputerLink as a means of delivering nursing intervention via electronic communication. The first trial involved 57 persons with acquired immunodeficiency syndrome (AIDS), and the second was carried out with 102 caregivers of people with Alzheimer's disease (AD). Separate ComputerLink networks were set up for each group, so only members of the same group could share information, and each group also had a condition-specific electronic encyclopedia. Most of the study subjects had no prior experience with a computer in the home, but about half had used them at work or school. The trials demonstrated that even people who were relatively to completely inexperienced could use ComputerLink. The communication services were used most often. AD caregivers tended to use the public features (the Forum) more often; the AIDS group tended to use private mail more often. Brennan reported that ComputerLink strengthened the decision-making confidence of users and improved some users' sense of receiving social support.

Brennan noted that if nurses are to use electronic communication effectively, they must tease out the "electronic equivalents" of unspoken communication that they would normally note in face-to-face or even telephone communication—body posture, pauses, loudness, and rate of speech. "Despite challenges of depersonalization and emotional distance, electronic communication appears surprisingly affective, purposeful, and particularistic" (Brennan, 1996, p. 100). Many of the messages posted were emotional, sometimes expressing despair, anger, frustration, and alienation. Electronic communication is purposeful, meaning that it requires the sender and receiver to turn on the computer and choose specific sections of ComputerLink. Electronic communication is "particularistic" because it was found that users developed unique patterns of using ComputerLink—some rarely, one person 1500 times in a 6-month period. Four user patterns were noted:

1. Early adopters used ComputerLink often, from the beginning to the end of their participation in the project.
2. Episodic users had long intervals (1 to 2 weeks) between log-ins.
3. Late adopters started slowly but increased their participation over time.
4. Negligible users made contact only a few times during the trial.

Overall, Brennan deemed the ComputerLink trials a success. She concluded:

Electronic networks hold great promise for nurses as they attempt to reach an ever-growing population in need of nursing care. . . . The demands of a society in need of nursing care can best be met by appropriate integration of technology into clinical practice. Technology that is congruent with nurses' core mission—interpersonal communication—is likely to be of greatest value. (Brennan, 1996, pp. 103–104)

Susan Grobe, another pioneer in nursing informatics, conducted a project at the University of Texas, Austin, to develop a taxonomy for classifying nursing interventions. The project was funded by the National Institute of Nursing Research and the National Library of Medicine. The use of nurses' natural language and the application of concepts and processes of linguistics were an important feature of her work. The resulting Nursing Intervention Lexicon and Taxonomy (NILT) consists of seven major intervention groups:

1. Care need determination
2. Care vigilance
3. Care environment management
4. Therapeutic care, general
5. Therapeutic care, psychosocial
6. Therapeutic care, cognitive understanding and control
7. Care information provision (Grobe, 1996).

Grobe (1996) has written about how NILT was used to describe patterns of care for patients receiving home care nursing. These patterns of care included nursing intensity, the frequency with which nursing interventions were carried out. The NILT intervention categories were used to define the focus of care. The comprehensiveness of care was reflected by the actual number of NILT categories recorded. Thus, in combination, these variables provided a means for quantifying patient care in a holistic way. The implications for documenting the nature and quality of nursing care delivered in the community so thoroughly and scientifically are exciting indeed. The availability of point-of-care technology such as portable computers, wireless technology, and database interoperability can make this kind of leap possible (Grobe, 1996; Andrew, 1995).

Roy Simpson (1996) has posed another exciting possibility regarding the potential impact of computer information systems in the context of community health: the probability that the Internet can supplant community health networks. He thinks this will happen. Issues of the security of identification and information, the accountability of users, and access have yet to be resolved, but he believes that will happen and that the Internet will serve as the central infrastructure for not only a community health information network but a global health information network. This suggests that the opportunities for nurses to extend their services widely into the community and educate specific populations are almost endless in the information age that carries us into the 21st century (Simpson, 1996).

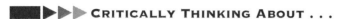 CRITICALLY THINKING ABOUT . . .

How can the Internet be used to help nurses carry out their tasks? Give two examples.

Bureaucratization and Nursing

As discussed earlier, a characteristic of bureaucratization is that organizations become increasingly complex in the activities they perform. This leads naturally to the creation of complex networks of organizational linkages to carry out activities efficiently and effectively. We see an example of this bureaucratization within health care as the rapid growth of managed care systems (see Chap. 10). Although hospitals have been the highly bureaucratized cores of the health care network, that is changing rapidly, and all segments of the care delivery system—health care workers, patients, and the public at large—are feeling the effects. Instead of having a single-unit focus (the hospital), the health care bureaucracy is developing rapidly into a complex, multiunit, multilevel system of health service delivery. There is no longer any "one-stop health care shopping."

Many physicians, nurses, and patients find this organizational shift troublesome. Many also have had experience with the negative aspects (listed earlier) that ever-more-complex bureaucracies can fall victim to.

In the name of efficiency and cost savings, managed care systems also contribute to a shifting of the nature of the relationship between the patient and the health care provider. This relationship has been a highly communal one throughout the history of American health care. In the past, patients chose their own physicians and often even their own specialists; that choice has been highly valued in our society. Physician–patient and nurse–patient relationships were highly personal, emphasizing the comfortable traditional roles of "dependent patient" and "all-knowing caregiver." As managed care systems become the dominant aspect of the health care landscape, the communal nature of the relationship is becoming more associational, and roles are shifting uncomfortably. For example, when a person is hospitalized, instead of being treated by his or her personal physician, he or she will probably be treated by one or more of the 30 or 40 physicians who are approved providers in a given health maintenance organization or practice—none of whom he or she has even seen before.

Although Americans may be uncomfortable with the increasingly complex bureaucracy of the health care system and the attendant transition from communal to associational relationships within that environment, managed care is here to stay. Admittedly, it causes problems for many nurses, but it also provides opportunities and challenges for nurses to find new and better ways of doing things and to develop new roles and talents.

Interactive Planning

Hospital nurses are facing a challenge brought on by the combination of delivering nursing care in a managed care environment, ever-expanding technology, and consumer concerns regarding the quality and cost of care. These have had the effect of requiring nurses to assimilate more accurate, reliable scientific knowledge into patient-centered care within a very limited time. "Nurses are expected to document [care] planning in an environment in which a written plan of care quickly becomes obsolete" (Foust, 1994, p. 129).

The planning of nursing care has been associated with the nursing process as a problem-solving approach. However, some have questioned its universal applicability because this approach does not include critical aspects of good clinical nursing practice, including intuitive, creative, and practical aspects. Others have argued that a nursing care plan is too limited to support holistic nursing practice (Foust, 1994). A viable alternative that has been suggested is a process of **interactive planning** that is founded on "a developmental perspective of people learning through planning in complex situations and environments of continuous change" (Foust, 1994, p. 129).

Three principles underlie interactive planning. First, no one in isolation can effectively plan for another person. Thus, effective planning must involve the patient, and the planning process becomes one of assuming shared responsibility for the outcomes. Second, planning is a continuous process, and revisions are part of planning. Finally, the underlying principle of holism dictates that information be drawn together from many sources. Thus, planning for care is a developmental activity for all participants.

A nurse who engages in interactive planning helps a patient and family plan for themselves. This represents a significant shift from the traditional "nurse-as-expert" role. The final product is the patient's plan, not the nurse's plan. This is highly appropriate in a time of increasingly shortened hospital stays because the patient and family will have a much more active role to play in the patient's full recovery. The nurse, while acting as a facilitator, also becomes a learner. Foust concluded that a "concerted focus on effective care planning by nurses will have the dual benefit of contributing to individualized patient care and our own professional future" (Foust, 1994, p. 131).

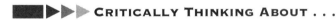 **CRITICALLY THINKING ABOUT . . .**

> How realistic do you think it is for a nurse in a hospital setting to engage in interactive planning with patients?

Nurse Case Manager Roles

It is clear that there has been a major shift in the health care paradigm from a system that was a patient-driven fee-for-service system to one that is a payer-driven, capitated managed care system. As noted earlier, a goal of this change has been to improve efficiency and increase accountability—two common goals of bureaucracies. To date, the shift has been a financial success. However, it still has some of the same limitations of the previous system because it still focuses on acute heath care needs. Thus, it is still inefficient and ineffective in dealing with the clients at the highest risk for requiring the most costly care—clients with highly complex or extended health care needs.

Roberta Conti, a faculty member in nursing administration, has proposed that case management using experienced nurses is the approach of choice for such clients.

Case managers can be employed by insurance companies or health maintenance organizations. Their recommendations and decisions take into account both the client's needs and the payer's policy. The case manager changes the plan of service whenever necessary but does not provide any direct care or treatment (Conti, 1996).

The role of the nurse case manager is a relatively recent one, so appropriate role behaviors and knowledge have yet to emerge. Conti, using the conceptual framework of "symbolic interactionism" developed by early sociologists, conducted a study to identify and understand the behaviors of nurse case managers. She first interviewed four practicing nurse case managers who worked for two national case management corporations in and around Washington DC. Using data from the interviews, Conti developed a questionnaire and mailed it to 100 other nurse case managers, 57 of whom returned completed forms.

Based on the interviews and surveys, Conti identified 16 "cluster labels" that were representative of nurse case manager roles (Box 13-2). She concluded that this is a relatively new job for nurses and requires nurses to assume multiple, complex roles for which they usually have not been prepared in their formal education. She predicted that the demand for nurse case managers will increase as more health care delivery systems turn to managed care. Clearly, these nurse case managers must be willing to "step out of traditional nursing roles and into one with minimal role definition" (Conti, 1996, p. 78). Thirteen of the 16 roles are typically not considered integral to nursing practice. In addition to their clinical knowledge, nurse case man-

---

Box 13-2
Cluster Labels as Representative of Nurse Case Manager Roles

Cluster Label Roles	Survey Respondents' Percent Selection Rate*
Public relator	100
Educator	99
Expeditor	98
Monitor	98
Problem solver	98
Explainer	98
Negotiator	97
Planner	97
Communicator	95
Contactor	92
Recommender	91
Broker	88
Researcher	88
Assessor	84
Documenter	82
Coordinator	82

*Selection rate = the frequency choice selection scores for the combination of choices "A" (almost all) and "B" (most). (From Conti, 1996, p. 78)

agers must understand business practices, must know how to integrate efficiency and effectiveness into the care of complex, long-term patients, and must have influential communication skills.

Conti cited Bureau of Labor Statistics projections that case management will be one of the fastest-growing positions within the health care professions—an increase of 250% by the year 2003. This means that the "nurse case manager will have significant application to health care reform policy and to the paradigm of managed care" (Conti, 1996, p. 79).

Nursing Managers in the Managed Care Future

For nursing to play a significant and positive role in the emerging managed care environment, there must be a radical change in the role of nurse managers. Nurse managers will still need the basic elements of nursing preparation, including strong preparation in the basic sciences, coursework to develop psychosocial and communication skills, and understanding of human values and ethics, and the practical, hands-on experience afforded by clinical internship. However, additional skills must be mastered, including budget development, cost accounting, and strategic planning. Anyone who expects to be a key player in the managed care system must know how to integrate financial and clinical knowledge. "Nurse managers must now make cost as well as care decisions, and too often they are ill-trained to confront money issues" (Moss, 1996, p. 132).

Mae Taylor Moss, a prominent nurse executive consultant, has written that the best preparation for nurses who are interested in moving into management and administration is a combination of a master's degree in nursing and a master's degree in business administration. Effective managers in service environments, such as health care institutions, must have skills that contribute to smooth transactions with their consumers (patients), their colleagues, ancillary area professionals, administrators, and the medical staff (Moss, 1996). Nurse managers will no longer function as "Lone Rangers" in their units; rather, they must assume a new role involving new relationships. "These new relationships can be summarized in the word 'teamsmanship'—the ability to function as a team with other stakeholders, with the single goal of providing enhanced patient care based on maximized resource utilization" (Moss, 1996, p. 132).

Moss identified a "core orientation" curriculum for nurse managers (Box 13-3) that looks very different from the traditional preparation for leadership in nursing. For many years, we assumed that by the time a nurse had reached managerial status, he or she was well equipped for the job by way of experience and clinical expertise. However, in managed care, that assumption is no longer valid. The new environment demands new skills and at the same time presents new opportunities for nursing leadership. Nurses must become proactive in looking for ways to streamline costs while continuing to provide quality and cost-effective care (Sherman & Jones, 1995; Nowicki, 1996). Nursing managers and administrators have the opportunity and responsibility to lead the way in this endeavor, because if nursing doesn't take responsibility for cutting nursing costs, someone else will.

Opportunities at the Crossroads

In 1996, Sister Rosemary Donley, a prominent nursing leader, presented an articulate, thought-provoking discussion of the crossroads to which the American health care system has come since the end of World War II. She suggested that there are three possible directions to travel.

Box 13-3
Core Orientation Curriculum for Nurse Managers

  I. Communications skills
 II. Changes in the workplace
   A. Mastering change
   B. Diversity
   C. Dealing with generation gaps in the workplace
III. Leadership in the workplace
   A. Training for the trainers
   B. Project management
   C. Leading people
   D. Nonmoney motivations
 IV. Problem solving and decision making
  V. Conflict management
 VI. Budget, finance, and accounting
VII. Effective personnel interviewing
VIII. Patient care in the 21st century
 IX. Ethics in managed care
  X. Computer skills
 XI. Benchmarking
XII. Strategic planning
   A. Mission
   B. Performance goals
   C. Strategies
   D. Action plans

(Moss MT, 1996)

The first path—the safest and most predictable—is the path that is most congruent with the driving forces of bureaucratization, and thus is the path that most nurses will be following into the 21st century. This path is a continuation of the road we are already traveling on—the merging of traditional and managed care philosophies. On that broad road, there is room for many alternative delivery plans to emerge. In multi-unit, multilevel systems, the development of information systems will become a key element in the smooth functioning of the integrated health delivery network, and nurses must play a key role in developing those information and communication systems.

The second road that Donley foresaw leads to an alternative health care system where "people are encouraged, inspired, and taught to bear responsibility for their well-being . . . [These] travelers . . . elect more than a health care system. They espouse a discipline and a way of life" (Donley, 1996, p. 328).

The third road leads to a community-based system of health care delivery similar to that in the United Kingdom. Such a system is supported by conservative attitudes about therapy. Indeed, "tertiary care is a last resort, not a first intervention . . . Conservative treatment and watchful waiting replace intrusive and radical treatments" (Donley, 1996, p. 329).

Donley acknowledged that there is a fourth alternative—simply staying in the middle of the crossroads, choosing no path at all. However, she observed, "given the dissonance and turmoil, it is hard to believe that one can stand very long in the crossroads" (Donley, 1996, p. 329).

Donley described the differences in practice emphasis for nurses opting for these different paths. Nurses who continue onto the first path—the merging of traditional and managed care (and that will be most nurses)—will be required to assume different roles than they have before. Nurses will still be practitioners, but they also will be health care team directors, information analyzers, and system managers. All nurses functioning in an integrated care delivery network, not just nursing administrators, must have more marketing and business insights, greater facility with data systems, and skills in implementing research programs to test the success of cost-containment measures and to measure the quality of care delivered (Donley, 1996, p. 329).

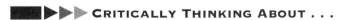 **CRITICALLY THINKING ABOUT . . .**

Do you think the crossroads analogy is appropriate to discuss changes in health care?

Urbanization and Nursing

Two of the major features of urbanization are social diversity and multiculturalism.

Social diversity involves a multiplicity of lifestyles based on differences among people in socioeconomic status, commitment to traditional family values and forms, and philosophies about what things are socially appropriate and what things are not. In cities, we find such diverse lifestyles as the gay community, traditional families with mothers staying at home, families with mothers working, childless couples, and aging seniors. There also are highly varied social worlds such as those of bodybuilders, symphony musicians, stamp collectors, Ironman competitors, and rock groupies. Further, the city is home to an array of social worlds that are deviant, and, in some cases, criminal: violent gangs, drug traffickers, and organized crime. In addition to all these, occupational groups have their own social worlds. Bankers, laborers, and elementary teachers seldom have much in common and spend little time together, choosing rather to be with "their own kind."

Cities are also multicultural. **Multiculturalism** means there are many ethnic groups, each with its own lifestyle, values, concerns, and philosophies. In Los Angeles, for example, more than 100 languages are spoken. The degree of variability in language alone poses a significant challenge to health care workers in the urban environment. Highly varied ethnic groups often come into competition and conflict with each other over jobs, housing, and services from the local government. For a city to function reasonably, these groups must work out accommodations with each other; otherwise, chaos and disorder rule. Groups need to view each other as significant elements in the complex mosaic that is the city. In Toronto, the most ethnically heterogeneous city in the world, residents proudly celebrate the ethnic diversity of their city.

Earlier in the 20th century, the concept of the "melting pot" was a dominant theme. According to adherents of the melting-pot concept, the differences between new Americans coming from vastly different cultures would eventually be erased because a fundamental goal of immigrant populations was to become acculturated into the dominant American culture. In other words, it was very important to them to speak, act, and look like Americans rather than Italians or Germans or Irish. The melting pot idea seemed to work for the immigrants from Europe. However, since the 1940s, the United States has received an increasingly large share of immigrants from Asia, Latin America, the Caribbean, and the Pacific Rim. It has become increasingly clear that the melting pot theory works only partly today. Instead of melting, more recent immigrant groups are maintaining a unique identity while participating to varying degrees in the mainstream economy and politics of American society.

More than 75% of Americans live in metropolitan communities, and there is little reason to suggest that this rural-to-urban shift of the population will abate. Moreover, immigrants to this country typically cluster in cities, adding even further to the urban character of the United States. Thus, most nurses will be working in urban environments. Those who work in the city itself will work in an environment characterized by a high degree of social diversity and multiculturalism. The demands of working in such diverse settings have significant implications for nursing education and clinical practice.

Nursing Education and Culturally Competent Care

Nursing educators bear a significant responsibility for preparing nurses who can provide **culturally competent care** to an increasingly multicultural clientele. In the early 1990s, three major nursing organizations (the American Nurses Association, the American Association of Colleges of Nursing, and the National League for Nursing) together developed strategies that colleges of nursing could use to develop and implement curriculum innovations that would help meet that goal. They urged that cultural diversity be more broadly defined beyond the inclusion of the traditionally defined minority groups such as Asians, Hispanics, Native Americans, or African-Americans. Instead, the term should also include women when they experience minority status and men in nursing and their related issues. Minorities also should mean groups of people with lifestyles that vary from those of the dominant population due to, for instance, their religion, employment status, or sexual orientation (Princeton, 1993). All these factors affect the development of nursing curricula that maximize students' opportunities to develop the knowledge and skills necessary for providing culturally competent care.

This call for action prompted many colleges of nursing to develop and implement curricular changes that would contribute to multiculturalism (Lindquist, 1990; Smith, Colling, Elander, & Latham, 1993). Lorraine Culley, an English nurse educator, cautioned nurse educators everywhere not to be casual or cavalier about the development of meaningful content and experiences. She pointed out that if health care is to be truly nonracist, nurses and other health care workers must understand the broader concepts of culture and cultural differences, as well as the ways in which services can be made more accessible to minority groups. She noted that nurses must be aware of the dangers of attributing cause directly to ethnicity alone (Culley, 1996).

Nursing educators and administrators also bear responsibilities for recruiting and retaining larger numbers of minority students to meet the care needs of America's increasingly racially diverse population (this was discussed in Chapter 7 as one of the challenges facing contemporary nursing education). Karine Crow, a transcultural nurse consultant, notes that the culture of nursing is transmitted through nursing education and academia. The world view of nursing education and academia is largely the same as that of the culture that is dominant in America—the Anglo middle-class culture. Thus, the educational focus of nursing education and academia is congruent with the overall values of Anglo middle-class culture. In other words, the focus is linear, sequential, and time-ordered—one is expected to maintain thoughts that are orderly (linear) and logical (sequential), and one adheres to schedules to be considered responsible (time-ordered). The Anglo middle-class culture also values individualism, competition, and dualism and has a commitment to the domination of nature. Thus, people who strike out on their own (individualism) and achieve success by competing with others (competition) are admired. From this perspective there is only right or wrong, each question has only one correct answer (dualism), and people try to master their own environment.

This entire orientation is completely at odds with the world view of people from many other cultures. Crow contrasts this world view with that of Native Americans to show how students who are not acculturated into this world view can be at a serious disadvantage in nursing education. One example is a difference in time orientation. Academia is highly time-ordered: events are scheduled and ruled by clock time. Things start at a given time and end at a given time. Being responsible means showing up on time. The Native American world view, however, is one of event orientation: the appropriate time to start an event is when everyone has arrived, and everyone stays until the event is complete. Clock time is irrelevant. Thus, in a class or clinical setting, a student who has an event orientation may be late according to clock time, but will stay after the scheduled amount of time has passed because he or she has not yet experienced complete learning. Cultural mismatches such as this can put a student's success in jeopardy.

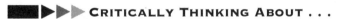 **CRITICALLY THINKING ABOUT . . .**

What do you think would be the best way for nursing programs to include multiculturalism throughout the curriculum?

Culturally Competent Care In Nursing Practice

Nurses' knowledge about and attitudes toward patients who are culturally different from themselves can be an important factor in the extent to which they can provide culturally competent care. Linda Rooda (1993) examined the knowledge and attitudes regarding patients of diverse cultural backgrounds among 274 nurses who practiced in a community rich in cultural diversity. The entire respondent group contained 11% nonwhite nurses, but their small numbers did not permit meaningful statistical analysis, so the nurses whose data were reported were all white. Almost 97% of the nurses were women, and the average length of time in nursing practice was 15 years. Rooda administered the Cultural Fitness Survey to the nurses and reported four major findings:

1. The nurses knew more about the culture and health care practices of Asian-Americans than those of Hispanics and African-Americans.
2. Their knowledge about culturally different patients differed by educational preparation. Baccalaureate graduates had less knowledge about minority patients than did associate degree or diploma graduates.
3. The nurses expressed different attitudes toward the cultures and health practices of these ethnic groups. Ranging from most to least positive, the ranking was whites, African-Americans, Asian-Americans, and Hispanics.
4. The nurses' cultural biases seemed to be consistent with their knowledge about the different minority groups. Associate degree graduates were less biased toward Hispanics than either diploma or baccalaureate graduates.

Margaret Andrews and Joyceen Boyle (1997) identified strategies practicing nurses can use to develop their ability to evaluate and anticipate culture-based differences in patient behavior. They identified four important components of effective transcultural nursing care: cultural assessment, understanding culture values, communicating with family members and significant others, and overcoming communication barriers. **Cultural nursing assessment** means systematically appraising people, groups, and communities in relation to their cultural beliefs, values, and practices. This will help the nurse determine the specific needs and intervention practices that are suitable within the patient's cultural context. Cultural assessment consists of both process (verbal and nonverbal communication and the order in which data are gathered) and content (the actual data gathered about patients). They identify three cultural assessment tools that could be used, but the one they describe most fully is Bloch's assessment guide (Box 13-4). Within the Bloch guide, each data category also contains questions and instructions.

To provide excellent nursing care that is culturally competent, the nurse must examine **culture values**, the "powerful, persistent, and directive forces that give meaning, order, and direction to the individual's, group's, family's, or community's actions, decisions, and lifeways, usually over a span of time" (Andrews & Boyle, p. 16AAA). For example, loyalty to one's group is the highest value among many Asian, Islamic, and tribal societies; accordingly, the welfare of an individual is subservient to whatever is best for the group. In contrast, as noted earlier, the dominant American culture emphasizes the rights of the individual.

Box 13-4
Assessment Guide for Ethnic and Cultural Variation

Cultural Data Categories

Ethnic origin
Race
Place of birth
Relocations
Habits
Customs, values, beliefs
Behaviors valued by culture
Cultural sanctions and restrictions
Language and communication
    processes
Healing beliefs and practices
Nutritional variables or factors

Psychological Data Categories

Self-concept
Mental and behavioral processes
Religious influences
Psychological responses to illness
Cultural responses to illness

Sociologic Data Categories

Economic status
Educational status
Social network
Family as supportive group
Supportive institutions in community
Institutional racism

Biologic and Physiologic Data Categories

Racial anatomic characteristics
Growth and development patterns
Variations in body systems
Skin and hair physiology
Diseases prevalent in ethnic group
Disease resistance in ethnic group

(Bloch B, 1991)

Andrews and Boyle pointed out variability in culture values in such diverse areas as orderliness, cleanliness, the nature of truth and deception, and stealing. It is also understood that a nurse who delivers culturally competent care is aware of his or her own cultural values, attitudes, beliefs, and practices (Andrews & Boyle, 1997).

Sensitivity and skill in communication with family members and significant others is critical in providing culturally competent care. There is a great deal of variation among cultures as to exactly who makes up a patient's significant others and who may be responsible for making the decisions regarding his or her health care. In a culture in which familism—an orientation that emphasizes interdependence (rather than independence), affiliation (rather than confrontation), and cooperation (rather than competition)—is a dominant value, it may be understood that the family rather than the individual patient makes the decisions about care.

One should not even make assumptions about exactly who constitutes the family. The understanding of sibling relationships varies with cultures. In Anglo-American culture, siblingship is understood to be based on shared parentage, but in some Asian cultures, the sibling relationship means that they were breast-fed as infants by the same woman. The culturally competent nurse must be able to discern the nature of the relationships and understand them within the context of the patient's cultural stance (Andrews & Boyle, 1997).

To provide culturally competent care, nurses may have to overcome significant communication barriers. Andrews and Boyle pointed out that communication—really understanding what a patient's words and actions mean—involves much more than language differences. Much of the challenge of interpreting a patient's communications to nurses and other caregivers arises from the **sick-role orientation** to which persons have been socialized in different cultures. A sick-role orientation involves the expectations that everyone, including the patient, has regarding the proper way for a sick person to behave. People are socialized into their culture's sick role very early in life.

In our society, adherence to the sick role means undemanding compliance with care providers' directives, providing any information the provider requests (no matter how personal or demeaning), having a respectful attitude toward the provider, and performing the behaviors that are requested. A little (or even a lot) of deference toward authority figures (such as nurses and physicians) is the expectation.

Not all cultures view the sick role in the same way, so nurses must be wary of interpreting communication behaviors—both verbal and nonverbal—in light of the dominant American culture's version of the proper sick role. Within the illness episode, culturally acceptable sick-role behavior may range from being aggressive and demanding to being passive and silent (Andrews & Boyle, 1997).

Andrews and Boyle concluded that the greatest challenge in providing culturally competent care is to be fully aware of the great diversity in the expressions, meanings, and referents of care across diverse cultures. It is this awareness that permits—indeed, compels—the nurse to "see" the patient as a product of his or her culture and to respond to the care needs of that patient in the most sensitive, culturally appropriate, and efficacious manner.

 CRITICALLY THINKING ABOUT . . .

How important is it today for nurses to be fluent in two or more languages? Are you multilingual? Why or why not?

Globalization and International Nursing

As stated earlier, globalization is the process through which societies increasingly become networked together in a world system. Through this network, goods, materials, and people are exchanged regularly, as are diseases. This has been true since the time of the European traders visiting China, through the European conquests of the Americas, and into the current time. As global travel becomes faster and accessible to increasing numbers of people, the worldwide spread of diseases in a very short time becomes more of a threat. We read regularly of terrifying outbreaks of Ebola, dengue hemorrhagic fever, Hataan viruses, cholera, and other exotic diseases.

This trend has health officials struggling to understand the latest outbreaks of diseases that were thought to be sharply diminishing in scope and severity. These same officials now find themselves mobilizing resources to fight these ancient killers, generally known as **infectious parasitic diseases (IPDs)**. IPDs are a major cause of death and disability in low-income countries. In developed countries, IPDs are reemerging as a serious health problem. When smallpox was finally eradicated in the 1970s, many health experts believed that IPDs would be eradicated too, but obviously it did not work out that way (*Population Today*, 1997).

Public health workers and the general public were shocked in the 1980s with the discovery of the human immunodeficiency virus (HIV), which causes AIDS. Neither medical knowledge nor the organization of health care delivery systems of rich or poor nations could cope with this new, lethal, global disease. The emergence of AIDS and the discovery of new strains of cholera, hemorrhagic fever, meningitis, multidrug-resistant tuberculosis, and other bacterial infections has caused health officials and scientists in many countries to join in widespread international health campaigns such as those coordinated by the World Health Organization and UNICEF (Olshansky, Carnes, Rogers, & Smith, 1997).

Nursing leaders the world over recognize the importance of enhancing global health through global cooperation and communication on matters of shared concern. In June 1997, more than 5000 nurses from 120 countries met at the 21st Quadrennial Congress of the **International Council of Nurses** in Vancouver, British Columbia, to discuss the direction of health care internationally and the role of nurses worldwide. The more than 600 nurses making up the American contingent found that their concerns were similar to those expressed by nurses from other countries: the use of unlicensed assistive personnel, declining financial resources, the debate over euthanasia, and the care of persons with HIV/AIDS.

A main theme of the congress was a call for nurses to exercise their leadership abilities as they advocate for high-quality care across the globe. The keynote speaker, Gloria R. Smith, a nurse who serves as vice president for programs at the Kellogg Foundation, told the attendees:

> Your leadership is essential, first, because the healthcare system and the health of people are dependent on the nurse as on no other profession. Your leadership is essential, second, because nurses have the resourcefulness, the flexibility in the face of challenge, and the critical thinking skills to discover and mobilize rich resources that others may have overlooked. (Helmlinger, 1997, p. 24)

In reporting on the congress, Connie Helmlinger of the American Nurses Association noted that nurses are working worldwide to break down barriers to health care. They are expanding into new territory to ensure continuity of care for patients.

Barbara Vaughn, program director of the United Kingdom's Kings Fund, described nurse-led clinics that deal with a range of health problems, including breast cancer, rheumatology, services for groups such as the homeless, and contraception use and HIV/AIDS among adolescents.

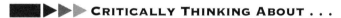 **CRITICALLY THINKING ABOUT . . .**

Have you visited health care delivery sites in other countries? If so, how do they compare to ours?

Rationalization and Nursing

At the heart of the process of rationalization is the idea that when people confront problems or new challenges, they do not automatically rely on traditional formulas. Instead, they engage in a process of **critical thinking**, which involves the following:

1. When confronted with an unusual or unique situation, one attempts to identify all its elements clearly.
2. One searches the professional literature in one's field and that of others to see what past reactions to the problem have been.
3. One identifies the variety of underlying beliefs held by people about the situation.
4. One identifies the reasons that support the beliefs.
5. One identifies values that are in conflict or in agreement with the situation.
6. One assesses the resources that are relevant and available to solve the problem.
7. One reaches a plan of action after evaluating alternatives.
8. One translates the plan of action into a series of behaviors aimed at solving the problem.
9. One evaluates the consequences of the actions and reformulates the plan of action accordingly.

It is through countless repetitions of this process that nursing knowledge, nursing science, and nursing practice have evolved to their current state. In a nursing context, critical thinking has been defined as "reflective and reasonable thinking about nursing problems without a single solution and focused on deciding what to believe and do" (Kataoka-Yahiro & Saylor, 1994, p. 352). Critical thinking has become a valued part of the nursing process and the development of sound clinical judgment (Oermann, 1997). It also is the foundation for the development of nursing knowledge and the growth of nursing research.

In addition to its application to the nursing process and clinical decision making, critical thinking underlies the entire process of the professionalization of nursing. Florence Nightingale was one of the preeminent critical thinkers of her time. Her heritage lives today in the actions of professional nursing organizations who rightly question and challenge current health care delivery decisions and propose new and creative alternatives to improve patient care. Because critical thinking is such an important part of the professionalization process, nursing students must understand the process and have regular opportunities to engage in it to hone their skills.

▶ CHAPTER SUMMARY

A great social transformation is occurring all over the world and will continue to develop well into the 21st century. Five primary societal forces are converging to affect all elements of American society, including the health care system in general and nursing in particular: industrialization, bureaucratization, urbanization, globalization, and rationalization. Taken together, these forces are reshaping societies the world over from being communal societies (characterized by an emphasis on tradition, informal and highly personalized relationships, and a consensus on important values) to being associational societies (characterized by an emphasis on rational thought, highly formalized and impersonalized relationships, and conflict over fundamental values).

Social change is continually creating new problems and issues for nursing to deal with. To confront these challenges successfully, nursing must mobilize its resources, must engage in creative critical thinking, and must use its collective power to effect positive, lasting changes in the health care system. The essence of this process is the day-to-day cooperation among nurses in confronting these challenges in a way that mobilizes their talents and magnifies the efforts of all. Through their joint activities in working toward common goals, the professionalization of nursing is advanced, and nursing itself becomes increasingly identified in the public eye as a significant health care profession contributing to the well-being of all.

KEY POINTS

▶ 1 **A great social transformation is occurring worldwide and will continue. Five primary forces are converging to affect all elements of American society, including the health care system and nursing in particular. Communal societies (characterized by an emphasis on tradition, informal and highly personalized relationships, and a consensus on important values) are evolving into associational societies (characterized by an emphasis on rational thought, highly formalized and impersonalized relationships, and conflict over fundamental values).**

▶ 2 **Industrialization is the force that brings about the reorganization of a society's economic base so that it becomes built on assembly line, mass production, production in large factories, a work force characterized by a highly specialized division of labor, and highly mechanized methods of transportation and communication.**

▶ 3 **Bureaucratization is the process through which human organizations grow, develop a complex division of labor, create a hierarchical power and decision-making structure, develop explicit and written rules for worker performance, develop a reward system for workers based on job performance, and create an extensive system of performance records.**

▶ 4 **Urbanization is the process through which, over time, an increasingly larger percentage of the population lives in cities due to rural-to-urban migration and immigration from other countries.**

▶ 5 **Globalization is the process through which people and societies become knit together through economic and political ties. A global society is one** that engages in trade with other societies, holds memberships in regional and worldwide political pacts, and exchanges people and goods with many countries.

▶ 6 Rationalization means that society's members come to place an emphasis on rational thought rather than on tradition in understanding the world, in identifying problems to be solved, and in planning actions to be undertaken.

▶ 7 A fundamental property of bureaucratization is that organizations become increasingly complex in the activities they perform, thereby leading to the creation of complex networks of organizational linkages to carry out activities efficiently and effectively. Within health care, this is evidenced by the rapid growth of managed care systems. Instead of having a single-unit focus (the hospital), the health care bureaucracy is developing rapidly into a complex, multi-unit, multilevel system of health service delivery. New nursing roles are emerging, and existing nursing roles are changing in terms of their nature and importance.

▶ 8 The industrial society gave us the hospital industry as we have known it—large-scale, high-tech, and physically centralized. Our society is moving from the industrial into the postindustrial period. Among the consequences of this change for nursing is the nucleation of the health care service delivery system and the increasing importance of high-tech communication, which is needed to link the nucleated units. The delivery of care in the community will gain greater importance, as will the role of nursing information technologies. Both of these trends are inextricably linked.

▶ 9 Two of the major features of urbanization are social diversity and multiculturalism. Nursing educators bear a significant responsibility for preparing nurses who can provide culturally competent care to an increasingly multicultural clientele. Culturally competent care has four important components: cultural assessment, understanding culture values, communicating with family members and significant others, and overcoming communication barriers.

▶10 Globalization has a significant impact on health in that the threat of worldwide epidemics is considerably greater than when societies were relatively isolated from each other. World health officials must be ever-vigilant. Nursing leaders the world over recognize the importance of enhancing global health through global cooperation and communication on matters of shared concern. They have formed the International Congress of Nursing to exercise their leadership abilities as they advocate for high-quality care around the globe.

▶11 At the heart of the process of rationalization is the idea that when people confront problems or new challenges, they do not automatically rely on traditional formulas. Instead, they engage in a process of critical thinking. Critical thinking is a key to professionalization: it is the responsibility of truly professional nurses to question and challenge current health care delivery decisions and propose new and creative alternatives to improve patient care.

REFERENCES

Andrew WF (1995). Applied information technology: A clinical perspective. Feature focus: The continuum of interoperability. *Computers in Nursing, 13*, 38–40.

Andrews MM, Boyle JS (1997). Competence in transcultural nursing care. *AJN, 97*(8), 16.

Baldwin JH (1995). Are we implementing community health promotion in nursing? *Public Health Nursing, 12*, 159–164.

Bloch B (1991). Cultural influences. In G. Cole (Ed.), *Basic Nursing Skills and Concepts* (pp. 75–79). St. Louis: Mosby–Year Book.

Bramadat IJ, Chalmers K, Andrusyszyn MA (1996). Knowledge, skills and experiences for community health nursing practice: The perceptions of community nurses, administrators, and educators. *J Advanced Nursing, 24*, 1224–1233.

Brennan PF (1996). The future of clinical communication in an electronic environment. *Holistic Nursing Practice, 11*(1), 97–104.

Brinkerhof DB, White LK, Riedmann AC (1997). *Sociology* (4th ed.). Belmont, CA: Wadsworth Publishing Company.

Conti RM (1996). Nurse case manager roles: Implications for practice and education. *Nursing Administration Quarterly, 21*, 67–80. *J Advanced Nursing, 23*, 564–570.

Culley L (1996). A critique of multiculturalism and health care: The challenge for nurse education. *J Advanced Nursing, 23*, 564–570.

Curry T, Jiobu R, Schwirian K (1997). *Sociology for the 21st Century*. Upper Saddle River, NJ: Prentice-Hall.

Donley R (1996). Nursing at the crossroads. *Nursing Economics, 14*(6), 325–331.

Fondiller SH, Nerone BJ (1996). Preparing for nursing's future. *AJN, 96*(9), 16.

Foust JB (1994). Creating a future for nursing through interactive planning at the bedside. *Image: J Nursing Scholarship, 26*, 129–132.

Graves JR, Corcoran S (1988). Identification of data element categories for clinical nursing information systems via information analysis of nursing practice. In *Proceedings of the 12th Annual Symposium on the Computer Applications in Medical Care*. Los Alamitos, CA: IEEE Computer Society Press.

Grobe SJ (1996). The nursing interventions lexicon and taxonomy: Implications for representing nursing care data in automated patient records. *Holistic Nursing Practice, 11*, 48–63.

Helmlinger C (1997, July–August). International meeting focuses on nursing's role in next century. *American Nurse*, 24.

Hoult TF (1969). *Dictionary of Modern Sociology*. Totowa, NJ: Littlefield, Adams Co.

Infectious diseases continue to threaten world health (1997). *Population Today: News, Numbers, and Analysis, 25*(7/8), 1–2.

Johnson J (1992). Computers in nursing in the year 2000. *Computers in Nursing, 10*, 143–144.

Korpman RA (1994). Integrated patient-centered computing: Operations optimization for the 21st century. *Topics in Health Information Management, 14*, 11–23.

Kuennen J, Moss VA (1995). Community program planning: A clinical outcome. *J Nursing Ed, 34*, 387–389.

Lindquist GJ (1990). Integration of international and transcultural content in nursing curricula: A process for change. *J Professional Nursing, 6*, 272–279.

Moss MT (1996). Perioperative nursing in the managed care era. Preparing nurse managers for a managed care future. *Nursing Economics, 14*, 132–133.

Nowicki CR (1996). 21 predictions for the future of hospital staff development. *J Continuing Education in Nursing, 27,* 259–266.

Olshansky SJ, Carnes B, Rogers RG, Smith L (1997). Infectious diseases—new and ancient threats to world health. *Population Bulletin, 52,* No. 2.

Ozbolt J (1988). Knowledge-based systems for supporting clinical nursing decisions. In Ball M, Hannah K, Gerdin-Jelger U, Peterson H (Eds.), *Nursing Informatics: Where Caring and Technology Meet.* New York: Springer-Verlag, pp. 274–285.

Princeton JC (1993). Promoting culturally competent nursing education. *J Nursing Education, 32,* 195–197.

Rooda LA (1993). Knowledge and attitudes of nurses toward culturally different patients: Implications for nursing education. *J Nursing Education 32*(5), 209–213.

Schardin KE (1995). Creating an environment for positive patient outcomes: An interview with Beverly Malone. *ANNA Journal, 22,* 289–293.

Sherman JJ, Jones CB (1995). The bottom line: Determining costs to allocate nursing resources. *Nursing Policy Forum, 1*(4), 14.

Simpson RL (1995). To retool the workplace, you'd better have the right technology tools. *Nursing Administration Quarterly, 20,* 87–89.

Simpson RL (1996). Technology: Nursing the system. Will the Internet supplant community health networks? *Nursing Management, 27*(2), 20–23.

Smith BE, Colling K, Elander E, Latham C (1993). A model for multicultural curriculum development in baccalaureate nursing education. *J Nursing Education, 32,* 205–208.

Thompson CB (1996). Research to support holistic nursing taxonomies. *Holistic Nursing Practice, 11,* 31–38.

Turley J (1996). Nursing decision making and the science of the concrete. *Holistic Nursing Practice, 11,* 6–14.

Wallerstein I (1979). *The Capitalist World Economy.* New York: Cambridge University Press.

Willson D, Neiswanger M (1996). Information system support of changes in health care and nursing practice. *Holistic Nursing Practice, 11,* 84–96.

Woolery L (1990). Expert nurses and expert systems. *Computers in Nursing, 8,* 23–28.

RECOMMENDED READINGS

Andrews MM (1997). Competence in transcultural nursing care. *AJN, 97*(8), 16.

Bulger RJ (1996). Old wine in new bottles—nursing in the 21st century. *J Professional Nursing, 12,* 338–348.

Donley R (1995). Advanced practice nursing after health care reform. *Nursing Economics, 13,* 84–88.

Graves JR, Corcoran-Perry S (1996). The study of nursing informatics. *Holistic Nursing Practice, 11,* 15–24.

Hillestad EA, Hawken PL (1996). Nursing in the year 2000. *J Professional Nursing, 12,* 127–128.

McCrone SH (1996). The impact of the evolution of biological psychiatry on psychiatric nursing. *J Psychosocial Nursing and Mental Health Services, 34*(1), 38–49.

Wells M (1994). The future perioperative role. *Nursing Management, 28,* 32E.

INDEX

Note: Page numbers in *italics* indicate illustrations; those followed by *t* indicate tables; and those followed by *b* indicate boxed material.

A

Abdellah, Faye, 36t
Aber, C.S., 38
An Abstract for Action, 23
Accountability, 294
Accreditation, 120, 166–170
  by American Association of Colleges of Nursing, 168–170
  changes in, 168–170
  definition of, 166
  government requirements for, 168–169
  by National League for Nursing, 167–169
  voluntary, 166–167
Acquired immunodeficiency syndrome (AIDS), bioethical issues in, 298–300
An Activity Analysis of Nursing, 22
Adaptation theory, 42
Admitting privileges, for advanced practice nurses, 280, 281
Advanced nursing practice, 143–151, 215–235
  admitting privileges in, 280, 281
  barriers to, 225–226, 280–281, 285
  certified registered nurse anesthetists in, 145t, 149, *217,* 218–219
  challenges to, 225–226
  client teaching in, 233
  clinical nurse specialists in, 145t, 147–148, *217,* 220–222, 225–226
  culturally sensitive care in, 229–231
  educational preparation for, 142–143, 150–151
  evolution of, 218–225
  general systems theory in, 232
  for high-risk and vulnerable populations, 229–231
  knowledge base for, 232–234
  managed care and, 251–253, 258
  models of, 226–229
  number of nurses in, 145t, *217*
  nurse-managed workplace care in, 227–229
  nurse-midwives in, 145t, 148–149, *217,* 219–220
  nurse practitioners in, 145t, 145–147, *217,* 222–225, *224*
  pathways for, *145,* 150–151
  patient-clinician partnership in, 227
  political action for, 280–281, 285
  prescriptive authority in, 223–225, *224,* 281
  primary care in, 227–229
  professionalization in, 215–235
  regulation of, 223–225, *224,* 280
  reimbursement in, 223, 225, 285
  role responsibilities in, 231, 232b
  role theory in, 233
  salaries for, 145t
  scope of practice in, 223–225, *224,* 280–281
  teaching-learning theory in, 233
Advocacy, 49, 295

African-Americans. *See* Racial minorities
AIDS, bioethical issues in, 298–300
Almshouses, 191
Alster, Kristine, 249, 250
Ambulatory care settings, 196–199
American Academy of Nursing, 19
American Association of Colleges of Nursing (AACN), 12, 163–164
  accreditation by, 168–170
American Association of Nurse Anesthetists (AANA), 218
American College of Nurse-Midwives (ACNM), 148–149, 220
American Journal of Nursing (AJN), 63
  patient care survey of, *247,* 247–249, 248t
American Nurses Association (ANA), 17–19
  American Nurses Credentialing Center of, 147
  Code of Ethics of, 292–293, 293b
  collective bargaining by, 12, 18
  Committee on Education of, 23
  credentialing and, 24
  entry into practice and, 23–24, 125, 161–162
  health care reform task force of, 276–280, 278b
  initiatives of, 18–19, 19b
  membership of, 18
  Men Nurses Section of, 20
  nursing definition of, 104
  nursing information classification systems and, 104
  nursing research and, 66–67
  Nursing's Agenda for Health Care Reform, 278b, 278–279
  Political Action Committee of, 19–20
  political activity of, 19–20, 268–269, 273–274, 276–280
  position statements of, 19b, 23
    on entry into practice, 23–24, 125
  report card study of, 251, 285
  social policy statements of, 274
  standards of practice and, 104
American Nurses Credentialing Center, 147
American Nurses Foundation (ANF), 19, 66
Amos, Linda, 169
ANA. *See* American Nurses Association (ANA)
ANA-PAC, 279
Anderson, Carole, 145–146
Andrews, Margaret, 336, 337
Anesthetists, certified registered nurse, 145t, 149, *217,* 218–220. *See also* Advanced nursing practice
Anesthetizers, 218
Annual Review of Nursing Research, 68
Anonymity, of research subjects, 305
Asian-Americans. *See* Ethnic minorities
Assessment, cultural, 336, 336b
Assessment skills, for community care, 321
Assisted suicide, 293–294

Associate degree education, 121t, 122t, 126–128. *See also* Nursing education
entry into practice and, 162, 164
Associate degree nurse, 128
Associational societies, 314–316
Autonomy, 14–15, 294
definition of, 14
diminished, 304
threats to, 14–15

B

Baccalaureate programs, 121t, 122t, 124–126. *See also* Nursing education
entry into practice and, 23–24, 125–126, 164
Baldwin, J.H., 322
Beckstrand, J., 43
Beland, I.L., 36t
Beletz, E., 38
Belmont report, 302–303
Beneficence, 295
in research, 303
Benner, Patricia, 249, 271–272
Bennett, D.N., 178, 179
Bergren, M.D., 38
Bernard, Sister Mary, 149
Betts, Virginia Trotts, 276, 278, 279, 282, 283
Beyers, Marjorie, 129
Bigbee, J., 222
Binder, Leah, 254
Bioethics, 296–300. *See also* Ethics
AIDS and, 298–300
decision making in, 297b, 297–298
definition of, 297
Biologic science theory, nursing theory and, 40
Blegen, Mary, 90, 96, 97, 98
Blue Cross, 242
Bonner, Carolyn, 255
Boundary-spanning roles, 97
Boyd, Barbara, 255
Boyle, Joyceen, 336, 337
Breckinridge, Mary, 148, 200b–201b, 220
Brewster, Mary, 200b
Brooten, Dorothy, 194
Brown, Esther Lucille, 22
Buerhaus, Peter, 245, 251, 252, 258
Bulechek, Gloria, 105
Bureaucracies, professions and, 7
Bureaucratization, 317–318
in nursing, 328–333
Burgess, May, Ayres, 21
Butts, Jimmie, 227, 228

C

Campbell, A.R., 175
Campbell, C., 206
Campbell-Heider, N., 38
Cancer nursing, managed care and, 257
Career opportunities, 189–212. *See also under* Nursing
in acute-care hospitals, 191–196
in advanced practice nursing, 215–235
in ambulatory care settings, 196–199
in community nursing, 199–208
in long-term care facilities, 208–210
Care plans, 329

Carnegie, Elizabeth, 65–66
Case manager, 329–331, 330b
care orientation curriculum for, 331, 332b
in managed care, 331
Castiglia, Patricia, 174
Catalano, Joseph, 274
Centering, 50
Certification, 166
of clinical nurse specialists, 147
of nurse practitioners, 146
Certified nurse-midwife (CNM), 145t, 148–149, 217, 219–220. *See also* Advanced nursing practice
Certified registered nurse anesthetist (CRNA), 145t, 149, 217, 218–219. *See also* Advanced nursing practice
Chang, Soon Bok, 71–72
Cherney, Nathan, 293
Chinn, P.L., 49
Civil law, 307
Clarifying, 49
Clark, Carolyn, 89
Client teaching, in advanced nursing practice, 233
Clinical nurse specialist (CNS), 145t, 147–148, 220–222. *See also* Advanced nursing practice
challenges to, 222, 225–226
number of, 145t, 217
role definition for, 225–226
Clinical trials, exclusion of women and minorities from, 301
Clinton, Bill, 245, 257, 273, 279, 282
Clinton, Hillary Rodham, 269
Codes of ethics, 292–293, 293b. *See also* Ethics
elements of, 294–295
law and, 308–309
values and, 294–295
Collaborative research, 95–96
Collective bargaining, by ANA, 12, 18
Committee on the Grading of Nursing Schools, 21–22
Common law, 307
Communal societies, 314–316
Community care, trend toward, 165, 321–322
Community health centers, 198–199
Community nursing, 199–208
culturally sensitive, 229–231
for high-risk and vulnerable populations, 229–231
history of, 200b–201b
home health care in, 199–202
hospice care in, 202–203
for immigrants and refugees, 229–231
managed care and, 255, 256–257
nursing information systems in, 326–328
nursing skills for, 321–322
occupational health care in, 204–205
parish, 207–208, 208b
school, 205–207, 206b
trend toward, 165, 321–322
Competencies, in differentiated practice, 164–165
Computerized nursing taxonomies, 323
ComputerLink, 326–327
Computers
in community care, 326–328

Computers (*continued*)
  in hospital-based care, 324–326
  in nursing, 322–328
Computer skills, teaching of, 134
Confidentiality, for research subjects, 305
Congressional representatives, communication
    with, 283
Consent, of research subjects, 303–305, 304b, 306
Conti, Roberta, 329–331
Core nations, 319
Correlational quantitative research, 71t, 72–74
Cranford, Robert E., 297
Credentialing, ANA position on, 24
Credentialization, 166
Crimean War, 60
Criminal law, 307
Critical Challenges: Revitalizing the Health Pro-
    fessions for the 21st Century (Pew Com-
    mission), 130–131, 131b
Critical thinking skills, 132–133, 339
Cronenwett, Linda, 35
Crow, Karine, 334, 335
Culley, Lorraine, 334
Cultural Fitness Survey, 335
Culturally competent care, 229–231, 334–337
  nursing education for, 334–335
  in nursing practice, 335–337, 336b
Cultural nursing assessment, 336, 336b
Cultural values, 336b, 336–337

D
Davis, S.M., 175
Decision making, bioethical, 297b, 297–298
Declaration of Helsinki, 302
Deductive nursing theories, 42–45
Descriptive quantitative research, 71t, 71–72
Developmental theories, 42
Diagnosis-related groups (DRGs), 199–202
Dickoff, James P., 43
Diers, D., 43
Differentiated nursing practice, 163–165
Diminished autonomy, 304
Diploma programs, 121t, 121–124, 122t. *See*
    also Nursing education
  entry into practice and, 161–162
  history of, 116–119
Diversity
  definition of, 171
  in nursing, 170–171
  in nursing education, 120, 171–180. *See also*
    Nursing education, diversity in
  social, 333
Doberneck, B., 47
Dock, Lavinia, 62, 63t
Doctoral programs, 66, 120, 151–156
  degrees offered in, 152, 180
  doctor of nursing science, 154
  doctor of philosophy, 66, 120, 153–154
  doctor of science in nursing, 154
  nursing doctorate, 154–155
  postdoctoral training and, 155
  professional doctoral degree, 154–155
Doctor of nursing science (DNS), 154
Doctor of philosophy, 66, 120, 153–154
Doctor of science in nursing (DSN), 154
Documentation, managed care and, 257–258
Donley, Sister Rosemary, 331–333

Dorman, R.E., 178, 179
Draper, E., 194
Drugs, prescribing of, by advanced practice
    nurses, 224, 224–225, 281
Drug trials, exclusion of women and minorities
    from, 301

E
Education
  medical, Flexner report on, 20–21
  nursing. *See* Nursing education
  vs. training, 62
Educational Preparation for Nurse Practitioners
    and Assistants to Nurses (ANA), 125
Education for All Handicapped Children Act of
    1975, 207
Elderly, long-term care for, 208–210, 209b
Ellis, J.R., 191
Empirical knowledge, 34
Employees, industry-sponsored comprehensive
    care for, 227–229
Engaging, 51
Entry into practice, 160–166
  ANA position on, 23–24, 125, 161–162
  associate degree programs and, 127, 162, 164
  baccalaureate programs and, 23–24, 125–126,
    164
  competencies and, 164–165
  for differentiated practice, 163–165
  diploma programs and, 161–162
  ethical aspects of, 160
  Pew Commission report on, 163
  post-baccalaureate programs for, 155
  recommendations for, 163, 165–166
Envisioning, 51
Esthetics, 50–51, 51t
Ethical codes, 292–293, 293b
  elements of, 294–295
  law and, 308–309
  values and, 294–295
Ethics, 48–49, 51t, 291–306
  biotechnology and, 296–300. *See also* Bioethics
  conflicts in, 296
  definition of, 292
  everyday, 295, 296
  health care workers and, 296
  law and, 308–309
  research, 301–306
  technical, 295–296
  types of, 295–296
Ethnic minorities
  culturally competent care for, 333–337
  exclusion of from drug trials, 301
  in nursing education, 171–175, 172, 173. *See*
    also Nursing education, diversity in
Ethnographic studies, 76–78, 77t
Ethnologic studies, 77t
Euthanasia, 293–294
Everyday ethics, 295, 296
Experimental quantitative research, 71t, 74–75
Expert systems, 324

F
Factory production system, 320
Faculty, 64–65, 120
  educational preparation of, 153–154

research by, 153–154. *See also* Nursing research
  role of in increasing diversity, 175–179
  service opportunities for, 154
Fagin, Clair, 254
Farr, William, 61
Faust, Shotsy, 229
Fawcett, J., 43
Fee-for-service model, 243
Fidelity, 294
Flexner, Abraham, 4–5, 20
Flexner report, 20–21
Flying nurses, 196
Ford, Loretta, 145, 222, 223
Freud, Sigmund, 221
Frontier Nursing Service, 148, 200b–201b, 220

G
Gender, power and, 270, 272
General systems theory, 232
  nursing theory and, 40, *41*
Gillies, Dee An, 89
Ginzberg, Eli, 16
Globalization, 319
  international nursing and, 338–339
Goldmark report, 21, 63t
Goodrich, Annie, 63t
Gordon, Marjory, 104
Gordon, Suzanne, 246
Graduate nursing programs, 66, 120, 142–157.
   See also Nursing education
  development of, 64–66
  doctoral degree, 66, 120, 151–156. *See also*
    Doctoral programs
  entry into practice and, 155
  master's degree, 142–151. *See also* Master's
    degree programs
  need for, 141–142
  pathways for, *145,* 150–151
  post-master's degree, 147
Great social transformation (GST), 314–340
  bureaucratization in, 317–318
    nursing and, 328–333
  communal, associational, and transitional societies in, 314–316
  forces of change in, 316–320
  globalization in, 319
    nursing and, 338–339
  industrialization in, 317
    nursing and, 320–328
  nursing in, 320–339
  rationalization in, 320
    nursing and, 339
  uniqueness of, 316
  urbanization in, 318–319
    nursing and, 333–337
Grobe, Susan, 323, 327
Grounded theory, 77t

H
Hadley, Elizabeth, 243, 257
Hamner, Jenny, 72–74
Hart, C.A., 38
Hartley, C.L., 191
Hawkins, J.W., 38

Health care
  reimbursement for. *See* Health care reimbursement
  trends in, 245b. *See also* Managed care
Health care reform. *See also* Managed care
  ANA involvement in, 276–280
  failure of, 284
  goals of, 284
  media coverage of, 276, 282
  nursing professionalization and, 284–285
  problem identification for, 276–278, *277*
Health care reimbursement, 241–243
  for advanced practice nurses, 223, 225, 285
  fee-for-service model for, 243
  government-funded, 242–243, 244
  history of, 241–243
  managed care and. *See* Managed care
  private insurance for, 241, 242
  prospective payment for, 243
Health care system
  history of, 241–243
  identification of problems in, 276–278, *277*
Health care workers, ethics and, 296
Health insurance, 242–243. *See also* Health care
   reimbursement
  government-funded, 192, 242–243
Health maintenance organizations (HMOs),
   202, 244. *See also* Managed care
Health Professions Education for the Future:
  Schools in Service to the Nation (Pew Commission), 130
Health Security Act of 1993, 280
Healthy America: Practitioners for 2005 (Pew
   Commission), 130
Healy, Bernadine, 283
Helmlinger, Connie, 338
HELP, 324–325, 325b
Helsinki Declaration, 302
Henderson, Virginia, 36t, 44t, 65
Henry Street Settlement House, 200b
Hicks, Carolyn, 89
Hill, Martha, 71–72
Hill-Burton Act, 192, 209
Hinshaw, Ada Sue, 68, 155
Hispanics. *See* Ethnic minorities
History, migration, 230
HIV infection, bioethical issues in, 298–300
HMOs (health maintenance organizations), 202,
   244. *See also* Managed care
Hodgkins, Agatha, 218
Hogstel, Mildred, 62
Holt, Frieda, 225
Home health care classification, 108
Home health nursing, 199–202
  managed care and, 255
Hornsby, J.A., 177
Hospice care, 203–204
Hospital(s)
  evaluation of as workplaces, 193–196
  growth of, 191–193
  magnet, 193–196
Hospital care
  cost containment for, 246, 246b. *See also*
    Managed care
  history of, 191–193
  nursing information systems in, 324–326
  trends in, 165, 190, 321–322. *See also* Managed care

Hospital nursing
    career opportunities in, 190–196
    selection of workplace in, 193–196
    temporary staffing opportunities in, 196
Hospital training schools, 121t, 121–124, 122t
    entry into practice and, 161–162
    history of, 116–119
Human immunodeficiency virus (HIV) infection,
    bioethical issues in, 298–300
Hungler, B.P., 91

I

Immigrants. *See also* Ethnic minorities
    community care for, 229–231
    culturally competent care for, 333–337
Inductive nursing theories, 45–47
Industrialization, 317
    nursing and, 320–328
Industry-sponsored comprehensive care, for em-
    ployees, 227–229
Infectious parasitic diseases, 338
Information. *See also under* Nursing information
Information technology, 322–328
Informed consent, of research subjects,
    303–305, 304b, 306
Inouye, Daniel, 286
Institute of Medicine (IOM) study, 128–129
Insurance, 242–243. *See also* Health care reim-
    bursement
    government-funded, 192, 199–202, 225, 233,
    242–243, 244, 285. *See also* Medicare
Interactive planning, 328
International Council of Nurses, 338
International Council of Nurses' Code for Nurses,
    294
International nursing, 338–339
Internet, 328
Intuiting, 51

J

James, P., 43
Jenny, J., 47
Joel, Lucille, 119, 120, 169, 207
Johns, Ethel, 22
Johnson, Dorothy E., 34, 37, 42–43, 44t
Johnson, Ted, 146
Journal of Nurse-Midwifery, 220
Journals, 67, 67t. *See also specific journals*
Justice, 294
    in research, 305

K

Kalisch, Beatrice, 38, 60
Kalisch, Philip, 38, 60
Katz, F., 14
Keepnews, David, 284, 285
Kelly, Lucy Young, 119, 120, 169
Kelly, N.R., 178
Ketefian, Shake, 180, 297
King, Imogene, 44t
Knaus, W., 194
Knowledge. *See also* Nursing knowledge
    empirical, 34
    types of, 34

Knowledge base
    for advanced nursing practice, 232–234
    specialized, 13–14
Kramer, Marlene, 49, 194, 195

L

Lang, Norma, 102, 248
Latent power, 270
Law, 306–309
    civil, 307
    common, 307
    criminal, 307
    definition of, 306
    ethics and, 308–309
    statutory, 306–307
    tort, 307–308
    types of, 306–308
Leadership skills, teaching of, 133–134
Leavitt, J.K., 283
Legal issues, 306–309
Legislators, communication with, 283
Leininger, Madeleine, 44t, 276
Length of stay (LOS), 199–202
Levine, Myra, 44t, 88
License, 166
    autonomy and, 14
    NCLEX for, 119
Linton, Ralph, 41–42
Lobbying, 258–259. *See also* Political activity
    by advanced practice nurses, 280–281
    by ANA, 19–20, 273–274, 276–280
    by nurses, 258–259
Logan, J., 47
Long-term care facilities, 208–210, 209b
Lysaught reports, 23

M

Magaw, Alice, 218
Magnet hospital studies, 193–196
Male nurses, 176–179, *177, 178*
Malone, Beverly, 321
Managed care, 239–262
    advanced nursing practice and, 251–253, 258
    advantages of, 253
    ANA report card study of, 251
    bureaucratization and, 328–333
    community care and, 255, 256–257
    definition of, 243
    disadvantages of, 253
    documentation and, 257–258
    downsizing in, 246–249
    economic forces behind, 241
    effects of on patient care, 247–249, 248t, 251
    elements of, 243–245
    health maintenance organizations in, 202, 244
    history of, 241–243
    home health care and, 255
    job loss in, 247–249
    nurse managers in, 331
    nursing in, 245–253
        suggestions for, 257–259
    nursing model of care and, 254
    oncology nursing and, 257
    overview of, 240–241, 245b
    patient care survey and, *247,* 247–249, 248t

perioperative nursing and, 255–256
political action and, 258–259
preferred provider organizations in, 244
prospective payment in, 243
staffing in, 247–251
succeeding in, 254–259
use of unlicensed assistive personnel in,
249–251
utilization review in, 243–244
Managed care organizations (MCOs), 243–244
Management skills, teaching of, 133–134
Manuel, Patricia, 249, 250
Martin, A., 36t
Marullo, Geri, 284, 285
Master of science (MS) degree, 143
Master of science in nursing degree, 143
Master's degree programs, 142–151
advanced practice roles and positions for graduates of, 143
basic requirements of, 143
for certified registered nurse anesthetists, 149
for clinical nurse specialists, 147–148
course content of, 143
development of, 142
for nurse-midwives, 148–149
for nurse practitioners, 145–147
student guidelines for, 144b
Matheney, R.V., 36t
Mayo, Ada, 204
McCloskey, Joan C., 105
McManus, Louise, 126
Mead, George Herbert, 41
Media
nursing coverage in, 276, 281–283
politics and, 281–283
Medicaid, 192, 242–243, 244
reimbursement for nursing services by, 223,
225, 285
Medical education, Flexner report on, 20–21
Medicare, 192, 242–243, 244
diagnosis-related groups and, 199–202
length of stay and, 199–201
reimbursement for nursing services by, 223,
225, 285
Meleis, Afaf, 45
Men, in nursing, 176–179, *177, 178*
Mental health nursing, 221
managed care and, 256–257
Merton, Robert S., 98
Mexican-Americans. *See* Ethnic minorities
Middle-range theory, 98–100, 99b
Midwives, 148–149. *See also* Nurse-midwives
Migration history, 230
Military, male nurses in, 177–178
Minorities
culturally competent care for, 333–337
exclusion of from drug trials, 301
in nursing education, 171–175, *172, 173. See
also* Nursing education, diversity in
Minority Academic Advising Program, 171,
174–175
Model, vs. theory, 45
Moloney, M.M., 160–161
Montag, Mildred, 126, 127, 162
Moreno, Jacob, 41, 42
Morse, J.M., 47
Moss, Mae Taylor, 256, 331

Multiculturalism, 333–334
culturally competent care and, 229–231,
334–337

N
NANDA (North American Nursing Diagnosis
Association), 104
taxonomy of, 105, 106t
National Advisory Council on Nurse Education
and Practice, 190
National Association of Colored Graduate
Nurses, 20
National Center for Nursing Research (NCNR),
68, 129
National Commission on Nursing (NCN) study,
129–130, 163
National Council Licensing Examination
(NCLEX), 119
National Hospice Organization, 203
National Institute of Nursing Research (NINR),
68–69, 155
National Institutes of Health (NIH), research
ethics and, 301
National League for Nursing (NLN), 19
accreditation by, 167–169
National Nursing Research Agenda (NNRA),
68–69
National Student Nurses' Association, 19
Nations
core, 319
periphery, 319
semiperiphery, 319
Negligence, 307
Networking, 274–275
Neuman, Betty, 44t
Nickel, Jennie, 95
Nightingale, Florence, 17, 36t, 59–61, 90, 117,
177, 257, 275
Nightingale school, 117, 117b
1965 Nurse Training Act, 221
1971 Nurse Training Act, 221, 278
1993 Nursing Summit, 279
Norris, D.M., 220
North American Nursing Diagnosis Association
(NANDA), 104
taxonomy of, 105, 106t
Notter, Esther Lucille, 63
Nuremburg Code, 302
Nurse(s)
advanced practice, 216–218. *See also* Advanced
nursing practice
associate degree, 128
delegation by, 250
flying, 196
job attrition among, 247–251, 248t. *See also*
Managed care
male, 176–179, *177, 178*
media portrayal of, 38
political action by. *See under* Political; Politics
registered, qualifications of, 119
replacement of by unlicensed assistive personnel, 247, 248, 249–251
restricted supply of, 16–17
shortage of, 128–129
technical, 126
work orientation of, 25

Nurse activists, 283
Nurse anesthetist, 145t, 149, *217,* 218–219. *See also* Advanced nursing practice
Nurse case manager, 329–331, 330b
  care orientation curriculum for, 331, 332b
  in managed care, 331
Nurse citizens, 282–283
Nurse-managed community health center, 198–199
Nurse-managed employee health center, 227–229
Nurse manager, 329–331
  care orientation curriculum for, 331, 332b
  in managed care, 331
Nurse-midwives, 145t, 148–149, *217,* 219–220. *See also* Advanced nursing practice
Nurse politicians, 283
Nurse practice acts, 12, 224, *224,* 306–307, 308–309
Nurse practitioner(s) (NP), 145t, 145–147, *217,* 222–225, *224. See also* Advanced nursing practice
  culturally sensitive care by, 229–231
  in managed care, 252–253
  merger of with clinical nurse specialists, 226
  number of, *217*
The Nurse Practitioner, 252
Nurse Training Act of 1965, 221
Nurse Training Act of 1971, 223, 276
Nursing
  advanced practice. *See* Advanced nursing practice
  ambulatory care, 196–199
  autonomy in, 14–15
  bureaucratization and, 328–333
  career opportunities in, 189–212
  community, 199–208. *See also* Community nursing
  in community health centers, 198–199
  culturally competent, 229–231, 334–337, 335–337, 336b
    nursing education for, 334–335
  definitions of, 35–36, 36t, 104
  disunity and divisiveness in, 24–25
  diversity in, 120, 170–180
  future trends in, 313–340
  great social transformation and, 320–339
  home health, 199–202
    managed care and, 255
  hospital, 190–196
  industrialization and, 320–328
  international, 338–339
  in long-term care facilities, 208–210, 209b
  in managed care environment, 245–253. *See also* Managed care
  media coverage of, 276, 281–283
  men in, 176–179, *177, 178*
  occupational health, 204–205
  on occupation-profession continuum, 11t, 11–12
  office practice, 196–197
  oncology, managed care and, 257
  in outpatient surgical centers, 197–198
  parish, 207–208, 208b
  perioperative, managed care and, 255–256
  power in, 269–275. *See also* Power
  powerlessness in, 272–273
  prestige of, 38
  professionalization of, 4, 10t, 11–25. *See also* Professionalization
  psychiatric, 221
    managed care and, 256–257
  rationalization and, 339
  rehabilitation, 210
  salaries in, 145t, 246, 246t
  school, 205–207, 206b
  as scientific discipline, 37
  society's view of, 37–39
  specialized knowledge base for, 13–14
  trifurcation of, 86, 87–90
  urbanization and, 333–337
  in urgent care centers, 197
Nursing assessment, cultural, 336, 336b
Nursing care plans, 329
Nursing competencies, 164–165
Nursing data, standardized, 101
Nursing doctorate, 154–155
Nursing education, 115–183
  academic, transition to, 64
  accreditation in, 166–170. *See also* Accreditation
  advanced, 140–157. *See also* Nursing education, graduate
  ANA position paper on, 23–24, 125
  associate degree, 121t, 122t, 126–128
  baccalaureate degree, 121t, 122t, 124–126
  challenges in, 180
  commonalities in, 119–120
  costs of, 119
  for critical thinking skills, 132–133
  for culturally competent care, 334–335
  for differentiated practice, 164–165
  diploma programs in, 121t, 121–124, 122t
  history of, 116–119
  diversity in, 120, 170–180
    faculty role in, 175–179
    means of increasing, 174–175
    men and, 176–179
    Minority Academic Advising Program for, 174–175
    pathways model for, 175
    racial and ethnic minorities in, 171–175, *172, 173*
  doctoral programs in. *See* Nursing education, graduate
  early traditions in, 116
  entry into practice and, 23–24, 125–126, 127, 160–166. *See also* Entry into practice
  faculty in, 64–65, 120
    educational preparation of, 153–154
    research by, 153–154. *See also* Nursing research
    response of to diversity, 175–179
    service opportunities for, 154
  Goldmark report on, 21
  graduate, 66, 120, 142–156, 142–157
    development of, 64–66
    doctoral programs in, 66, 120, 151–156. *See also* Doctoral programs
    entry into practice and, 155
    master's degree programs in, 142–151. *See also* Master's degree programs
    need for, 141–142
    pathways for, *145,* 150–151
    postdoctoral programs in, 155
    post-master's degree programs in, 147

growth of, 62
history of, 116–119
Institute of Medicine study on, 128–129
issues and challenges in, 160–183
for leadership and management skills,
133–134
men in, 176–179
National Commission on Nursing Study of,
129–130
new directions in, 131–134
Nightingale school for, 117, 117b
for nursing informatics utilization skills, 134
nursing research in, 65, 66–67
Pew Commission reports on, 130–131,
131b
re-entry programs in, 125
sites of, 120
studies and reports on, 21–24, 128–131
vs. training, 62
types of, 119–128, 121t, 122t
for university faculty roles, 64–65
Nursing ethics. *See* Bioethics; Ethics
Nursing for the Future (Brown), 22
Nursing homes, 209b, 209–210
Nursing informatics, 323
in community care, 326–328
in hospital-based care, 324–326
teaching of, 134
Nursing information classification systems
(NICS), 86, 100–108
ANA support for, 104
criteria for, 102–104
development of, 102–104
Nursing Minimum Data Set for, 102–104,
103b
nursing taxonomies and, 104–107, 106t
purpose of, 100–101
utility of, 101–102
Nursing information systems, 323
in community care, 326–328
in hospital-based care, 324–326
Nursing Intervention Lexicon and Taxonomy
(NILT), 327
Nursing interventions classification taxonomy,
105–107, 327
Nursing journals, 67, 67t. *See also specific journals*
Nursing knowledge, 34–39, 85–109
for advanced nursing practice, 232–234
classification of, 48, *48*, 51t
for community care, 322
definition of, 34
development and use of, 86–108
fostering of, 100–108
empirical, 48, *48*, 51t
esthetic, *48*, 50–51, 51t
ethical, *48*, 48–49, 51t
growth of, 34–35
personal, *48*, 49–50, 51t
practice-based, 46–47
society's view of, 37–39
theory for, 39–47. *See also* Nursing theory
Nursing leaders, 12–13
Nursing Minimum Data Set (NMDS), 102–104,
103b, 323
Nursing model, vs. nursing theory, 45
Nursing model of care, managed care and, 254
Nursing Organization Liaison Forum, 18

Nursing organizations, 17–20. *See also specific
organizations*
membership levels in, 273–274
political action by, 258–259, 273–274
power of, 273–274
Nursing practice. *See also* Nursing
differentiated, 163–165
as separate from research and theory, 87–90
Nursing report card, 251, 285
Nursing research, 58–81. *See also* Research
ANA support for, 66–67
by baccalaureate nurses, 66
changing focus of, 65–66
clinical focus in, 65–66
collaborative, 95–96
correlational
descriptive, 71t, 72–74
experimental, 71t, 74–75
development and progress of, 59–69, *70*
from 1870–1950, 61–64, *70*
from 1950–1980, 64–67, *70*
from 1980 to present, 67–69, *70*
in Nightingale era, 59–61, *70*
early leaders in, 62–63, 63t
educational preparation for, 153–154
ethical issues in, 301–306
foundations of, 59–61
by graduate nurses, 66–67
hiatus in, 61–64
incorporation of research into, 96–100
literature of, 67, 67t
Nightingale's contributions to, 61–62
qualitative, 75–81
ethnographic, 76–78, 77t
ethologic, 77t
grounded theory, 77t
phenomenologic, 77t, 78–81
quantitative, 69–75, 81
correlational, 71t, 72–74
descriptive, 71t, 71–72
experimental, 71t, 74–75
as separate from theory and practice, 87–90
teaching of, 65
types of, 69–81
utilization of, 90–95
barriers to, 94–95
guidelines for, 91
institutional support for, 91–92
Iowa model for, 92, *93*
Nursing roles, boundary-spanning, 97
Nursing's Agenda for Health Care Reform
(ANA), 278b, 278–279, 284
Nursing Schools: Today and Tomorrow, 22
Nursing shortage, 128–129
Nursing's Social Policy Statement, 35–36
Nursing staffing agency, 196
Nursing students. *See also* Nursing education
diversity of, 120, 171–179. *See also* Nursing
education, diversity in
male, 176–179, *177, 178*
Nursing taxonomies, 104–107, 106t
computerized, 323
home health care classification, 108
NANDA, 105, 106t
nursing interventions classification, 105–107,
327
Omaha problem classification system, 107–108

Nursing theory, 39–48
  adaptation theory and, 42
  biologic science theory and, 40
  classification of, 39
  deductive, 42–45
  developmental theories and, 42
  general systems theory and, 40, *41*
  imported, 40–42
  incorporation of into research and practice,
    96–100
  inductive, 45–47
  middle-range, 98–100, 99b
  vs. nursing model, 45
  prescriptive, 43
  proponents of, 44t
  role theory and, 41–42
  as separate from research and practice, 87–90
Nutting, Adelaide, 63t

O

Occupation, vs. profession, 4
Occupational health, industry-sponsored com-
    prehensive care for, 227–229
Occupational health nursing, 204–205
Occupational Safety and Health Administration
    (OSHA), 205
Occupation-profession continuum, 6–7, *7*
  nursing's place on, 11t, 11–12
O'Connell, Muriel, 95
Office practice, 196–197
Omaha problem classification, 107–108
Oncology nursing, managed care and, 257
Opening, 50
Organizational theory, 233
Orlando, Ida Jean, 44t
Outpatient surgical centers, 197–198

P

Page, Gayle, 74–75
Parish nursing, 207–208, 208b
Parse, Rosemarie Rizzo, 43–44
Pathways model, 175
Patient care survey, by *American Journal of
    Nursing, 247,* 247–249, *248*
Patient-clinician partnership, 227
Pavalko, Ronald, 11
Payment. *See* Reimbursement
Pearson, Linda, 252
Pender, Nola, 45
Peplau, Hildegard, 36t, 44t, 46, 220, 221
Perioperative nursing, managed care and,
    255–256
Periphery nations, 319
Perkins, J.L., 178, 179
Personal knowing, *48,* 49–50, 51t
Pesthouse, 191
Peters, T.J., 194, 195
Peterson, C., 283
Pew Commission reports, 130–131, 131b, 142,
    163, 165
Pfefferkorn, Blanche, 22
PhD programs, 66, 120, 153–154. *See also* Doc-
    toral programs
Phenomenologic studies, 77t, 78–81
Picella, David, 226

Pike, Adele, 273
Planning, interactive, 328
Policy
  definition of, 283–284
  nursing's influence on, 268–269. *See also
    under* Political; Politics
Polit, D.F., 91
Political activity
  of ANA, 19–20, 273–274, 276–280
  electoral, 280–281
  media and, 281–283
  nonelectoral, 281
  by nurses, 258–259, 275–283
    in advanced practice, 280–281
    evaluation of, 286
    goals of, 286
    for improved patient care, 285
    levels of, 282–283
    strengths and weaknesses in, 275–276
  problem identification for, 276–278, *277*
  for professionalization, 283–284
Political power. *See also* Power
  of nurses, positive and negative forces for,
    275–276
Politics, 267–287, 275–283
  definition of, 275
  media and, 281–283
Politics of Nursing, 286
Porter, Eileen Jones, 78–80
Postdoctoral training, 155
Postindustrialization, 317
Post-master's degree programs, 147
Power, 269–275. *See also under* Political; Politics
  definition of, 269, 270
  gender and, 270, 272
  latent, 270
  nature of, 269–270
  networking and, 274–275
  nursing excellence and, 272b
  of professional organizations, 273–274
  sources of, 270–271
  unity and, 273–274
  ways to increase, 273–275
Power base, 271
Powerlessness, in nursing, 272–273
Power orientation, 271
Power struggles, 273
Practice acts, 12, 224, *224,* 306–307, 308–309
Practice-based nursing knowledge, 46–47
Preferred provider organizations (PPOs), 244
Prescriptive theory, 43
Prestige, professional, 5, 6b, 14
Primary care, 227–229
Proctor, Fletcher D., 204
Profession(s)
  autonomy in, 14–15
  characteristics of, 4–5
  definition of, 64
  ethical codes of, 292–295. *See also* Ethical
    codes
  impact of bureaucracies on, 7
  level of commitment in, 16
  limitations on membership of, 16–17
  monopoly over services of, 15–16
  nursing as, 4
  vs. occupation, 4. *See also* Occupation-profes-
    sion continuum

prestige of, 5, 6b, 14
self-regulation of, 5, 8
specialized knowledge base for, 13–14
Professional(s), 7–8
definition of, 16
limitation of number of, 16–17
Professional codes of ethics, 292–295, 293b,
308–309
Professional doctoral degrees, 154–155
Professionalism, 8
Professionalization, 4, 7, 8–11, 10t, 11–25
in advanced nursing practice, 215–235
barriers to, 24–25
challenges to, 13–17
health care reform and, 284–285
milestones in, 17–24
monopoly over services and, 15–16
policy and, 283–284
politics and, 267–287
power and, 267–287
process of, 9–11, 10t
progress in, 12–13
Professionalizers, 25
Professional journals, 67, 67t. *See also specific
journals*
Professional organizations, 17–20
power of, 273–274
Prospective payment, 243
Psychiatric nursing, 221
managed care and, 256–257
Public policy, 283–285
nursing's influence on, 268–269. *See also
under* Political; Politics

Q

Qualitative research, 75–81. *See also* Nursing re-
search
Quality assurance, 285
Quantitative research, 69–75, 81. *See also* Nurs-
ing research
Quetelet, Adolphe, 60

R

Racial minorities
culturally competent care for, 333–337
exclusion of from drug trials, 301
in nursing education, 171–175, *172, 173.* See
also Nursing education, diversity in
Rationalization, 320
nursing and, 339
Realizing, 50
Reed, Pamela, 46
Re-entry programs, 125
Refugees. *See also* Ethnic minorities
community care for, 229–231
culturally competent care for, 333–337
Registered nurse. *See also* Nurse(s)
qualifications of, 119
Rehabilitation nursing, 210
Reimbursement, 241–243
for advanced practice nurses, 223, 225, 285
fee-for-service model for, 243
government-funded, 192, 199–202, 223, 225,
242–243, 244, 285. *See also* Medicare
history of, 241–243

managed care and. *See* Managed care
methods of, 241–243
private insurance for, 241, 242
prospective payment for, 243
Report card study, 251, 285
Research
beneficence in, 303
collaborative, 95–96
ethical, nurses' responsibilities in, 305–306
ethical issues in, 301–306
informed consent for, 303–305, 304b, 306
nursing. *See* Nursing research
respect for persons in, 303–305
rights of subjects in, 301–305
vulnerable populations in, 304–305
Research studies, 20–24. *See also* Nursing research
Goldmark report, 21
Research subjects
anonymity of, 305
confidentiality for, 305
diminished autonomy of, 304–305
informed consent of, 303–305, 304b, 306
rights of, 301–305
nurses' protection of, 305–306
Research utilization program, 91–92, *93. See also*
Nursing research, utilization of
Resnick, Barbara, 76–78
Richards, Linda, 118
Richardson, Elliott, 223
Robb, Isabel Hampton, 4, 63t
Rogers, Lina L., 205
Rogers, Martha, 4, 36t, 44t, 87
Role(s), 8
of advanced practice nurses, 231, 232b
boundary-spanning, 97
sick, 337
Role/self merger, 8
Role theory, 232
nursing theory and, 41–42
Rooda, Linda, 335
Roy, Sister Callista, 44t, 72

S

Saba, Virginia, 108
Salaries
of advanced practice nurses, 145t
as factor in rising health care costs, 246, 246t
Salsberry, Pamela, 95
SAS Health Care Center, 227–228
Saunders, Dame Cicely, 203
Sayner, Nancy, 62
Schmalenberg, Claudia, 194, 195
Schmidt, R.E., 177
School nursing, 205–207, 206b
Seedhouse, David, 296
Self-concept, 8
Semiperiphery nations, 319
Semiprofessionals, characteristics of, 14, 16
Semmelweis, Ignaz, 61
Senators, communication with, 283
Service opportunities, for faculty, 154
Shoemaker, M., 178
Sick-role orientation, 337
Sigsby, L.M., 206
Silver, Henry, 145, 223

Simpson, Roy, 327–328
Sluzki, Carlos, 230
Smith, C., 256
Smith, Gloria, 338
Smith, Janet E., 291
Smoyak, Shirley, 220
Snow, John, 61
Social diversity, 333
Social policy statements, of ANA, 274
Society
    associational, 314–316
    communal, 314–316
    transitional, 314–316
Sosne, Diane, 249
Sowell, P.M., 256
Staffing, in managed care, 247–251, 248t
Standards of practice, 104
State nurse practice acts, 12, 224, *224,* 306–307,
    308–309
Statutory law, 306–307
Steele, T., 178
Stereotypes, of nurses, 38–39
Stewart, Harriet, 204
Stewart, Isabel, 63
Stigma, 299
Stigmatization, of AIDS, 299–300
Student nurses. *See also* Nursing education
    diversity of, 120, 171–179. *See also* Nursing
        education, diversity in
    male, 176–179, *177, 178*
*The Study of Credentialing in Nursing: A New
    Approach* (ANA), 24
Styles, Margretta, 24
Suburbanization, 319
Suicide, assisted, 293–294
Sullivan, Harry Stack, 221
Surgery
    managed care and, 255–256
    outpatient, 197–198
Systems theory, nursing theory and, 40, *41*

T
Tanner, Christine, 174
Taxonomies, nursing, 104–107, 106t
    computerized, 323
    home health care classification, 108
    NANDA, 105, 106t
    nursing interventions classification, 105–107,
        327
    Omaha problem classification system, 107–108
Teaching, 64–65, 120
    educational preparation for, 153–154
Teaching-learning theory in, 233
Technical ethics, 295, 296
Technical nurse, 126
Technological development, 320
Telephone triage, 257
Temporary nursing service, 196
Theory
    middle-range, 98
    vs. model, 45
    nursing. *See* Nursing theory

Third party payments. *See also* Reimburse-
    ment
    for nursing services, 223, 225, 285
Thompson, C.B., 297, 323
Thompson, H.O., 297
Thompson, J.B., 297
Titler, Marita, 90, 92, 94
Tort law, 307–308
Traditionalizers, 25
Training, vs. education, 62
Transitional societies, 314–316
Tripp-Reimer, Toni, 90, 96, 97, 98
Tuskegee study, 302
Twenty Thousand Nurses Tell Their Story, 22,
    66

U
Unlicensed assistive personnel (UAP), 247, 248,
    249–251
Urbanization, 318–319
    nursing and, 333–337
Urgent care center, 197
Utilization review, 243–244
Utilizers, 25

V
Values. *See also* Ethics
    codes of ethics and, 294–295
    cultural, 336b, 336–337
Valuing, 49
Vaughn, Barbara, 339
Veracity, 295
Vulnerable populations, in research studies,
    304–305

W
Wagner, D., 194
Wald, Lillian, 62, 63t, 200b, 205
Waterman, R.H., 194, 195
Watson, Jean, 44t
Werley, Harriet, 102, 103, 104
Westberg, Granger, 207
Wilensky, H., 9, 14
Williams, P.W., 256
Women
    exclusion of from drug trials, 301
    power and, 270, 272
Work orientation, 25
Workplace, employer-sponsored comprehensive
    care in, 227–229

Y
Yoder, Marilyn, 176

Z
Zakrzewska, Marie, 118
Zimmerman, J., 194
Zorn, C., 103